GUIDELINES FOR NURSING PROCEDURES

As you provide nursing care you want to communicate through your actions that you are a competent and caring nurse. Through developing systematic work habits you can communicate organization and efficiency that will not only save you time but are consistent with competency and help you focus on the client rather than the procedure. Plan your activities to include CDC Standard Precautions.

As you practice the procedures in this book, include the following activities in each procedure.

PRELIMINARY ACTIONS

Before you perform a procedure, always:

Confirm physician's order. When a nursing procedure is part of medical therapy or the implementation of medical therapy you need to confirm that a physician's order is written and that you are familiar with any guidelines the physician has provided.

Gather equipment. Planning the procedure and gathering the equipment will allow you to work efficiently. You want to gather all the supplies you will need to avoid repeated trips to the supply storage area. However, choose the items wisely. In the hospital setting you cannot replace supplies to a clean storage area after you have taken them to a client's room.

Confirm client's identity. Clients in an inpatient setting are identified with an armband. Check the client's armband against the chart or computer-generated worksheet. This check is especially important when the client's level of consciousness is altered or when you are working from a work station where items (especially medications) for multiple clients are stored. Asking the client to state his or her name is considered more reliable identification than asking, "Are you John Smith?"

Explain procedure to client. Form the habit of introducing yourself to the client and explaining what you are going to do. Explain in terms the client can understand. Avoid using medical or nursing jargon.

Arrange the work area. This activity may include raising the bed to a comfortable working height, clearing the over-the-bed table to provide a work surface, and placing the trash can in a convenient place.

Perform hand hygiene. You should perform hand hygiene before every procedure. Washing your hands in the client's presence adds to the client's confidence that you are providing for safety.

Provide for privacy. In a health care setting the client has the right to privacy. Close the door, pull a curtain around the bed, and drape the client if needed to avoid exposing usually private body parts.

COMPLETION ACTIONS

After you finish a procedure, always:

Make the client comfortable. Straighten the bed linens, adjust the pillow, and assist the client to a position of comfort. Lower the bed, raise one or more rails according to client need, and position the call light. Place water and personal items within easy reach.

Perform hand hygiene. You should perform hand hygiene after every procedure.

Document the care. Document the time of the procedure. Document the indication for the procedure, what was done, how it was done, supplies used, and pertinent observations made during the procedure.

OTHER CONSIDERATIONS

If you are unfamiliar with the agency policies and procedures, you should access the policy and procedure manual for guidelines specific to the agency. If you are assisting with an invasive procedure, confirm the agency's requirement for written informed consent.

Study Guide for

*F*undamentals of Nursing

Caring and Clinical Judgment

Third edition

Mary E. Stassi, RN, C
Health Occupations Coordinator
Adjunct Faculty
St. Charles Community College
St. Peters, Missouri

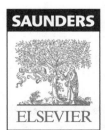

SAUNDERS

ELSEVIER

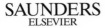

SAUNDERS
ELSEVIER

11830 Westline Industrial Drive
St. Louis, Missouri 63146

Notice

Knowledge and best practice in this field are constantly changing. As new research and experience broaden our knowledge, changes in practice, treatment and drug therapy may become necessary or appropriate. Readers are advised to check the most current information provided (i) on procedures featured or (ii) by the manufacturer of each product to be administered, to verify the recommended dose or formula, the method and duration of administration, and contraindications. It is the responsibility of the practitioner, relying on their own experience and knowledge of the patient, to make diagnoses, to determine dosages and the best treatment for each individual patient, and to take all appropriate safety precautions. To the fullest extent of the law, neither the Publisher nor the Author assumes any liability for any injury and/or damage to persons or property arising out or related to any use of the material contained in this book.

The Publisher

Executive Editor: Susan R. Epstein
Senior Developmental Editor: Maria Broeker
Publishing Services Manager: John Rogers
Project Manager: Beth Hayes

Working together to grow
libraries in developing countries

www.elsevier.com | www.bookaid.org | www.sabre.org

ELSEVIER　　BOOK AID International　　Sabre Foundation

Printed in the United States of America

Last digit is the print number:　9　8　7　6　5　4　3　2　1

This *Study Guide* is dedicated to all of students I have had the opportunity to work with over the years. Your hard work and committment is truly an inspiration.

To C from M for believing in fairy tales and happily ever after.

Acknowledgments

This *Study Guide* is the result of the hard work of many dedicated and talented individuals. I gratefully acknowledge all of the individuals who devoted their time and energy to make this book a reality.

I am especially grateful and appreciative of the efforts by:

Suzi Epstein, executive editor at Elsevier, who gave me the opportunity to participate in the project.

Maria Broker, senior developmental editor for nursing at Elsevier, who allowed me to ask as many questions as it took to bring the project to successful completion and kept everyone on schedule.

Helen Harkreader, Mary Ann Hogan, and Marshelle Thobaben, authors of the text, who permitted me to join their team.

All of the contributors and reviewers who worked on the third edition of the text and provided a wonderfully complete manuscript from which to work.

PREFACE

The *Study Guide* for Harkreader, Hogan, and Thobaben's *Fundamentals of Nursing: Caring and Clinical Judgment* was developed to assist you, the nursing student, to understand and apply the important concepts presented in the textbook. As a beginning nursing student, you will be presented with a tremendous amount of material in a relatively short time. The *Study Guide* was written to help you make good use of your valuable study time.

The front of the *Study Guide* contains Guidelines for Nursing Procedures. These Guidelines are activities that should be performed before beginning a procedure as well as after you have finished the procedure. The guidelines will help you develop systematic work habits and allow you to focus on caring for the client rather than the procedure itself. The Guideline itself is referenced in the procedure as appropriate; however, the individual steps are not repeated. It is important that you familiarize yourself with these activities and incorporate them into each procedure you perform. In some procedures, such as handwashing, the preliminary actions are not necessary.

Each *Study Guide* chapter follows a specific format:

- **Purpose:** Each chapter begins with a brief purpose statement that summarizes in a few sentences the content of the corresponding textbook chapter.
- **Matching:** Matching exercises allow you to test your recall of basic terminology from each chapter.
- **True or False:** True or false exercises allow you to test your understanding of factual information presented in the text of the chapter. The answer key at the end of the book corrects the false statements.
- **Fill in the Blanks:** Fill in the blanks exercises help you master comprehension of important fundamental concepts and apply them in a specific context.
- **Exercising Your Clinical Judgment:** "Exercising Your Clinical Judgment" sections use the case study presented in the textbook chapter and NCLEX®-style multiple-choice questions to

give you practice in applying clinical reasoning skills.
- **Test Yourself:** The "Test Yourself" sections present a series of freestanding NCLEX-style multiple-choice questions to give you practice in test-taking and help you prepare for exams.
- **Prioritization:** Select chapters contain prioritization type questions that require you to to evaluate or weigh each option to determine which problems or needs require immediate action and which ones could be delayed until a later time because they are not urgent.

The answers to all of the exercises are provided at the end of the book for immediate feedback on the degree to which you have mastered the chapter contents.

Following the answer section, you will find **Performance Checklists** that correspond to the Procedures in the textbook. Each one presents the essential elements of the corresponding Procedure beginning with the *Performed Preliminary Actions* and ending with the *Performed Completion Actions*. The checklists are designed to be used in two ways. First, you may use them for individual review as you practice performing procedures. Second, an instructor may use them to test your mastery of the procedures. The format allows the instructor not only to rate your performance, but also to provide specific comments that will enhance your learning and help you to refine your skills.

I hope you find the *Study Guide* to be not only useful but also enjoyable for study. I also wish you success as you begin your career, and anticipate that you will quickly discover all the richness, fulfillment, and satisfaction that nursing has to offer!

Happy Learning,
Mary

Mary E. Stassi RN, C

CONTENTS

THE NURSING PROFESSION

PURPOSE

This chapter provides a broad overview of the nursing profession. It describes significant events in history and how they have affected the evolution of the nursing profession. The chapter also examines the various roles you will have as a nurse, professional nursing practice standards, advanced education options, and current issues of concern to those in the nursing profession.

MATCHING

1. _____ autonomy
2. _____ client
3. _____ health
4. _____ holistic care
5. _____ Licensed Vocational Nurse (LVN)/Licensed Practical Nurse (LPN)
6. _____ National Council Licensure Examination for Registered Nurses (NCLEX-RN®)
7. _____ nursing
8. _____ profession
9. _____ Registered Nurse
10. _____ standards of nursing practice

a. the protection, promotion, and optimization of health and abilities, prevention of illness and injury, alienation of suffering through the diagnosis, and treatment of human response, and advocacy in the care of individuals, families, communities, and populations

b. an individual's ability to make decisions using critical-thinking skills to solve problems and decide behaviors based upon a wide knowledge and expertise from which to make an accurate choice

c. nursing care that goes beyond physical needs to include spiritual, cultural, and psychological needs to help an individual achieve health

d. an individual who participates with health care workers in the planning and implementation of one's own health care

e. a set of nursing actions constituting safe and effective client care and generally agreed upon by groups of nurses in their area of nursing

f. a nurse who is registered to practice nursing in a particular state after graduating from a state-approved educational program and passing the NCLEX-RN examination

g. a diverse group of individuals who use a specialized body of knowledge to provide an essential service to society; has a theoretical body of knowledge, requires relative independence in decision making in practice, requires specialized education, and has a code of ethics for behavior of its members

h. physical, social, spiritual, and mental well-being

i. a computer-adapted examination that tests the graduate of diploma, associate, or bachelor's degree in nursing program's ability to meet client needs and reflects questions on leadership, priority setting, delegation, and all areas of nursing care

j. a licensed member of the health care team that assists in the delivery of care to clients under the direction of the professional registered nurse

TRUE OR FALSE

11. _____ Nursing has been defined in many different ways, but the caregiving focus has remained humanistic and holistic.

12. _____ Nursing as a profession is under the domain of medicine and is regulated by medicine.

13. _____ The American Nurses Association is the representative professional association for nurses in the United States whose members are the state nurses organizations.

14. _____ Florence Nightingale is considered by many to be the founder of nursing education.

15. _____ Isabel Hampton Robb was the cofounder of the *American Journal of Nursing*.

16. _____ A doctoral degree program is considered entry-level education in nursing.

17. _____ A nurse who is planning the best method of care delivery for a client is engaged in the nursing role of rehabilitator.

18. _____ Specialty nursing organizations often offer certification for nurses practicing in that specialty.

19. _____ A client's cultural beliefs must be understood and incorporated into the plan of care to achieve an acceptable outcome.

20. _____ Today's nurse must learn scientific principles and apply them to all possible circumstances in the clinical setting.

FILL IN THE BLANKS

21. The nursing process is identified as the following phases of care: _____, _____, _____, _____, and _____.

22. _____ _____ was a war nurse, publisher, and nurse theorist who was the founder of modern nursing education.

23. The newest role of the nurse, called _____ _____, focuses on coordinating care based on technologic regulation and dispensing of care at the bedside.

24. The first nurse to be appointed a university professorship at Columbia University Teachers College was _____ _____ _____.

25. In 1893, Lillian Wald founded _____ _____ nursing when she opened the Henry Street Settlement Service in New York City.

26. Two prominent cultural influences on the development of nursing today include the characteristics and beliefs that have evolved from the _____, _____, and _____ cultures within the border of the United States.

27. A nurse practitioner, nurse educator, or nurse administrator often completes a 2-year _____ _____ program.

28. Continuing education is mandatory in some states to maintain _____ _____.

29. The Nurse Practice Act defines the scope of nursing practice in a _____.

EXERCISING YOUR CLINICAL JUDGMENT

Kate Lorraine is a 22-year-old nursing graduate. She has just taken her first job in a subacute unit of a local rehabilitation nursing center. Kate is highly motivated to grow in her professional practice and to deliver quality nursing care to her clients.

30. To be aware of her specific legal responsibilities in her daily nursing practice, Kate should become familiar with which of the following?
    1. State Nurse Practice Act
    2. National League for Nursing (NLN) accreditation criteria
    3. Association of Rehabilitation Nurses (ARN) guidelines
    4. American Nurses Association (ANA) standards of nursing practice

31. As Kate is working on the evening shift, she observes one client looking through the bedside table drawer of another client. Kate intervenes, knowing that the following nursing role assumes the highest priority:
    1. Caregiver
    2. Communicator
    3. Client advocate
    4. Manager

32. Kate takes a dinner break with a nursing colleague. They talk about the flyers for continuing education programs that are hanging on the break room bulletin board. Kate begins to think about the importance of acquiring continuing education units (CEUs) to maintain which of the following?
    1. Opportunities for future pay increases
    2. Professional licensure
    3. Status among her colleagues
    4. Membership in the ANA

33. Kate overhears that another nurse has just received Nursing Administration certification from the American Nurses Credentialing Center (ANCC). She is aware that this nurse has which of the following as a minimum educational degree?
    1. Associate's degree
    2. Bachelor's degree
    3. Master's degree
    4. Doctorate degree

TEST YOURSELF

34. Nursing can best be defined as a discipline that focuses on which of the following?
    1. Human responses to health and illness
    2. A wide variety of disease states
    3. The interaction between nurses and other disciplines
    4. The women's movement in the United States

35. What impact has the increase in the aging population had on health care?
    1. Increased money is available for health care needs
    2. Social security is able to meet the retirement needs of this generation of workers
    3. The average age of doctors, nurses, and health care educators is the mid-50s
    4. The aging population is less informed about their health care choices than previous generations

36. Which of the following is the official publication by the American Nurses Association for registered nurses?
    1. *RN*
    2. *American Journal of Nursing*
    3. *Nursing*
    4. *Nursing Research*

37. With the changing health care delivery system, which of the following settings for nursing practice is experiencing a decline in the number of patient care days?
    1. Rehabilitation centers
    2. Home health care
    3. Private duty nursing
    4. Hospitals

38. Which challenge must a nurse in today's health care field be prepared to meet?
    1. Developing standardized plans of care to control costs
    2. Teaching clients to become more dependent on their health care provider
    3. A focus on nursing that will revert back to illness rather than health
    4. Using evidence-based practice skills as much as possible in daily care

LEGAL AND ETHICAL CONTEXT OF PRACTICE

PURPOSE

This chapter discusses the legal foundation for nursing practice and explores the theories and principles of ethics. It provides information about the legal and professional regulation of nursing practice, client rights, quality of care improvement initiatives, and methods to safeguard your nursing practice against legal threats. It also provides guidelines for ethical decision making that can be applied systematically to nursing practice.

MATCHING

1. ____ accreditation
2. ____ administrative law
3. ____ advance directive
4. ____ assault
5. ____ autonomy
6. ____ battery
7. ____ beneficence
8. ____ certification
9. ____ civil law
10. ____ common law
11. ____ confidentiality
12. ____ contract
13. ____ credentialing
14. ____ criminal law
15. ____ defamation
16. ____ defendant
17. ____ durable power of attorney for health care
18. ____ ethics
19. ____ false imprisonment
20. ____ fidelity
21. ____ fraud
22. ____ informed consent
23. ____ invasion of privacy
24. ____ justice
25. ____ law
26. ____ liability
27. ____ license
28. ____ living will
29. ____ malpractice
30. ____ morals
31. ____ negligence
32. ____ nonmaleficence

33. ____ plaintiff
34. ____ procedural law
35. ____ professional misconduct
36. ____ public law
37. ____ registration
38. ____ statutory law
39. ____ substantive law
40. ____ tort
41. ____ values
42. ____ values clarification
43. ____ veracity

a. includes standards and rules applicable to our interactions with one another that are recognized, affirmed, and enforced through judicial decisions
b. the individual against whom a lawsuit is filed
c. involves the legal right of a client to receive adequate and accurate information about their medical condition and treatment
d. acts of negligence by a professional person as compared with the actions of another professional person in similar circumstances
e. violations of a Nurse Practice Act that can result in disciplinary action against a nurse
f. the client's right to privacy in the health care delivery system
g. a process that monitors an educational program's ability to meet predetermined standards for students' outcomes
h. can occur when a nurse unreasonably intrudes upon a client's private affairs
i. occurs when harm or injury is caused by an act of either omission or commission by a layperson
j. adhering to the truth
k. law enacted by the state or federal legislative branch of government
l. a written document that provides direction for health care when a person is unable to make treatment choices
m. an agreement between two or more individuals that creates certain rights and obligations in exchange for goods or services
n. a body of rules of action or conduct prescribed by a "controlling authority"
o. the party bringing a lawsuit who alleges certain facts and outcomes

p. a process by an applicant that provides specific information to the state agency administering the nursing registration process

q. an attempt or threat to touch another person unjustly

r. the methods by which the nursing profession attempts to ensure and maintain the competency of its practitioners

s. standards of conduct that represent the ideal in human behavior to which society expects its members to adhere

t. a document that designates a person to make decisions about a client's medical treatment in the event that the client becomes unable to do so

u. involves the restraining, with or without force, against a person's wishes

v. a civil wrong by one person against another person or his or her property

w. the actual willful touching of another person that may or may not cause harm

x. defines specific behaviors determined to be inappropriate in the orderly functioning of society

y. establishes the manner of proceeding used to enforce a specific legal right or obtain redress

z. implies a legal obligation for which a nurse can be held responsible and accountable

aa. a voluntary process by which a nurse can be granted recognition for meeting certain criteria established by a nongovernmental association

bb. either a false communication or a careless disregard for the truth that results in damage to one's reputation; can take two forms—libel and slander

cc. grants an owner formal permission from a constituted authority to practice a particular profession

dd. the false representation of a fact with the intention that it will be acted upon by another person

ee. regulates disputes between individuals and/or individuals and groups

ff. refers to a person's right to make individual choices; to self-determine

gg. ideals, beliefs, and patterns of behavior that are prized and chosen by a person, group, or society

hh. the branch of philosophy that attempts to determine what constitutes good, bad, right, and wrong in human behavior

ii. the promotion of good

jj. a document that provides written instructions about when life-sustaining treatment should be terminated

kk. requires the practitioner to do no harm

ll. allows you to identify your personal values and develop self-awareness

mm. rules and regulations established through specific hearings and rule-making procedures by state or federal administrative agencies

nn. honoring agreements and keeping promises

oo. moral rightness, fairness, or equity

pp. a part of law that actually stipulates one's rights and duties including the nurse's obligations as a professional nurse

qq. a law that regulates the relationship of individuals to government agencies and is applicable to a whole group of persons such as annual tuberculosis testing for health care workers

TRUE OR FALSE

44. _____ A nurse who was overheard making vicious untrue comments about a co-worker could be charged with defamation.

45. _____ False imprisonment does not include refusing to let clients leave the hospital against their wishes, as long as it is in their best interest to stay.

46. _____ A person who has been declared incompetent by the court is considered to lack the capacity for entering into a contract.

47. _____ A nurse who diverts and sells narcotics can be tried in the court system under civil law.

48. _____ Failing to practice within legal boundaries of nursing practice could result in professional discipline, civil or criminal lawsuits, or employer disciplinary action.

49. _____ The American Nurses Association is the body that has the power to change a Nurse Practice Act.

50. _____ A nursing school that is accredited meets predetermined standards for student outcomes.

51. _____ The process of registration or the renewal of registration helps to ensure that a state has the most current information about a person granted a nursing license.

52. _____ Values shape decisions in everyday life, from the clothes we wear to the movies we prefer.

53. _____ Maintaining client confidentiality means not discussing client issues in hallways, elevators, hospital parking lots, or at home with family and friends.

54. _____ An example of applying the principle of veracity is not telling a terminally ill client his or her prognosis.

55. _____ When two or more principles are in conflict or when choices are favorable, you have an ethical dilemma.

56. _____ In the United States, the American Nurses Association Code for Nurses is the document governing ethical nursing practice.

57. _____ A common ethical problem you may encounter is unit staffing patterns that negatively influence the provision of safe nursing care.

FILL IN THE BLANKS

58. A nurse who administers an injection to a client despite the client's refusal has committed _____.

59. A nurse who is threatened with loss of license is given the right to a fair hearing under _____ law.

60. A nurse who sits for an examination administered by a specialty nursing organization is seeking _____.

61. The process whereby a union negotiates with an employer for nurses' salaries is termed _____ _____.

62. Before undergoing an invasive procedure, the client must give _____ _____.

63. By avoiding conversations about clients in elevators and hallways, a nurse is protecting the client's right to _____.

64. A nurse would fill out an _____ _____ if a client slipped and fell on a wet floor on the nursing unit.

65. The study of _____ entails the examination of human behavior in terms of what ought to be done in the course of human interactions, and it seeks to provide guidelines or principles as a way to direct human interaction.

66. Values are learned behaviors that are influenced by _____, ethnicity, education, and _____ _____.

67. Confidentiality means maintaining another's _____ by safeguarding information that is entrusted to you.

68. _____ is the complement of beneficence.

69. Durable powers of attorney for health care and living wills are both included in a client's _____ record.

EXERCISING YOUR CLINICAL JUDGMENT

A registered nurse has arrived on the clinical unit in the hospital to begin a shift. The nurse will be assigned to a group of seven clients and has been designated as the charge nurse for the day.

70. While beginning to listen to intershift report at the nurses' station, a nurse notes that a client is within earshot. The client states that he would like a cup of coffee until the meal trays arrive. The most appropriate action by the nurse would be to:
    1. ask the client to wait until after report.
    2. tell the client that coffee is unavailable at this time.
    3. ask a nursing assistant to bring coffee to the desk for the client, and continue with report.
    4. ask someone to bring coffee to the client's room, and continue with report after the client leaves.

71. A nurse receives a telephone call stating that a client will be admitted with suspected tuberculosis in the infectious stage. The nurse would plan care for this client using infection-control guidelines from the:
    1. Centers for Disease Control and Prevention.
    2. Occupational Safety and Health Administration.
    3. State Nurse Practice Act.
    4. American Nurses Association.

72. A nurse is documenting care given to an assigned client. The nurse would do which of the following to make an appropriate legal entry in the client's medical record?
    1. Use descriptive words such as *good* or *angry*.
    2. Record measurable and factual information about the client's condition.
    3. Use correcting fluid after making a mistake.
    4. Sign each entry using initials and license number.

TEST YOURSELF

73. You and your classmate discuss your clients in the parking lot. You think that others are not listening to your conversation. Which of the following principles did you breach?
    1. Autonomy
    2. Fidelity
    3. Confidentiality
    4. Beneficence

74. You tell your client that you will give her pain medication at 10 AM. You follow through and give the medication when you stated. You are supporting which ethical principle when you follow through on your commitment?
    1. Autonomy
    2. Beneficence
    3. Nonmaleficence
    4. Fidelity

75. Your client, who has a terminal illness and is expected to live for 6 months, is alert, oriented, and competent. She has very definite wishes about when life-sustaining treatment should be terminated. To support the client's self-determination, the best advice to give her is to:
    1. tell her primary care provider about her wishes.
    2. have a living will.
    3. have a durable power of attorney.
    4. talk with the institution's ethics committee.

76. A nurse is being charged with malpractice. The element of malpractice that is proven by determining that the nurse did not meet the standard of care is:
    1. duty.
    2. breach of duty.
    3. causation.
    4. damages.

77. A nurse is admitting a client who wishes to have "do not resuscitate" status. The nurse determines whether the client has a copy of which of the following items to add to the client's record?
    1. Letter of intent
    2. Physician letter of approval
    3. Advance directive
    4. Last will and testament

78. A nurse is uncertain whether a client understood information about an upcoming invasive diagnostic procedure as presented by a physician. Which of the following factors may invalidate this client's consent?
    1. Emotional status only
    2. Intelligence
    3. Educational level
    4. Emotional or physical barriers

79. A nurse who works with a client population with a high incidence of hypertension (high blood pressure) attends a full-day workshop providing information on nursing management of this disorder. This nurse is striving to maintain which of the following types of competency in nursing practice?
    1. Technical
    2. Cognitive
    3. Interpersonal
    4. Global

80. Three components of a moral conflict include:
    1. personal values, uncertainty, and distress.
    2. choosing, prizing, and acting.
    3. uncertainty, dilemma, and distress.
    4. identifying, examining, and evaluating solutions.

81. You answer a client's questions about his or her diabetes, even though it would have been more comfortable for you to tell the client "not to worry" about the disorder. Which ethical principle applies in this situation?
    1. Autonomy
    2. Virtue
    3. Veracity
    4. Beneficence

82. Using the six-step ethical decision-making process, step 2 is gathering pertinent data. Which of the following questions should you ask to attempt to gather data about an ethical dilemma?
    1. Do institutional values and systems support the nursing decisions made?
    2. With whom must the final decision be made, and is that person competent or empowered to make decisions?
    3. Is the situation truly an ethical dilemma?
    4. What is the effect on those involved?

83. The American Hospital Association's Patient Care Partnership supports the client's right to refuse a recommended treatment or plan of care to the extent permitted by law and hospital policy. Which ethical principle does the bill of rights support?
    1. Nonmaleficence
    2. Autonomy
    3. Beneficence
    4. Veracity

Chapter 7

CULTURAL CONTEXT OF PRACTICE

PURPOSE

This chapter discusses concepts of culture and ethnicity as they relate to nursing care. It provides an overview of transcultural nursing and gives suggestions for performing a transcultural assessment. It also explores basic aspects of selected cultures and their effect on the successful delivery of nursing care.

MATCHING

1. _____ cultural competence
2. _____ culture
3. _____ diversity
4. _____ ethnic
5. _____ ethnicity
6. _____ ethnocentrism
7. _____ humanistic care
8. _____ multicultural society
9. _____ stereotyping
10. _____ transcultural nursing
11. _____ universality

a. groups of persons of the same race or national origin within a larger cultural system who are distinctive based on traditions of religion, language, or appearance
b. culturally competent nursing care focused on differences and similarities among cultures, with respect to caring, health, and illness, based on the client's cultural values, beliefs, and practices
c. a society composed of more than one culture or subculture
d. the assumption that an attribute present in some members of a group is present in all members of a group
e. having enough knowledge of cultural groups that are different from your own to be able to interact with a member of a group in a manner that makes the person feel respected and understood
f. reflects the characteristics a group may share in some combination
g. a common mode or value of caring, or a prevailing pattern of care across cultures
h. the belief that one's own ethnic beliefs, customs, and attitudes are the correct and thus superior

i. a patterned behavioral response that develops over time as a consequence of imprinting the mind through social and religious structures and intellectual and artistic manifestations
j. the differences in modes or patterns of care between cultures, including specific patterns of care within cultural groups
k. includes understanding and knowing a client in as natural or human a way as possible while helping or guiding the client to achieve certain goals, make improvements, reduce discomfort, or face disability or death

TRUE OR FALSE

12. _____ One benefit of providing care within the framework of the client's culture is that it can improve compliance with the health regimen.
13. _____ The majority of Asian Americans would prefer acupuncture to Western approaches to analgesia.
14. _____ The nurse who wishes to provide culturally competent care must have a willingness to compromise with the client about some aspects of care.
15. _____ The cultural phenomenon of space in the transcultural assessment model refers to personal space.
16. _____ A person who is future-oriented in terms of time often has difficulty accepting a plan of care that conflicts with traditional treatments.
17. _____ When communicating with a client from another culture, it is helpful to use eye contact, touch, and seating arrangements that are comfortable for that client.
18. _____ The African-American culture as a group values religion and the power of prayer.
19. _____ Mexican Americans are more likely to perceive life as being under the influence of a divine will.

20. _____ Husbands and elders have authority over wives and children in the family/social structure of the Chinese-American culture.
21. _____ Native Americans subscribe to the germ theory of medicine.

FILL IN THE BLANKS

22. A nurse who helps a client to continue an important cultural practice during illness is engaged in cultural care _____ or _____.

23. A nurse who changes personal behavior or actions to be more fully understood or accepted by the client is engaged in cultural care _____ or _____.

24. _____ is the attribute of cultural competency in which a health care provider recognizes the values and beliefs of both the client and self.

25. _____ _____ is the element of transcultural assessment that indicates clients' beliefs about their ability to control disease.

26. The _____-American cultural group tends to be acutely aware of time and prefers to work efficiently and accomplish tasks in a timely manner.

27. Sickle cell disease is a genetic disorder that is prevalent in the _____-American population.

28. The strength of the nuclear family (parents and children) is the foundation of the _____-American community.

29. The cultural group that adjusts personal diet to meet the yin-yang quality of a disease is the _____-American group.

30. Type 2 diabetes mellitus has high prevalence and tends to occur in the teens and 20s among the _____-_____ group.

31. In traditional Navajo culture, health reflects living in total _____ with nature and having the ability to survive under extremely difficult circumstances.

EXERCISING YOUR CLINICAL JUDGMENT

Mrs. Haygood is a 50-year-old African-American client who has been hospitalized for cardiovascular surgery. She has three grown children and works part time as a receptionist for a local business. A nurse has been assigned as the primary nurse for this client during her postoperative course of recovery.

32. A certified nursing assistant (CNA) tells the nurse that the client speaks "black English" when conversing with family and friends, and reverts to standard English when speaking with nursing staff. The nurse helps the CNA to understand this behavior by indicating that it most likely represents:
    1. a rejection of American culture by the client.
    2. a dislike of American school systems and the standard English language.
    3. a means of maintaining cultural identity.
    4. a permanent learning disability due to uncertain socioeconomic background.

33. Using knowledge of the family/social structure of the African-American culture, the nurse places highest priority on accommodating visits to Mrs. Haygood by which of the following individuals?
    1. A religious leader
    2. A local politician
    3. A new coworker
    4. A friend of a cousin

TEST YOURSELF

34. Which of the following is not a characteristic usually shared by persons within an ethnic group?
    1. Religious faith or faiths
    2. Language or dialect
    3. Food preferences
    4. Loose or distant ties to others in the group

35. A culturally competent practitioner has which of the following attributes?
    1. Lack of awareness
    2. Sensitivity
    3. Lack of respect
    4. Ability to hold firm to one's viewpoint

36. A nurse who is speaking with a client from a different culture would find which of the following communication strategies to be *least* helpful?
    1. Asking the client about the meaning of health, illness, and planned care
    2. Finding out how the illness is likely to affect life, relationships, and self-concept
    3. Trying to anticipate the client's responses
    4. Asking the client how he or she prefers to manage the illness

37. A Mexican-American client tells the nurse about seeking the help of a *curandero* before coming to the health clinic. The nurse understands that, in the Mexican-American culture, this type of folk healer is a:
    1. holistic healer.
    2. healer who uses only herbs.
    3. male witch.
    4. female witch.

38. A hospitalized Chinese-American client states a preference for eating foods that have a yang quality. The nurse would offer the client which of the following food items?
    1. Cucumbers
    2. Oranges
    3. Watermelon
    4. Warm milk

THE HEALTH CARE DELIVERY SYSTEM

PURPOSE

As you begin your professional career in nursing, you will need to identify the components of the health care delivery system, identify the roles of members of the health care team, and understand the effects of social and political forces that will affect your practice. In this chapter you will be introduced to the providers, services, and financing methods that make up the health care delivery system in the United States. You will also explore some of the issues and opportunities facing health care delivery in the twenty-first century. You will want to further explore these issues as you learn more about health care delivery.

MATCHING

1. _____ access
2. _____ capitation payment system
3. _____ diagnosis-related groups (DRGs)
4. _____ exclusive provider organization (EPO)
5. _____ health maintenance organization (HMO)
6. _____ health promotion
7. _____ illness prevention
8. _____ managed care
9. _____ Medicaid
10. _____ medical model
11. _____ Medicare
12. _____ preferred provider organization (PPO)
13. _____ prospective payment system
14. _____ rehabilitation
15. _____ retrospective payment system (PPS)
16. _____ supportive care
17. _____ unlicensed assistive personnel (UAP)

a. involves the use of modalities such as immunizations and medications that avert disease or detect diseases in their earliest, most treatable stages

b. a complex construct representing the personal use of health care services and the structures or processes that facilitate or impede that use

c. a means to modify a client's knowledge, attitudes, and skills to adopt behaviors leading to a healthier lifestyle thus achieving a higher level of wellness from any point on a continuum from health to illness

d. a system of classification or grouping of clients according to medical diagnosis for purposes of paying hospitalization costs

e. a type of group health care practice in which enrollees are restricted to a list of preferred providers of health care called "exclusive providers"

f. a type of group health care practice that provides basic and supplemental health maintenance and treatment services to voluntary enrollees who prepay a fixed periodic fee that is set without regard to the amount or kind of services received

g. payment for health care services as an arrangement between the purchaser of care and the provider in which the provider receives a flat fee to provide a defined level of care

h. has the goals of restoration of function, maintenance of the remaining levels of physical and mental function, and prevention of further deterioration

i. a system that combines the functions of health insurance and the actual delivery of care in a way that controls utilization and costs of services by limiting unnecessary treatment

j. a grant program providing partial health care services for indigent people: supported jointly by federal and state governments

k. a federally funded national health insurance program in the United States for persons over 65 years of age and some chronically ill persons

l. an organization of physicians, hospitals, and pharmacists whose members discount their health care services to subscribers (clients); may be organized by a group of physicians, an outside entrepreneur, an insurance company, or a company with a self-insurance plan

m. a payment system in which the amount paid for for a specific service, is predetermined

n. traditional method of reimbursement; insurance paid based on the services that are received

o. medical, nursing, psychological, and social services aimed at helping a client manage a chronic illness, disability, or terminal illness when rehabilitation or restoration is not a realistic goal

p. health care delivery in which the identification and treatment of an illness or disease is the focus of care

q. an unlicensed individual who is trained to function in an assistive or supportive role to the licensed nurse in the provision of direct client care or peripheral activities that have been delegated by the nurse

TRUE OR FALSE

18. _____ Nurses focus on health promotion and disease prevention and are major care providers for sick and injured clients.

19. _____ Advanced practice nurses include nurse practitioners and physician assistants.

20. _____ Alternative practitioners are irrelevant to a discussion of health practices in the United States.

21. _____ Because of the strict regulation of hospitals, all Americans have equal access to high-quality hospital services.

22. _____ Long-term care (LTC) describes a range of health and housing services provided to persons who are unable to care for themselves independently or in need of assistance to maintain their independence.

23. _____ Paramedics and emergency medical technicians are often the first persons at the scene of an accident or sudden illness and are trained to provide critical early treatment both on site and in transit.

24. _____ Respite care is potentially cost-effective because it helps those who need long-term care to stay at home.

25. _____ The U.S. government has only a limited role in the financing of health care.

26. _____ A health maintenance organization is a means of financing health care for its members but has no influence on the quality of care provided.

27. _____ Health care rationing is associated only with countries that have a national health care system.

28. _____ The fastest-growing segment of the population is persons over the age of 85.

29. _____ There will be a growing demand for health care providers who speak languages other than English and who understand the health needs of a multiethnic society.

30. _____ More than 14% of the U.S. gross national product is consumed by health care.

31. _____ As a nurse, you are primarily concerned with quality of care rather than with cost of care.

FILL IN THE BLANKS

32. _____ are the largest group of health care professionals in the United States.

33. _____ dispense medications and assist physicians in making appropriate drug choices.

34. The term _____ describes a client who receives care in the context of an overnight stay in a hospital or other health care facility.

35. An example of a first tier of the hospital system that offers more limited scope of services is a _____.

36. _____ is a service offered to clients who need restorative services or treatment to recover from an injury or illness.

37. _____ is a method of care that regards both the client and the family as the unit of care.

38. A _____ is the primary site for the delivery of physician services.

39. _____ is a daytime program that provides a wide range of health and recreational services to frail (usually elderly) adults who require supervision and care while family members are away at work.

40. The _____ _____ spends more money per person on health care than any other country in the developed world.

41. A _____ _____ _____ may be organized by a group of physicians, an outside entrepreneur, an insurance company, or a company with a self-insurance plan.

42. Medicare finances health care for _____, _____, and _____.

43. In _____ (country) the government finances health care, but private providers deliver health care services.

44. _____% of American households with children under the age of 18 include a married couple.

EXERCISING YOUR CLINICAL JUDGMENT

You are working on a cardiac unit in a community hospital. Your client is a 58-year-old male who has had a minor heart attack. You are working with this person to plan for care after discharge. The following questions address the needs you and the client have identified.

45. The client has smoked a pack of cigarettes a day for 42 years. He knows he needs to quit but has been unsuccessful despite multiple attempts. He wants to join a support group. Which source is most likely to provide access (financial support) to a support group?
    1. A preferred provider organization
    2. A health maintenance organization
    3. Catastrophic health insurance
    4. Medicare

46. Your client would like to try the cholesterol-reducing medication that has recently been advertised on television. You would suggest that he ask his:
    1. pharmacist.
    2. physician.
    3. respiratory therapist.
    4. managed care organization.

47. The physician has recommended a cardiac rehabilitation program for the next 6 months. You are reviewing a pamphlet about the program with the client. He asks, "What does *rehabilitation* mean? I thought that was for persons who were paralyzed." Your best answer would be:
    1. "*Rehabilitation* is any long-term care service for persons who need additional therapy or treatment to recover from an illness or injury."
    2. "Using that term is a way to get your insurance to pay for the services."
    3. "*Rehabilitation* only refers to the exercise program that will be designed by a physical therapist."
    4. "Any service outside a hospital is rehabilitation."

TEST YOURSELF

48. Your client is being discharged after having a growth removed from her abdomen. The doctor has assured her that the tumor was benign and that no further treatment is indicated. She says, "My neighbor uses an Ayurveda practitioner. She had cancer 15 years ago and it never returned. What do you think?" Your most appropriate response would be:
    1. "It sounds like a good idea to me. You never know what will work."
    2. "I don't think it's safe to use alternative medicine. None of it is proven."
    3. "You should learn more about it before trying it. Let me get you a pamphlet that gives some suggestions for evaluation of alternative practices."
    4. "Ayurveda therapy won't prevent the recurrence of cancer. You need to stick with your medical doctor."

49. Your client tells you that his insurance company will allow him to see any physician he chooses, but the fees are better if he chooses a physician from a list provided by the insurance company. He is most likely describing:
    1. a health maintenance organization.
    2. a managed care organization.
    3. Medicaid coverage.
    4. a preferred provider organization.

50. If you could make a change in the delivery of health care for the growing number of Hispanic Americans, which would be most likely to result in integrating cost control and improved quality?
    1. Targeting genetically transmitted diseases that only affect Hispanics
    2. Increasing the number of Hispanic health providers
    3. Ensuring access to health care for Hispanic persons
    4. Targeting the most common health problems for Hispanic persons

51. A 95-year-old male client is admitted to a nursing home after an episode of heart failure. The doctor has given him the option to have a heart valve replacement, but the client prefers conservative treatment. The nursing home will monitor his medication and will help him achieve a balance of rest and activity, maintain a low-salt diet, and maintain his relationship with his family. This type of care is best labeled:
    1. illness prevention.
    2. acute care.
    3. rehabilitation.
    4. supportive care.

PURPOSE

This chapter introduces of the importance of nursing theory. It compares and contrasts the leading nursing theories, including the concepts of person, environment, health, and nursing as the most recognized organizing realities of nursing theory. It helps you recognize how and when you use your ciritcal thinking skills and enables you to improve the use of these skills. It also introduces the nursing process, a patterned way of thinking used in making nursing judgments, decisions, and diagnoses. You will be able to identify how multiple thinking strategies apply to each phase of the nursing process.

MATCHING

1. _____ abstract
2. _____ Benner's stages of skill acquisition
3. _____ caring
4. _____ clinical judgment
5. _____ concept
6. _____ critical thinking
7. _____ decision making
8. _____ diagnostic reasoning
9. _____ empirical
10. _____ nursing process
11. _____ problem solving
12. _____ theory
13. _____ T.H.I.N.K. model

a. the process of clustering assessment data into meaningful sets and generating hypotheses about a client's human responses
b. a critical thinking framework that includes decision making, diagnostic reasoning, problem solving, and clinical judgment; it is composed of five interrelated parts: assessment, diagnosis, planning, intervention, and evaluation
c. defining a problem, selecting information pertinent to its conclusion (recognizing stated and unstated assumptions), formulating alternative solutions, drawing a conclusion, and judging the validity of the conclusion.

d. purposeful self-regulatory judgment that gives reasoned and reflective consideration to evidence, contexts, conceptualizations, methods, and criteria
e. choosing between two or more options as a means to achieve a desired result
f. a conclusion or an opinion that a problem or situation requires nursing care
g. an idea, thought, or notion conceived in the mind
h. a group of propositions used to describe, explain, or predict a phenomenon
i. concepts that can be observed or experienced through the senses
j. to be attentive or watch over the needs of another person
k. concepts that are not observable such as caring and hope
l. a critical thinking model that incorporates total recall, habits, inquiry, new ideas and creativity, and knowledge of how you think simultaneously or in combination
m. the five levels of proficiency a nurse passes through while moving from novice to expert

TRUE OR FALSE

14. _____ Theories are important to nurses because they interpret and explain the reality of nursing, thus guiding practice, education, and research activities for nursing as a profession.

15. _____ A nursing theory is unacceptable when the consensus of the nursing profession is that the theory provides an adequate description of reality.

16. _____ Roy believed that caring is the central theme in nursing knowledge and practice.

17. _____ The T.H.I.N.K. model is based on the idea that you use different elements of thinking in different situations.

18. _____ Inquiry includes the quality of being curious or wondering about the meaning of information.
19. _____ Assessment means collecting answers to a predetermined list of questions.

FILL IN THE BLANKS

20. The concepts of _____, environment, health, and _____ are the most recognized organizing realities of nursing theory.

21. It is helpful for you to know more than one nursing _____ because what you observe, document, choose as an intervention, and evaluate depends on your theoretical perspective guiding nursing practice.

22. Orem's theory focuses on the role of the _____ in helping clients meet their needs.

23. Obstacles to critical thinking include _____, _____, _____, _____, _____, and _____.

24. In the planning phase, you set _____ and plan _____ care.

25. Dependent interventions are activities carried out under a _____ order.

26. NANDA stands for the _____ _____ _____ _____ _____.

TEST YOURSELF

27. Your client is Irish American who has had abdominal surgery. You recognize the client's pain and that her minimizing of the pain may be related to cultural ways. You stress to the client that if she has adequate pain relief she will be able to tend to all of her needs. You are applying which nursing theorist's theory?
    1. Hildegarde Peplau
    2. Faye Abdellah
    3. Dorothea Orem
    4. Madeleine Leininger

28. You are taking an admission history. You know the medical diagnosis, but the client's report of symptoms does not exactly fit the pattern of expected symptoms. Which action would be the *least* consistent with critical thinking?
    1. Explore the symptoms further.
    2. Record the symptoms as described by the client.
    3. Record only the symptoms you believe are pertinent to the diagnosis.
    4. Ask the client about his perception of the symptoms.

29. You have a new job as a home health nurse. You must perform a procedure in the client's home. Although you have done the procedure many times in the hospital, you do not have the same resources in the home. Which mode of thinking will be most useful to you?
    1. Total recall
    2. Habit
    3. Inquiry
    4. New ideas

30. A client complains of nausea. You know the physician has written an order for a medication to treat nausea if the client needs it. Using the nursing process to guide your thinking, you would first:
    1. ask the client to further describe the nausea.
    2. give the antinausea medication.
    3. plan to cancel the client's lunch.
    4. notify the physician.

31. Nursing theories do which of the following?
    1. Differentiate the focus of nursing from other professions and facilitate the continued growth and development of the profession
    2. Provide a conceptual diagram of the profession
    3. Are beliefs about phenomena
    4. Are relationship statements that are tested

32. Which nursing leader's theory is the primary basis for psychiatric nursing?
    1. Virginia Henderson
    2. Hildegarde Peplau
    3. Faye Abdellah
    4. Dorothea Orem

33. Which of the following nursing leaders emphasized that nursing is not something a person does, but a body of abstract knowledge and a learned profession that is both science and art?
    1. Virginia Henderson
    2. Hildegarde Peplau
    3. Faye Abdellah
    4. Martha Rogers

34. You assess your client and find that she has sluggish skin turgor, sunken eyeballs, and a low urinary output. You know that these are signs of dehydration and conclude that your client should drink more water. You have:
    1. made an interpretation of data.
    2. made an assumption.
    3. engaged in problem solving.
    4. recognized the purpose of thinking.

35. You are assigned to work with a staff nurse. When you and the staff nurse enter a client's room, you find the client slumped in bed. You assume that the client is sleeping, but the staff nurse turns on the call light and pages for a resuscitation team. Which of Benner's stages apply to the staff nurse?
    1. Advanced beginner
    2. Competent
    3. Proficient
    4. Expert

36. You are assigned to a different nurse on the following day. A client tells you that she does not need a laxative. The nurse tells you that a laxative is always given after the procedure the client has had, and you should insist that the client take it. This nurse is most likely in which stage?
    1. Novice
    2. Advanced beginner
    3. Competent
    4. Proficient

Chapter 6

CLIENT ASSESSMENT: NURSING HISTORY

PURPOSE

This chapter outlines the thinking skills associated with assessment and introduces a general pattern for taking a nursing history. You will learn additional information about nursing history with each clinical chapter you study.

MATCHING

1. _____ active listening
2. _____ active processing
3. _____ assessment
4. _____ biographical data
5. _____ cardinal signs and symptoms
6. _____ chief complaint
7. _____ closed question
8. _____ cue
9. _____ data
10. _____ database
11. _____ demographic data
12. _____ functional health patterns
13. _____ inference
14. _____ interview
15. _____ intuition
16. _____ leading question
17. _____ minimum data set
18. _____ nursing history
19. _____ objective data
20. _____ open-ended question
21. _____ orientation phase
22. _____ signs
23. _____ subjective data
24. _____ symptoms
25. _____ termination
26. _____ validation
27. _____ working phase

a. a phase of the interview process during which a client and nurse work together to review the client's health history and establish potential and actual problems that will be addressed as part of the care plan

b. subjective information supplied by the client that describes characteristics of disease or dysfunction

c. substantiating or confirming the accuracy of the information against another source or by another method

d. information that is provided by a client and cannot be directly observed

e. the problem that causes a client to seek health services, call the doctor, or request a visit from a nurse; a description of what a client thinks is the problem

f. a planned series of questions designed to elicit information for a particular purpose

g. any directly observable information about a client

h. the positive and negative behavior a person uses to interact with the environment and maintain health

i. a question designed to allow a client freedom in the manner of response

j. a process of reasoning from understanding the whole without having systematically examined the parts

k. a brief exchange to establish the purpose, procedure, and nurse's role in the interview process

l. objective data that are evidence of disease or dysfunction

m. a narrative of a client's past health and health practices that focuses on information needed to plan nursing care

n. the least information allowable to be collected on every client entering an institution or being admitted to a particular service within the institution

o. the process of attaching meaning to data or reaching a conclusion about data; based on a premise or proposition that supports or helps support a conclusion

p. a question that suggests a possible appropriate response from a client

q. information that identifies and describes a client, such as name, address, age, gender, religious affiliation, race, or occupation

r. a question that calls for a specific short response from a client

s. all of the information that has been collected about a client and recorded in the health record as a baseline for the initial plan of care

t. factual information that can be aggregated to describe populations of clients

u. the data of greatest significance in diagnosing a particular illness, disease, or health problem

v. an indicator of the presence or existence of a problem or condition that represents a client's underlying health status

w. participation in a conversation with a client in which the nurse attends to what the client says and has a part in helping the client clarify, elaborate, and give additional pertinent information

x. the process of gathering data about a client's health status to identify the concerns and needs that can be treated or managed by nursing care

y. pieces of subjective or objective information about a client or the signs and symptoms of disease

z. a systematic series of mental actions to analyze and interpret information about a client

aa. skillfully ending an interview so that the nurse and client feel satisfied that the purpose has been accomplished

TRUE OR FALSE

28. _____ When prevention is the focus of care, client assessment includes risk and lifestyle factors.

29. _____ When, how often, and how to assess a client is a nursing judgment based on individual client needs.

30. _____ It is always appropriate to gather data from a client's family.

31. _____ Collecting data in a systematic way is a standard of nursing practice.

32. _____ Grouping data into meaningful patterns helps you translate the data into a meaningful statement.

33. _____ For any client, the purpose of an admission interview is always to collect a standard set of data.

34. _____ The termination phase of an interview is limited to the last few minutes of the interview.

35. _____ Biographical data are collected only to help you know the client as a person.

36. _____ The medical history is not part of the nursing history.

37. _____ Beliefs about health and the ability to change health are a key element of the health perception–health management pattern.

38. _____ A functional health pattern includes both functional and dysfunctional patterns.

39. _____ The activity-exercise pattern includes only the musculoskeletal system.

40. _____ Only objective data are documented in the medical record.

41. _____ It is legally advisable to document the facts that lead to a conclusion or opinion rather than your own conclusion or opinion.

FILL IN THE BLANKS

42. To decide how often to assess a client, you need to anticipate the _____, _____, and _____ of change.

43. The seven general factors used to assess a symptom are _____, _____, _____, _____, _____, _____, and _____.

44. Questions describing the onset of symptoms, when symptoms occur, and the events surrounding symptoms are classified as _____.

45. A description of a client's dietary habits is included in the _____-_____ pattern.

46. A description of a client's tolerance for activity is included in the _____-_____ pattern.

47. A description of a client's perception of body image is included in the _____-_____-_____ pattern.

TEST YOURSELF

48. A female client who has four children, works full time, and volunteers at her church is admitted. She has peptic ulcer disease, an illness that is sometimes exacerbated by stress. Which of the following activities would you do to assess the coping-stress tolerance pattern?
   1. Assume that the illness is exacerbated by stress.
   2. Plan to teach the client stress-reduction techniques.
   3. Avoid discussion of the many stressors in the client's life.
   4. Validate the client's experience of stress by eliciting information about her perceptions.

49. Which of the following activities would you do to assess the self-concept pattern on every client?
   1. Ask a series of questions to elicit information about the self-concept.
   2. Observe, listen, and be sensitive to covert messages.
   3. Administer a standardized test for self-concept.
   4. Ask the client to rate his or her self-concept on a scale of 1 to 10.

50. A 55-year-old male client is hospitalized for heart disease. His doctor has suggested that he needs to retire. Which functional health pattern would you explore to help him through this experience?
    1. Sexuality-reproductive pattern
    2. Role-relationship pattern
    3. Coping-stress tolerance pattern
    4. Sleep-rest pattern

51. You are taking an admission history. The client tells you that he has pain in his leg. Which question is most pertinent to his safety in the hospital?
    1. "How long have you had the pain?"
    2. "Where is the pain located?"
    3. "Do you have any difficulty walking?"
    4. "What aggravates the pain?"

52. Your client has requested pain medication. If you could only ask one question for further assessment, which question would you choose?
    1. "Did the last pain medication relieve the pain?"
    2. "How long have you had the pain?"
    3. "What brought on the pain?"
    4. "Is your pain less than yesterday's pain?"

53. Select the statement that is true of assessment.
    1. Assessment means collecting data.
    2. Assessment includes analyzing data to determine the need for nursing care.
    3. Assessment does not include physical examination.
    4. Assessment is a separate activity from planning and implementing care.

54. Which of the following items provides the best description of the term *focused assessment?*
    1. Paying close attention to a client's needs
    2. Concentrating on an identified need, and getting more information
    3. Identifying a client's needs
    4. Using the acronym FOCUS

55. Which of the following items provides the best description of objective data?
    1. It is pertinent to an objective or goal.
    2. It can be gathered through the use of one of the five senses.
    3. It is elicited from a client in an objective manner.
    4. It is related to the objects in a client's room.

56. You are sharing information with a client's physician that the wife of the client has given you. The physician asks you if the wife is a reliable source. Which of the following data is the most useful to you in deciding whether or not the wife is a reliable source?
    1. The couple has been arguing about the nature of his symptoms.
    2. The husband has asked you to talk to his wife about his symptoms.
    3. The wife presents information factually and has kept a diary of the symptoms.
    4. The husband shows evidence of minor memory impairment.

57. *Fact:* Your client's antihypertensive medication prescription was filled 15 days ago with 60 tablets. He is supposed to take 2 tablets a day. He has 40 tablets left. *Premise:* There is a high incidence of failure to take blood pressure medications correctly among persons with hypertension because of side effects. Select the most accurate conclusion.
    1. The client does not understand how to take the medication.
    2. The client does not want to take the medication.
    3. The client has taken the medication incorrectly.
    4. The side effects have been intolerable for the client.

PURPOSE

The purpose of this chapter is to help you learn accurate techniques for measuring vital signs and to understand the physiological changes that affect vital signs. You will also begin the process of interpreting or attaching meaning to your findings.

MATCHING

1. _____ apical pulse
2. _____ auscultatory gap
3. _____ basal metabolic rate (BMR)
4. _____ bradycardia
5. _____ bradypnea
6. _____ diastolic blood pressure
7. _____ eupnea
8. _____ Korotkoff's sounds
9. _____ orthostatic hypotension
10. _____ oxygen saturation
11. _____ peripheral vascular resistance
12. _____ pulse deficit
13. _____ pulse oximeter
14. _____ pulse pressure
15. _____ systolic blood pressure
16. _____ tachycardia
17. _____ tachypnea
18. _____ thermogenesis
19. _____ thermolysis
20. _____ tidal volume

a. the condition of the apical pulse rate exceeding the radial pulse rate
b. the processes through which heat is dispersed from the body through radiation, conduction, convection, and evaporation
c. the generation of heat from the chemical reactions that take place in cellular activity
d. the heart rate counted at the apex of the heart on the anterior chest
e. the amount of energy needed to maintain essential basic body functions expressed as calories per hour per square meter of body surface
f. the difference between the systolic and diastolic blood pressures

g. normal quiet respirations with a rate of 12 to 20 breaths/minute in an adult at rest
h. the absence of Korotkoff II sounds; sometimes present in hypertension
i. a heart rate less than 60 beats/minute
j. a respiratory rate less than 12 breaths/minute
k. the pressure in the blood vessels that remains during relaxation of the ventricles
l. a heart rate greater than 100 beats per minute
m. the volume of air exchanged with each breath
n. five distinct sounds heard as a blood pressure cuff is deflated from total occlusion of the artery to complete free flow of blood
o. the pressure in the arteries produced by the cardiac output during contraction of the ventricle
p. a respiratory rate of more than 20 breaths/minute
q. the amount of oxygen in a client's arterial blood.
r. an electronic device that measures the amount of oxygen in a client's blood through a sensor unit or probe
s. the impediment of blood flow through the vascular system
t. a blood pressure drop of 20 mm Hg or more that occurs with a change in the client's position

TRUE OR FALSE

21. _____ The absolute value of vital signs is the basis for inferences about vital signs.
22. _____ How often you take vital signs is a nursing judgment.
23. _____ The body's cells work within a narrow range of normal temperature but can tolerate some changes for a brief period.
24. _____ High temperatures damage cells by inactivating proteins and enzymes.
25. _____ An oral temperature can be accurately measured by placing the thermometer anywhere in the mouth.
26. _____ You clean a glass thermometer by wiping from the bulb toward the end.

27. _____ A heart rate of 100 is always a cause for concern.
28. _____ Vomiting can cause bradycardia.
29. _____ Adrenalin increases the heart rate.
30. _____ Head injuries always increase the heart rate.
31. _____ The strength of the pulse wave is only a function of the strength of myocardial contraction.
32. _____ The carotid artery is the most common site for counting the pulse.
33. _____ The most accurate pulse count is obtained at the apex of the heart.
34. _____ The medullary control center for respiration responds to high levels of carbon dioxide.
35. _____ Sighing is a protective mechanism that periodically expands unused alveoli.

FILL IN THE BLANKS

36. _____ _____ are the signs of life.

37. The processes through which the body balances heat production and heat loss to maintain a temperature between 96.8° F and 99.4° F is called _____.

38. The _____ thermometer is inexpensive, easy to use, and easily disinfected; however, it frequently contains mercury, which is poisonous.

39. The _____ thermometer utilizes a heat-sensitive probe that is placed in the ear canal.

40. Children have a slightly _____ heart rate than adults do.

41. Adrenergic drugs (acting like adrenaline) cause the heart rate to _____ (increase, decrease).

42. When the pulse wave increases during inhalation and decreases back to normal during exhalation, the phenomenon is called _____ _____.

43. When blood vessels constrict, blood flow is impeded because the lumen of the vessels is smaller. The smaller diameter creates peripheral vascular _____.

44. The systolic blood pressure is created by the _____ (contraction, relaxation) of the ventricles.

45. The diastolic blood pressure is the pressure that remains during _____ (contraction, relaxation) of the ventricles.

46. The width of the blood pressure cuff should be about _____ _____ the length of the upper arm.

TEST YOURSELF

47. Your client has a temperature of 103° F, respiration of 30, and pulse of 50. She is cold and clammy, and her blood pressure is 100/60. Which conclusion is most consistent with these findings?
    1. The temperature has caused a decrease in her pulse rate. Correcting the temperature will fix the problem.
    2. The low pulse rate is causing a decrease in cardiac output, thus reducing the blood pressure. It may or may not be related to the temperature.
    3. The low pulse rate and blood pressure is a compensatory response to decrease the metabolic rate.
    4. The high temperature is consistent with the low pulse rate and blood pressure.

48. The physician tells you that the client has atherosclerotic vascular disease that is increasing peripheral vascular resistance. Which vital signs would be consistent with this information?
    1. Blood pressure 140/100, pulse 90, respiration 18
    2. Blood pressure 110/60, pulse 60, respiration 18
    3. Blood pressure 160/80, pulse 56, respiration 16
    4. Blood pressure 140/84, pulse 80, respiration 20

49. Your client's blood pressure is 180/106. You administer an antihypertensive drug and go to the room to recheck the blood pressure in 1 hour. You find the client in the bathroom, and she is pale, sweating, and feels faint. You get her back to bed and take her vital signs. Which of the following would you expect?
    1. Blood pressure is 180/106; the medication did not work.
    2. Blood pressure is 120/80; the sudden drop caused the symptoms.
    3. Blood pressure is 160/96; the medication is taking effect, but has made her sick.
    4. Blood pressure is 120/80; the medication has been effective, and the symptoms have another cause.

50. Digitalis is a medication that slows the heart rate and strengthens the contraction. Before giving digitalis, it is common practice to check the pulse. If the client's pulse has been averaging 80 for the last 3 days, which pulse rate would suggest that the expected result has become a toxic effect?
    1. Pulse 56
    2. Pulse 66
    3. Pulse 76
    4. Pulse 96

51. Your client was burned on the right arm while lighting a charcoal fire. He has an intravenous line in the left arm that was inserted with difficulty. Which action would you take related to vital signs?
    1. Because he is awake and alert, omit taking a blood pressure.
    2. Use a smaller-size cuff for the blood pressure.
    3. Take the blood pressure in the thigh.
    4. Assess the systolic pressure only by palpating the radial artery.

52. You have admitted a 16-month-old client with fever of unknown origin. The child's cheeks are red, and the skin feels warm to the touch. The tympanic thermometer reads 98.6° F. Which of the following would be the best action?
    1. Check the temperature in the room, and lower the thermostat for comfort.
    2. Ask the mother about the technique she used to take the temperature to determine if the reported fever was accurate.
    3. Straighten the ear canal, and recheck the temperature. Use another method if necessary to accurately measure the temperature.
    4. Recalibrate the thermometer, and check the temperature.

53. You take a client's temperature at 6 AM. It is 96.8° F. What is the most probable cause?
    1. A cold room
    2. Drinking ice water
    3. Circadian rhythms
    4. A faulty thermometer

54. Which of the following activities is appropriate when preparing to take an axillary temperature?
    1. Dry the axilla before inserting the thermometer.
    2. Lubricate the thermometer before insertion.
    3. Position the client in the side-lying position.
    4. Shave the axilla.

55. The client's rectal temperature is 100° F. After conversion, which of the following would be a comparable axillary temperature?
    1. 97° F
    2. 98° F
    3. 99° F
    4. 101° F

56. Nurses have some discretion in selecting the route to take a temperature. Which of the following represents the best judgment?
    1. Taking an oral temperature for a 12-month-old child
    2. Taking a rectal temperature for a confused 85-year-old man
    3. Taking an axillary temperature for a newborn
    4. Taking an oral temperature for a client who had oral surgery

57. Select the situation that may result in an inaccurate measurement of blood pressure.
    1. The width of the cuff is 20% greater than the diameter of the arm.
    2. The aneroid sphygmomanometer is viewed from the side.
    3. The meniscus of the mercury manometer is at eye level.
    4. The cuff is placed 1 inch above the fold of the elbow.

58. Which of the following should be recorded as the diastolic pressure in an adult?
    1. The first distinct beat that is heard
    2. The change in sound from a clear distinct tapping to a soft muffled sound
    3. The middle sound between the first and last beat that is heard
    4. The last sound that is heard

59. To obtain the most accurate blood pressure reading, the cuff should be inflated to:
    1. 30 mm Hg above the palpated systolic pressure.
    2. the systolic reading last recorded on the client's chart.
    3. 50 mm Hg above the last diastolic reading.
    4. 200 mm Hg in an adult client.

60. Which action might result in a falsely low systolic blood pressure reading?
    1. Allowing the client to cross the legs while blood pressure is being taken
    2. Deflating the cuff too rapidly while blood pressure is being auscultated
    3. Requiring the client to support the arm isometrically while blood pressure is being taken
    4. Having the client think relaxing thoughts

61. Select the inference that is most accurate without further assessment.
    1. A right radial pulse of 88 beats per minute indicates that the client has adequate oxygenation to the right hand.
    2. Respirations of 18 per minute indicate that the client is taking in sufficient amounts of oxygen.
    3. The auscultated blood pressure of 130/88 is a normal blood pressure for this particular client.
    4. When the apical pulse is 80 and the radial pulse is 60, the client has a pulse deficit.

62. A client has just been admitted with a lung infection. His vital signs indicate hypotension, tachycardia, and tachypnea. This information would be supported by which set of data?
    1. Blood pressure 150/105, pulse 123, respiration 12
    2. Blood pressure 90/40, pulse 110, respiration 28
    3. Blood pressure 120/80, pulse 50, respiration 40
    4. Blood pressure 115/80, pulse 100, respiration 30

63. A client had a temperature of 104° F at 10 AM. At 1 PM, the skin is warm and wet with perspiration. The nurse retakes the temperature. Select the finding that would be expected.
    1. A normal or near-normal temperature is found.
    2. The fever has not abated.
    3. The temperature has increased.
    4. The client is anxious.

64. For which of the following clients would you take a rectal rather than an oral temperature?
    1. A 10-year-old female client admitted with a urinary tract infection
    2. A 79-year-old male client with dentures who is NPO for surgery
    3. A 40-year-old male client admitted for new-onset confusion
    4. An 80-year-old female client admitted for a total hip replacement

65. A 45-year-old client has been in a motor vehicle accident (MVA). He was examined in the emergency room and transferred to your unit for observation. Vital signs are blood pressure 100/60, pulse 94, respiration 22, and temperature 98.6° F. Select the best conclusion concerning these findings.
    1. The vital signs may indicate impending shock; notify the physician.
    2. These are normal findings for this age; continue routine monitoring.
    3. These may be normal findings, but there is concern about the blood pressure; continue monitoring.
    4. The client probably received pain medication in the emergency room.

PURPOSE

This chapter provides information about the basic techniques of physical examination and the primary instruments used in physical assessment. You will also be introduced to some abnormal findings as a way to help you begin to compare normal and abnormal findings.

MATCHING

1. _____ accommodation
2. _____ auscultation
3. _____ bronchial
4. _____ bronchovesicular
5. _____ ecchymosis
6. _____ inspection
7. _____ lesion
8. _____ ophthalmoscope
9. _____ otoscope
10. _____ palpation
11. _____ percussion
12. _____ point of maximum impulse (PMI)
13. _____ precordium
14. _____ respiratory excursion
15. _____ tactile fremitus
16. _____ turgor
17. _____ vesicular

a. the area on the anterior chest overlying the heart and great vessels
b. the use of short, sharp strikes to the body surface to produce palpable vibrations and characteristic sounds
c. touching or feeling with the hand to obtain information regarding temperature, moisture, texture, consistency, size, shape, position, and movement
d. normal breath sounds heard over the right and left branch; a combination of sounds from the bronchi and alveoli
e. the process of listening to sounds generated within the body
f. a normal sound heard with a stethoscope over the main bronchus

g. the systematic visual examination of the client
h. a wound, injury, or a pathological change in the body
i. an instrument used to visualize the retina, including the optic disk, macula, and retinal blood vessels through the pupil
j. an instrument used to examine the external ear, the eardrum, and, through the eardrum, the ossicles of the middle ear; consists of a light, a magnifying lens, a speculum, and sometimes a device for insufflation
k. the point where the heart comes the closest to the chest wall at the apex of the heart
l. a reflection of the skin's elasticity measured as the time it takes for the skin to return to normal after being pinched lightly between the thumb and forefinger
m. a normal sound of rustling or swishing heard with a stethoscope over the lung periphery; characteristically higher-pitched during inspiration and falling rapidly during expiration
n. a blue-black skin discoloration, characterized by large irregularly formed hemorrhagic areas; changes to greenish brown or yellow during healing
o. adjustment of the eye for seeing objects at various distances
p. a vibration in the chest that is felt on the thorax while the client is speaking
q. the ability of the lungs to expand as evidenced by the degree to which the chest wall expands

TRUE OR FALSE

18. _____ You should always begin a physical examination with the client in the sitting position.
19. _____ The sagittal plane divides the body into right and left halves.
20. _____ The heart is located lateral to the midline on the right side.

21. _____ The advantage of using a balanced scale is accuracy because the scale can be balanced at zero with each use.

22. _____ If the client can tell you that the current time of day is after lunchtime, you may assume orientation to time.

23. _____ Damage to the facial nerve (cranial nerve VII) results in lack of control of the muscles needed to close the eye.

24. _____ Yearly eye exams are indicated for clients with bleeding disorders or those on anticoagulant therapy.

25. _____ PERRLA is checked on the unconscious client to determine visual acuity.

26. _____ Arteries are distinguishable as brighter than veins when checking the ocular fundus.

27. _____ You should angle the otoscope at a 90-degree angle to the ear to visualize the eardrum.

28. _____ The thyroid gland should feel smooth and hard.

29. _____ A cervical lymph node that is less than 1 cm with definite margins and is mobile and nontender is a normal finding.

30. _____ Assessing the breast for lumps includes assessing the axilla.

31. _____ Decreased respiratory excursion occurs with any condition that limits the expansion of the lungs.

32. _____ S_2 is associated with the closure of the pulmonic and aortic valves.

33. _____ An apical/radial pulse should be checked on every client with heart disease.

34. _____ A rapid rhythm with an S_3 sound is described as a ventricular gallop.

35. _____ A grade 6 murmur is barely audible.

36. _____ A bruit is normally heard at the carotid artery because of the vessel's large size.

37. _____ If you cannot feel a popliteal pulse, you should confirm its absence with a Doppler.

38. _____ Identifying hypoactive bowel sounds is a precise measurement of the volume and frequency of the sounds.

39. _____ A gastric bubble causes a tympanic sound with percussion over the right upper quadrant.

40. _____ The Babinski reflex should be absent in an adult.

FILL IN THE BLANKS

41. Use the technique of _____ _____ to identify and examine lesions or masses on the surface of the skin or immediately under the skin.

42. Use the physical assessment skill of _____ to tap on the abdomen to detect the presence of "gas" or flatus.

43. Using the technique of listening to the abdomen is called _____.

44. _____ _____ refers to patterns of thinking such as logic, relevance, organization, and coherence of thought.

45. Skin is best assessed in _____ light.

46. _____ is a crackling or rubbing sound heard during movement of joints, such as the temporomandibular joint.

47. A reported result of 30/60–2 on a visual acuity test means the client is able to read with _____ errors at a distance of _____ feet, a line of print that a client with normal vision can read at _____ feet.

48. The _____ test is a hearing test that compares air and bone conduction using a tuning fork.

49. A client with periodontal disease often has red, swollen gums indicating _____.

50. _____ respiration is the deep rapid breathing seen in diabetic ketoacidosis.

51. If you hear an abnormal breath sound in part of the cycle of respiration (such as with inspiration and not expiration), you would describe the sound as _____ (continuous, discontinuous).

52. _____ _____ reflexes are elicited by stretching a tendon by tapping with a reflex hammer.

53. The _____ _____ is a cytology test used to screen for cervical cancer.

54. A _____ can be felt as a string of beadlike nodules or "bag of worms" in the scrotum.

TEST YOURSELF

55. Your client is a 90-year-old female who is admitted to the hospital with a respiratory problem. She seems clean, well-groomed, and well-nourished, but is unsteady when walking, seems a little confused, and has pain in her chest. Circle all of the elements of the physical exam that you would consider essential.
    1. Assessment for adventitious sounds
    2. Formal mental status exam
    3. Assessment of all pulses
    4. Complete abdominal assessment
    5. Rectal examination
    6. Skin assessment
    7. Complete musculoskeletal assessment
    8. Inspection of the toenails
    9. Hearing and vision screening
    10. Assessment of rate and rhythm of the heart
    11. Listening for murmurs

56. Your client has returned from a cardiac catheterization. The catheter was threaded through the right femoral artery. You are checking for blood clots traveling from the artery to the lower leg. The dorsalis pedis pulse is strong. What would you do next?
    1. Check the popliteal pulse.
    2. Check the femoral pulse.
    3. Check the color and warmth of the toes.
    4. Conclude that the circulation is good.

57. Your client has an irregular heartbeat, and the apical/radial pulse is 80/60. Which of the following additional findings would you expect?
    1. Talkative, skin color pink, looking forward to visitors
    2. Blood pressure low, skin pale, feels weak
    3. Skin hot, face flushed, feels anxious
    4. Mentally alert, blood pressure 140/90, respiration 16

58. Which assessment data provides the nurse with the best information regarding the client's ability to perfuse distal tissues?
    1. Blood pressure, Homans' sign, and breath sounds
    2. Respiration, peripheral pulses, and skin turgor
    3. Capillary refill, peripheral pulses, and skin color
    4. Skin turgor, skin color, and quality of pulse

59. During lung auscultation, the nurse would ask the client to do which of the following?
    1. Breathe deeply with the mouth open
    2. Cough with each inhalation
    3. Hold the breath
    4. Breathe quietly and normally

60. During assessment, you cannot palpate a client's pedal pulses bilaterally. Which of the following would be the best nursing action?
    1. Palpate the femoral arteries.
    2. Immediately call the doctor.
    3. Assess the color and temperature of the client's feet.
    4. Ask the client to wiggle his or her toes.

61. A client's left radial pulse is assessed as irregular. Which of the following would be the best nursing action?
    1. Take an apical pulse for 1 full minute.
    2. Recount the radial pulse for 2 minutes to assess for regularity.
    3. Have another nurse check the right radial pulse while the first nurse recounts the left pulse.
    4. Record the finding without further assessment.

62. After auscultating a client's abdomen for 30 seconds, the nurse hears hypoactive bowel sounds in the RUQ and LUQ, and hears no bowel sounds in the RLQ and LLQ. Which of the following would be the best nursing action?
    1. Immediately report the information to the physician.
    2. Listen 1 to 3 minutes in each of the lower quadrants.
    3. Chart the information, and reassess in 4 hours.
    4. Assess for abdominal distention.

63. When the nurse elicits calf pain on dorsiflexion of a client's right foot, which of the following represents the best documentation?
    1. Complaint of cramping pain in the right calf
    2. Positive Homans' sign in the right leg
    3. Painful right leg bruit
    4. Deep vein thrombosis

64. A client is telling you about the difficult times he has had since the death of his wife. He is smiling and periodically interrupts his story with a giggle. You most likely use which of the following terms to describe his affect?
    1. Flat
    2. Inappropriate
    3. Nonplus
    4. Timorous

65. Your client's skin has a yellow cast, and you observe yellow color of the conjunctiva. Which of the following terms would you use to document this finding?
    1. Cyanosis
    2. Flushing
    3. Normal
    4. Jaundice

66. You ask the client to smile, frown, raise the eyebrows, or tightly close the eyes. Which cranial nerve are you testing?
    1. I
    2. III
    3. V
    4. VII

67. When you ask a client to read a newspaper or pamphlet, you are testing which of the following?
    1. Distance vision
    2. Near vision
    3. Discrimination
    4. Accommodation

68. To check the ocular fundus, begin with the ophthalmoscope approximately how many inches from the eye?
    1. 7 inches
    2. 6 to 10 inches
    3. 8 to 12 inches
    4. 16 to 18 inches

69. When you palpate the sinuses, you are primarily looking for which of the following?
    1. Changes in temperature
    2. Changes in color
    3. Tenderness
    4. Nodules

70. When examining the tonsils as part of an oropharyngeal assessment, you would expect to see which of the following?
    1. Tonsils somewhat darker than the rest of the oropharynx
    2. An irregular tonsillar surface
    3. Tonsils that do not protrude beyond the tonsillar pillar
    4. Tonsils that protrude between the pillars and the uvula

71. To palpate cervical lymph nodes, you feel on both sides of the neck at the same time. Which of the following represents the reason for this technique?
    1. To save time
    2. For bilateral comparison
    3. To prevent distortion
    4. To compress the neck

72. When you are assessing for breast symmetry, you would expect to find which of the following?
    1. Both breasts have perfectly equal symmetry.
    2. The right breast is larger in right-handed people.
    3. The breasts have the same general shape, with some minor variation.
    4. The breasts are of equal size.

73. To detect excess mucus in the bifurcation of the bronchi, you would listen in which of the following areas?
    1. At the third intercostal space on the right
    2. Over the sternum at the angle of Louis
    3. Over the sternum at the level of the fourth rib
    4. At the sternal angle

74. To assess the bases of the lungs, you would listen posteriorly over which of the following areas?
    1. Twelfth intercostal space
    2. Tenth intercostal space
    3. Eighth intercostal space
    4. Sixth intercostal space

75. The physician's physical examination report identifies a grade 3 holosystolic murmur. Which of the following would you expect to hear?
    1. A moderately loud muffled or nondistinct sound throughout S_1
    2. A moderately loud muffled or nondistinct sound throughout S_2
    3. A barely audible sound throughout S_1 and S_2
    4. A barely audible muffled or nondistinct sound throughout S_2

76. Even if a client has liver disease, the liver is not assessed every shift or even daily. The rationale for this action is that:
    1. nurses can't legally perform liver assessment.
    2. it involves deep palpation, causing unnecessary discomfort.
    3. there are other better signs of liver enlargement.
    4. liver enlargement is a normal finding in many clients.

77. Observing your client from the posterior, you notice an *S*-shaped curve to the spine. You would describe this finding as which of the following?
    1. Ankylosing spondylitis
    2. Lordosis
    3. Scoliosis
    4. Kyphosis

78. Screening for sexual abuse includes external inspection of the genitalia. In a 3-year-old girl, you would be less suspicious of sexual abuse if you made which of the following observations about the hymen?
    1. It is edematous.
    2. It is intact.
    3. It is absent.
    4. It is torn.

79. Which of the following findings is associated with scrotal edema?
    1. Slightly darker pigmentation than the rest of the body
    2. Absence of rugae
    3. The left testicle is lower than the right
    4. Presence of a varicocele

NURSING DIAGNOSIS

Chapter 9

PURPOSE

This chapter provides information about the process of making a nursing diagnosis. It also provides an overview of nursing diagnosis classification systems, diagnostic reasoning, and preventing nursing diagnostic errors.

MATCHING

1. _____ clinical judgment
2. _____ collaborative problem
3. _____ cue
4. _____ defining characteristics
5. _____ descriptor
6. _____ diagnostic label
7. _____ diagnostic reasoning
8. _____ differential diagnosis
9. _____ nursing diagnosis
10. _____ related factors
11. _____ risk factors
12. _____ "risk for" nursing diagnosis
13. _____ taxonomy
14. _____ wellness nursing diagnosis

a. a system of identification, naming, and classification of phenomena
b. the name of the nursing diagnosis
c. internal or external environmental factors that increase the vulnerability of a person, family, or community to an unhealthful event or state
d. a process of logical, flexible thinking to solve problems and plan nursing care that accounts for individual client needs and uses the individual strengths of the client and nurse to the fullest
e. factors that appear to show some type of patterned relationship with the nursing diagnosis
f. describes human responses that may develop in a vulnerable person, family, or community
g. a conclusion or opinion that a problem or situation requires nursing care and that determines the cause of the problem, distinguishes between similar problems, or discriminates among two or more courses of action

h. an indicator of the presence or existence of a problem or condition that represents a client's underlying health status
i. descriptions of a client's behavior that determine whether a nursing diagnosis is present and whether a particular diagnosis is appropriate or accurate
j. a clinical problem that cannot be solved by the nursing staff alone, but requires substantial nursing judgement
k. describes human responses to levels of wellness in an individual, family, or community that has the desire to move toward a higher state of being healthy
l. a clinical judgment about individual, family, or community responses to actual or potential health problems or life processes
m. the process of deciding among several possible diagnoses to most accurately describe the client's problem
n. a word, such as *impaired, decreased, ineffective, acute,* or *chronic,* that modifies or limits a nursing diagnosis, or gives it greater specificity

TRUE OR FALSE

15. _____ Nursing diagnosis is a problem for which nurses are accountable and can diagnose and treat independently.
16. _____ Nursing diagnosis is part of the nursing process.
17. _____ The American Nurses Association is the group that develops, refines, and promotes a taxonomy of nursing diagnoses.
18. _____ A benefit of nursing diagnosis is that it contributes to the autonomy and self-regulatory capacity of nursing.
19. _____ Using a shared diagnostic language places the emphasis on completing tasks in a timely manner to enhance quality of care
20. _____ Nurse diagnoses have not been developed or approved for testing with all combination of axes.

21. _____ A limitation of the current NANDA diagnosis group is that it does not adequately include wellness diagnoses, community health nursing diagnoses, or psychiatric diagnoses.

22. _____ A diagnostic label is a concise term or phrase that represents a pattern of related cues.

23. _____ The process of making a nursing diagnosis involves several interrelated steps.

24. _____ Nursing diagnoses should seldom, if ever, be discussed with a client.

FILL IN THE BLANKS

25. Nursing diagnosis is the _____ phase of the nursing process.

26. The _____ System has developed from 15 years of research and includes nursing diagnoses that reflect the home and community health setting.

27. The first part of a nursing diagnostic statement is the _____ _____.

28. *Family coping: potential for growth* is an example of a _____ nursing diagnosis.

29. After gathering nursing assessment data, the nurse _____ it to gain insight into the client's condition.

30. The nurse who is engaged in the nursing diagnosis step of _____ among possible diagnoses is narrowing the number of possible nursing diagnoses to identify the most appropriate one.

31. A _____ _____ is a descriptor of a client's behavior that determines whether a nursing diagnosis is present and appropriate or accurate.

32. The nursing diagnosis *Ineffective infant feeding pattern related to negligent mothering and maternal selfishness* written in a client's chart could be viewed as _____ _____.

33. Trying to include every possible nursing diagnosis that could ever apply to a client would be considered to be the nursing diagnosis error of _____.

EXERCISING YOUR CLINICAL JUDGMENT

Mrs. Marcus had her gallbladder removed in surgery earlier in the day, and has an incision in the right upper abdomen near the diaphragm. Her temperature is 98.8° F, pulse is 92, and respiration is 22/minute and shallow. Blood pressure is stable at 128/78 mm Hg. Mrs. Marcus has an intravenous line for fluid replacement and has an indwelling Foley catheter to drain urine from the bladder. She complains that it hurts to take a deep breath and exhibits guarding of the incision area. She says she feels "achy" from being immobilized on the operating room table. The last dose of a prn narcotic analgesic was given 3 hours ago and is now due. The nurse who admitted Mrs. Marcus from the postanesthesia care unit must formulate a list of nursing diagnoses and develop a plan of care.

34. Which of the following nursing diagnoses represents the most well-constructed nursing diagnostic statement about this client's pain?
    1. *Pain related to right upper abdominal incision and operative positioning*
    2. *Risk for pain related to frequency of ordered narcotic analgesic*
    3. *Pain related to insufficient pain medication frequency*
    4. *Risk for pain related to overall surgical experience*

35. If the nurse is considering the nursing diagnosis *Risk for urinary retention*, when should it be instituted?
    1. When the nurse writes the initial care plan
    2. When the Foley catheter is discontinued
    3. When the client's urine output falls below 30 mL/hour with the catheter in place
    4. When the client is ready for discharge to home

36. Which of the following would be the most appropriate nursing diagnosis for the client's respiratory status?
    1. *Risk for impaired gas exchange due to increased secretions*
    2. *Risk for ineffective breathing pattern related to subdiaphragmatic incision and guarding*
    3. *Ineffective airway clearance related to weak cough and shallow respirations*
    4. *Impaired gas exchange due to anesthesia and abnormal respiratory rate*

37. If the nurse considers the possibility that the client could develop an infection in the wound or because of invasive lines, the nursing diagnosis would be written as which of the following?
    1. An actual diagnosis
    2. A wellness diagnosis
    3. A medical diagnosis
    4. A "risk for" diagnosis

TEST YOURSELF

38. Which of the following is one of the limitations of the current NANDA system for classifying nursing diagnoses?
    1. It is specific to only a few nursing specialties.
    2. It is not well accepted in nursing education.
    3. It is endorsed by the American Nurses Association.
    4. It contains diagnoses at different levels of abstraction.

39. The part of the nursing diagnostic statement that contains a descriptor is called:
    1. a diagnostic label.
    2. a definition.
    3. the defining characteristics.
    4. the etiologic factors.

40. Which of the following is the broadest and highest level type of thinking that may be required for clinical nursing practice?
    1. Ordinary, logical thinking
    2. Clinical judgment
    3. Critical thinking
    4. Diagnostic reasoning

41. A nurse working in a community health setting would choose which of the following nursing diagnoses as the most realistic after taking into consideration the care setting?
    1. *Impaired home maintenance management*
    2. *Decreased cardiac output*
    3. *Ineffective thermoregulation*
    4. *Decreased adaptive capacity: intracranial*

42. For which of the following reasons is the nursing diagnosis *Ineffective airway clearance related to infrequent suctioning* most inappropriate?
    1. It is judgmental.
    2. It is derogatory.
    3. It suggests negligence.
    4. It suggests poor opinion of colleagues.

Chapter 10

PLANNING, INTERVENING, AND EVALUATING

PURPOSE

The purpose of this chapter is to introduce you to planning, intervention, and evaluation as phases of the nursing process. Although the chapter focuses on the individual, you will also consider planning, intervention, and evaluation for groups of clients who have a common set of needs. Planning and intervention are inherent parts of designing and delivering services to meet the needs of a client population. During evaluation, you will measure expected client outcomes and determine the degree to which an institution's external and internal standards are met.

MATCHING

1. _____ care plan conference
2. _____ case management
3. _____ clinical pathway
4. _____ collaboration
5. _____ computerized care plan
6. _____ consultation
7. _____ discharge planning
8. _____ evaluation
9. _____ expected outcomes
10. _____ goals
11. _____ individualized care plan
12. _____ long-term goal
13. _____ nurse-initiated intervention
14. _____ nursing care plan (NCP)
15. _____ nursing intervention
16. _____ Nursing Interventions Classifications (NIC)
17. _____ Nursing Outcomes Classifications (NOC)
18. _____ nursing-sensitive client outcome
19. _____ physician-initiated intervention
20. _____ short-term goal
21. _____ standardized care plan
22. _____ standards of care

a. broad, general statements about the desired results of nursing care
b. a care delivery system that focuses on the management of client care across an episode of illness
c. a standardized language to describe nursing activities used to develop a plan of care

d. a measurable client or family caregiver state, behavior, or perception that is conceptualized as a variable and is largely influenced by nursing interventions
e. a systematic and ongoing process of examining whether expected outcomes have been achieved and whether nursing care has been effective
f. written separately for each client who enters a health care facility; allows for the nurse to identify the unique problems of each client to decide on the outcomes to be achieved and to identify which nursing interventions will be appropriate to achieve those outcomes
g. suggests that the resolution of the nursing diagnosis can be accomplished in an hour, day, or week
h. within the independent scope of nursing practice and prescribed by the nurse independent of the physician
i. within the scope of nursing practice but requiring a physician's order for the nurse to implement
j. any treatment, based upon clinical judgment and knowledge, that a nurse performs to enhance client outcomes
k. the desired result from nursing care expressed in terms of measurable client behaviors
l. preparation for moving a client from one level of care to another within or outside the current health care agency
m. a multidisciplinary plan that projects the expected course of the client's progress over the hospital stay
n. a guide for health care that identifies client problems in need of nursing care, predicts outcomes sensitive to nursing care, and lists interventions that should result in the expected outcomes
o. a standardized language for measuring the effects of nursing care using indicators sensitive to nursing intervention
p. suggests that the expectation for resolution of the nursing diagnosis will take place in small measurable steps but may take a few weeks or months
q. authoritative statements that describe a competent level of clinical nursing practice

r. the act of two or more health care professionals, one being an expert or specialist, deliberating for the purpose of making decisions

s. a team effort that may include the client, family, and health care professionals who work cooperatively to achieve a common goal

t. the action of a group conferring to plan care for the client

u. a care plan written by a group of nurses who use their collective expertise to produce a plan for clients with specific medical diagnoses or undergoing special procedures

v. a care plan created by a computer program based on information written by expert clinicians that can be easily changed or updated using a computer software program

TRUE OR FALSE

23. _____ Planning occurs only at the beginning of the nurse-client relationship.

24. _____ A nursing care plan for clients who are undergoing a hysterectomy is sufficient for all hysterectomy clients.

25. _____ A nursing care plan does not include interventions performed by other team members, such as the dietitian.

26. _____ Planning includes projecting the desired outcomes of the care.

27. _____ Priorities are always based upon physiological needs first.

28. _____ Because needs are often interrelated, several problems may be grouped together as a priority.

29. _____ To use the Nursing Outcomes Classification system, the nurse must choose which measurement parameters are needed in a given client situation.

30. _____ Nursing interventions are clarified by indicating *who, what, when, how,* and *why.*

31. _____ Nursing practice that consistently upholds standards of care is important in achieving positive client outcomes.

32. _____ If client outcomes are not achieved, only the nursing interventions are revised.

33. _____ Nurses can determine a client's level of satisfaction with care by asking the opinions of other nurses assigned to that client.

34. _____ Formulating measurable and realistic client outcomes is a factor that facilitates attainment of those outcomes.

35. _____ Inadequate information about a client's disease, treatment, or care is a barrier that impedes attainment of expected outcomes.

36. _____ A nurse using a clinical pathway in the care of an assigned client would document the reasons for any variances in the client's medical record.

FILL IN THE BLANKS

37. The frequency of planning during a client's span of care depends on how often the client's condition _____.

38. Basic survival needs take first priority when a client has a threat to _____ _____.

39. Nursing diagnoses are documented in the health care record in the _____ care plan or the _____ care plan.

40. Through the development of expected outcomes, nurses can be held _____ for the results of nursing care.

41. In planning nursing care, you should choose outcomes that are _____ to nursing care.

42. To evaluate a client's progress, you will need to review the _____ _____ for each diagnosis.

43. A standardized language provides a common language for _____.

44. If a client has begun to achieve expected outcomes, but has not yet fully met them, the nurse would consider that the goals for this client have been _____ met.

45. A nurse whose evaluation shows that a client has fully met the expected outcomes for a nursing diagnosis would determine that the nursing diagnosis should be _____.

46. A factor that impedes the ability of a client to meet an expected outcome is considered to be a _____.

TEST YOURSELF

47. All of the following interventions are missing some of the five elements of *who, what, when, how,* and *why.* Select the one you think would be the most consistently carried out across all three shifts.
   1. Turn q2h
   2. Turn on even hours, side to back to side
   3. Turn as needed to prevent decubiti
   4. Instruct nursing assistant to turn client

48. You refer a client to AIDS Services (a local volunteer agency) for assistance in obtaining medication. Which domain of interventions (NIC) have you used?
    1. Physiological
    2. Behavioral
    3. Safety
    4. Health systems

49. Your client needs to learn to give an injection to himself on a weekly basis. Which of the following would be the most measurable client outcome?
    1. Understands the mechanics of the injection technique
    2. Demonstrates the correct injection technique before discharge
    3. Develops a procedure for injection suitable to his lifestyle
    4. Knows how to give his own injection

50. A client has a fractured ankle. He is learning to walk on crutches. Which of the following outcomes best reflects the client's long-term goal?
    1. Safely demonstrates stair climbing with crutches
    2. Can walk the length of the corridor correctly using a three-point gait
    3. Can use crutches independently at discharge
    4. Bears weight on ankle without pain

51. Which of the following nursing activities most clearly reflects a nurse-initiated intervention?
    1. Safely administers intravenous gentamicin (Garamycin)
    2. Establishes schedule for the administration of medication
    3. Observes for side effects of medication
    4. Teaches client to self-administer medication after discharge

52. Which of the following would be the most significant disadvantage of a computerized nursing care plan?
    1. Difficult care plan development and revision
    2. Low rating for readability
    3. Lack of individualization
    4. Lack of clarity of the terms used in planning

53. Select the statement that reflects an advantage to the NIC system for documentation of interventions.
    1. Each intervention is specific for a NANDA diagnosis.
    2. NIC provides ease of documentation of individualized care.
    3. NIC provides the specific details of the activities used for each client.
    4. NIC provides a short notation that implies the same set of activities to all who use the system.

54. Select the statement that best exemplifies the purpose of case management. It seeks to:
    1. ensure quality care in a health care system focused on cost control.
    2. expand the hospital's control beyond the acute care experience.
    3. increase the number of roles for professional nurses in acute care.
    4. ensure that clients get access to all possible services.

55. Which of the following statements best describes a clinical pathway?
    1. Describes the specifics of nursing care in measurable terms
    2. Is a multidisciplinary plan with criteria for daily progress of a client with a particular diagnosis
    3. Is a plan of care for an individual client
    4. Predicts the course of a client's illness based on the identification of that client's individual risk factors

56. There are multiple methods of documenting a nursing care plan (NCP). Which of the following is essential?
    1. Using a form developed for the agency for documentation of the NCP
    2. Using columns for expected outcomes, interventions, and resolution of the problem
    3. Documenting the elements of diagnosis, expected outcomes, and interventions
    4. Having the plan on a separate form from the documentation of care

57. A nurse who is facilitating a client's attainment of expected outcomes would:
    1. have a vague idea of the client's plan of care.
    2. assess the client thoroughly and accurately.
    3. not be overly concerned with revising the plan of care.
    4. consult with the family, but not the client, about expected outcomes.

58. The nurse would determine that a case management approach was most effective if the client:
    1. is approved by the insurance company to remain in the hospital an extra day or two.
    2. achieved a satisfactory clinical outcome and did not require rehospitalization.
    3. received every type of service available.
    4. incurred the least cost even if the outcome was less than desirable.

DOCUMENTING CARE

PURPOSE

This chapter explains the purpose, principles, and methods of documenting client care. It differentiates among the various charting formats and describes the usefulness of various types of flow sheets.

MATCHING

1. _____ admit note/admission note
2. _____ APIE (PIE) charting
3. _____ charting by exception
4. _____ computerized provider order entry (CPOE)
5. _____ critical or clinical pathways (care maps)
6. _____ discharge note
7. _____ documentation
8. _____ electronic health record (EHR)
9. _____ electronic medical record (EMR)
10. _____ electronic medication administration records (eMAR)
11. _____ flow sheet
12. _____ focus charting
13. _____ interval or progress note
14. _____ narrative charting
15. _____ problem-oriented medical records
16. _____ SOAP charting
17. _____ transfer note

a. an interdisciplinary note that reflects the circumstances surrounding the release of a client from a facility

b. a method of charting that addresses client problems or needs and includes a column that summarizes the focus of the entry

c. a method of charting that provides information in the form of statements that describe events surrounding client care

d. the first nurse's note acknowledging the arrival of a new client

e. a computerized account of a client's health information across several episodes of care and different facilities

f. the acronym that stands for assessment, problem identification, interventions, and evaluation

g. direct electronic documentation of orders by health care providers into a clinical information system

that are routed to the appropriate clinical area for action

h. a form of documentation originally designed to organize information according to identified client problems, with all members of the health care team documenting information sequentially

i. recording of information relevant to assessment, planning, implementation, and evaluation (client response) as a legal record that is permanent and retrievable for future purposes

j. forms used to document data that can be more easily followed in graphic or tabular form

k. provides documentation in progress notes only if data are significant or abnormal

l. interdisciplinary notes entered at various times during a shift that reflect any aspect of change in client condition, or anything affecting the client such as tests, STAT or prn medications, and procedures

m. a nursing note that reflects the movement of a client from one unit to another within the agency or to another agency

n. a format of charting used to record progress notes with problem-focused charting; it includes subjective data, objective data, assessment, and plan

o. a computerized account of a client's admission or care episode within a health care facility

p. may be recorded using an interdisciplinary approach or organized by health care discipline

q. a computerized version of a medication administration record

TRUE OR FALSE

18. _____ Client outcomes serve as the measure of quality and are monitored through complete and accurate documentation.

19. _____ Agencies do not chart errors in clients' charts to avoid being sued.

20. _____ Medical abbreviations are used consistently throughout the medical/nursing community.

21. _____ Charting should be done in complete sentences, using as much description of the situation as possible.

22. _____ You are responsible for charting how your client responds to your teaching, and whether the client and/or family can return-demonstrate a skill such as wound care or explain the instructions in their own words.

23. _____ Narrative charting is unstructured, providing you with flexibility in determining how information is recorded.

24. _____ The use of computer systems for documentation has raised concerns over confidentiality and security of client information.

FILL IN THE BLANKS

25. The primary purpose of _____ of a client's care is _____ among health team members, thus promoting continuity of care among departments, throughout 24 hours of care, and during the entire hospital stay.

26. Quality assurance focuses on providing care according to established _____.

27. _____ is the choice of color for charting, unless an agency has a different policy.

28. When you chart, you do not include the _____ name or the word _client_ or _patient_.

29. Copying a chart usually requires written consent by the _____ or responsible party.

30. Upon admission to a facility, documentation of a client's _____ to the facility should be made.

31. Nursing notes should state _____ rather than opinion.

EXERCISING YOUR CLINICAL JUDGMENT

32. You admitted Ms. Peters, the client from the chapter's case study, to your hospital unit. You charted: _68-yr-old female admitted to room 268A via stretcher from ER with dx FX L h P 92, BP 142/89, T 98. C/o pain to L hip from mid-thigh to greater trochanter area, marked bruising noted in same area._ The agency where you work is using which type of charting format?
    1. Narrative
    2. Focus
    3. APIE
    4. Charting by exception

33. You charted the following nursing note in black ink: _12:00 ate lunch; 7:30 AM prn medication given for pain; 1:00 transferred to X-ray via a stretcher, accompanied by aide._ What is incorrect about this entry?
    1. The prn medication should not have been recorded.
    2. The recording of the information is not done sequentially.
    3. Black ink is not the ink of choice for most institutions.
    4. The charting should have included the client's name.

34. Ms. Peters, the elderly client from the chapter's case study, has been on your unit for several days. You chart the following: _Dr. Warren visited with orders to d/c current meds. Neighbor notified and on the way. Home Health Nurse notified of discharge, and arrangement for first visit made. PT visited concerning walker and reinforced proper use._ This is an example of which type of nursing note?
    1. Progress
    2. Interval
    3. Discharge
    4. Assessment

TEST YOURSELF

35. Your client has his dressing changed every 4 hours. You forgot to chart the morning dressing change. You remembered the omission when you began to document your client's afternoon dressing change. The client's morning dressing had no drainage on it, and the wound was healing without any problems. How would you handle this situation?
    1. Chart the morning results with your afternoon charting.
    2. Call the physician, and report that you did not chart the dressing change in the client's chart.
    3. Add the information as an addendum to the afternoon charting.
    4. Do nothing; because the dressing is changed frequently, it is not necessary to add the morning dressing change to the client's chart.

36. You are about to chart and notice that the previous charting was not signed. How should you chart?
    1. Sign the previous nurse's charting, and then do your own charting and sign it.
    2. Have the head nurse sign the previous nurse's charting, and then do your own charting.
    3. No action is necessary; do only your own charting.
    4. Do not sign for the previous nurse; report it to the head nurse, and chart and sign your own charting.

37. You charted the following nursing note regarding your client's current condition: *Awake, alert and oriented × 3. Skin warm and dry. IV D_5W infusing in R lower arm at 100 mL/hr with 450 TBA. Site without redness or edema. Reports pain in L hip. States pain is 8 on scale of 1–10. Tylox tabs ii given PO*. Which type of nursing note is this?
    1. Admit note
    2. Change-of-shift note
    3. Assessment note
    4. Interval note

38. You chart a progress note on a client's condition using the same problem list as the client's other health care providers used. What type of medical record is your facility using?
    1. Source-oriented
    2. Problem-oriented
    3. Critical pathways
    4. Narrative

39. Which type of charting addresses client problems or needs and includes a column that summarizes the focus of the entry?
    1. Focus
    2. SOAP
    3. Narrative
    4. PIE

PURPOSE

This chapter will orient you to beginning theories, principles, and techniques of therapeutic communication related to the nurse-client interaction.

MATCHING

1. _____ acting-out behaviors
2. _____ active listening
3. _____ attending behaviors
4. _____ body language
5. _____ communication
6. _____ context
7. _____ decoder (receiver)
8. _____ empathy
9. _____ encoder (sender)
10. _____ feedback
11. _____ language
12. _____ message
13. _____ nonverbal communication
14. _____ paralanguage
15. _____ personal space
16. _____ sensory channel
17. _____ therapeutic rapport
18. _____ therapeutic relationship
19. _____ unconditional positive regard
20. _____ verbal communication

a. a helping relationship
b. a special bond that exists between a nurse and a client who have established a sense of trust and a mutual understanding of what will occur in their relationship
c. inappropriate or unexpected client behaviors that communicate the client's true or subconscious feelings and concerns
d. person who initiates a transaction to exchange information, convey thoughts and feelings, or engage another person
e. the content a sender wishes to transmit to another person (the receiver) in the process of communication
f. the means by which a message is sent
g. a person to whom a message is aimed
h. the condition under which a communication occurs

i. the process by which effectiveness of communication is determined
j. involves the use of words to convey messages
k. a set of words that have meanings that are comprehensible within a group
l. a set of behaviors that convey messages either without words or by supplementing verbal communication
m. refers to nonverbal communication behaviors that are accomplished by the movement of our bodies or body parts, by the presentation of ourselves to the world, and by the use of our personal space
n. refers to nonverbal components of spoken language
o. a private zone or "bubble" around our body that we believe is an extension of ourselves and belongs to us
p. shows that you are paying attention and listening to what the client is saying
q. term coined by psychologist Carl Rogers; describes respect for the client that is not dependent on the client's behavior
r. the accurate perception of the client's feelings
s. understanding not only the words spoken but also the feeling and intent behind the message
t. a complex process in which information is exchanged between two or more individuals

TRUE OR FALSE

21. _____ A therapeutic relationship is personal, client-focused, and aimed at realizing mutually determined goals.
22. _____ Peplau, a nurse theorist, believed that the nurse is a human being who is vulnerable to stereotypes, labels, and generalizations.
23. _____ Nonverbal communication includes body posture.
24. _____ Generally speaking, a person's personal space is similar for most cultures.
25. _____ A rule of thumb is to ask permission before touching a client.
26. _____ According to Torppa's theories, women expect relationships to be based on mutual dependence and cooperation, and men expect relationships to be based on independence and cooperation.

27. _____ To encourage a formulation of a plan of action, you should consider what might be the best thing to do in a future situation.

28. _____ Summarizing can help bring closure in the termination phase of a therapeutic relationship.

FILL IN THE BLANKS

29. Confidentiality is an _____ obligation to share a client's health care information only with other persons who have a _____ need to know his or her health status.

30. _____ feedback affirms your efforts to communicate by rewarding and reinforcing successful communication.

31. Personal appearance, conscious and unconscious changes in facial expressions, body posture and gestures, and the distances maintained from others are examples of common _____ _____ behaviors.

32. You can help the client who is experiencing a misperception of reality by using a technique called _____ _____.

33. If you are using therapeutic techniques correctly, your client will be doing most of the _____ as you listen and guide the interaction.

34. Many people (nurses and clients) are uncomfortable with _____ and will talk continuously about nothing in particular just to avoid it.

35. _____ listening is a means of "being with" the client and indicating acceptance and agreement by using verbal and nonverbal cues.

EXERCISING YOUR CLINICAL JUDGMENT

36. You say to Mr. Lewis, the client from the chapter's case study, "Why are you afraid of having the surgery?" This is an example of which type of nontherapeutic technique?
    1. Requesting an explanation
    2. Probing
    3. Challenging
    4. Testing

37. You say to Mr. Lewis, "Would you mind explaining more about what you mean so I can be more helpful?" You are using which therapeutic communication technique?
    1. Offering self
    2. Focusing
    3. Asking for clarification
    4. Reflecting

38. You say to Mr. Lewis, "Tell me what I can cover next about your surgery." This is an example of which therapeutic communication technique?
    1. Providing broad openings
    2. Focusing
    3. Summarizing
    4. Reflecting

TEST YOURSELF

39. "I don't know the answer right now. But I will find out and let you know in about an hour." This is an example of being honest with the client, which is an essential step in:
    1. developing a trusting relationship with the client.
    2. developing a friendship with the client.
    3. helping the client with termination issues.
    4. believing that you are a competent nurse.

40. During which phase of the nurse-client relationship do you complete nursing interventions that address expected nursing outcomes?
    1. Working phase
    2. Termination phase
    3. Orientation phase
    4. Therapeutic phase

41. "Hmm, I believe you are right," is an example of which type of paralanguage?
    1. Rate
    2. Pitch
    3. Quality
    4. Pause

42. You say to your adult client, "I have 30 minutes available to talk with you at 10 AM today." This is an example of which therapeutic communication technique?
    1. Offering self
    2. Presenting reality
    3. Focusing
    4. Testing

43. You say to your client who is 3 years old, "Do you want your Baby Lisa? Is she your doll?" Which therapeutic communication techniques are you using?
    1. Focusing
    2. Placing events in sequence
    3. Providing broad openings
    4. Seeking consensual validation

CLIENT TEACHING

PURPOSE

This chapter introduces you to the key concepts that you must understand to provide effective client teaching. It introduces teaching-learning theory and processes, and guides you to use the nursing process effectively in meeting clients' learning needs.

MATCHING

1. _____ affective learning domain
2. _____ cognitive learning domain
3. _____ learning
4. _____ learning contract
5. _____ learning objective
6. _____ psychomotor learning domain
7. _____ teaching
8. _____ teaching plan

a. includes physical and motor skills, such as giving injections
b. much like any business contract; each party (nurse and client) agrees to contribute certain things to the agreement
c. considered the "thinking" domain and includes acquiring knowledge, comprehending, and using critical thinking skills
d. a set of planned activities performed to impact knowledge, behavior, or skill
e. includes values, beliefs, feelings, and attitudes
f. acquisition of knowledge, behavior, or skill through experience, practice, study, or instruction.
g. describes the intended results of learning rather than the process of instruction
h. an organized, individualized written presentation of what the client must learn and how the instructions and information needed will be provided

TRUE OR FALSE

9. _____ JCAHO, the Joint Commission on Accreditation of Healthcare Organizations, includes client education within their nursing standards.

10. _____ Client education is a factor in quality control in that it ensures clients have the knowledge they need to provide self-care.
11. _____ The client must reach the synthesis level of learning about his or her health care problem to be successful.
12. _____ In the United States, literacy is not a concern for those who provide client education.
13. _____ A child's imagination may create greater fear than the truth, told directly and simply.
14. _____ For the adult learner, you should assume that the learner has some knowledge you can use to build on to enhance education.
15. _____ In a hospital setting, the best method of teaching is verbally providing information in a one-on-one situation with the client.
16. _____ It is safe to assume that all clients want to learn about their health problems.
17. _____ *Deficient knowledge* is the only nursing diagnosis used for client learning needs.
18. _____ Teaching from the simple to the complex is a principle of teaching.
19. _____ Writing specific measurable objectives helps to clarify your teaching plans.

FILL IN THE BLANKS

20. The advantage of _____ instruction is pacing and customizing to meet an individual client's needs.

21. The advantage of _____ instruction is economy of teaching time and sharing of experiences.

22. The advantage of _____ materials is that they are affordable and can be used to teach or reinforce a learning experience.

23. Repetition is used to _____ _____.

24. Discussion allows the learner to be an _____ _____ in learning.

25. Evaluation has two types of goals. Assessing the client's ability to repeat the information is a _____-_____ goal.

26. Assessing for a change in lifestyle at a 3-month follow-up is a _____-_____ goal.

EXERCISING YOUR CLINICAL JUDGMENT

27. Mrs. Avery, the client from the chapter's case study, is going to go home on a new medication to control her diabetes (insulin). Based on the axiom that adult learners learn best when there is a need to know, which of the following would you emphasize?
    1. How the medication works in the body
    2. The need to memorize all side effects
    3. The importance of maintaining the prescribed dose schedule
    4. The possible complications of diabetes

28. Which of the following is most likely true of Mrs. Avery as an adult learner?
    1. Prefers the nurse to identify what knowledge is needed
    2. Is bored with being shown how to perform a skill
    3. Likes to know why knowledge is needed
    4. Likes role playing as a method of learning

29. Mrs. Avery indicates that she has the greatest motivation to learn when she does which of the following?
    1. Asks questions about giving herself insulin.
    2. Thanks the nurse and says she will read the information provided
    3. Talks about the difficulties of giving herself insulin
    4. Tells the nurse to talk to her granddaughter about the insulin injections

TEST YOURSELF

30. Your client has just been admitted with an asthma attack. This is the third admission in 6 months, and the client is highly anxious. You suspect that the client does not fully understand the preventive measures recommended by the physician. You would:
    1. review the measures while the client is waiting for the medications to take effect.
    2. gather limited information at this time and postpone teaching.
    3. give the client written information to be read later.
    4. use the opportunity to emphasize the importance of prevention.

31. The physician has recommended that your client follow a low-fat diet and wants you to introduce the topic to the client. Knowing that you should teach from the simple to the complex, you would start with the topic of:
    1. a general list of foods to avoid.
    2. pathophysiology of the formation of fatty plaque in arteries.
    3. planning menus.
    4. maintaining a diet that is less than 30% fat based on grams of fat in common foods.

32. Early discharge for hospitalized clients has changed client teaching by:
    1. increasing the client's need for information.
    2. shifting the responsibility for teaching from the hospital nurse to the home health nurse.
    3. reducing the need for teaching because complications are reduced.
    4. allowing hospital nurses to focus only on acute physical needs.

33. Quality care is improved when:
    1. the client and family are active participants in restoring health.
    2. clients do what they are told without asking questions.
    3. the physician is in control of all decision making.
    4. clients have absolute faith in health care providers.

34. Which behavior represents the complex overt response level of psychomotor learning?
    1. Performs the skill precisely following the steps as taught
    2. Performs the skill correctly while visiting with a friend
    3. Modifies the skill to meet lifestyle needs
    4. Creates a new way of performing the skill

35. Your client is a shy 7-year-old. She is learning to use an asthma inhaler. Her asthma attacks occur no more frequently than once a week. Her mother has received permission from the school for the child to have the inhaler with her in the classroom, but the child says she cannot use it in front of her friends. Which teaching activity would you select?
    1. Tell her that her friends won't care
    2. Role-play asking the teacher if she can be excused from the room to use her inhaler
    3. Get the prescription changed to a tablet taken four times a day
    4. Tell her mother that she has to do it whether she likes it or not

36. Your client is having surgery and expects to be in the hospital for 4 days. The postoperative care will involve complex wound care after discharge. The best time to start the teaching is:
    1. preoperatively.
    2. on the first day after surgery.
    3. on the day of discharge.
    4. after the client is at home.

37. Select the client who would most likely need repetition to ensure learning.
    1. A 90-year-old client using insulin injections for the first time
    2. A 20-year-old client who needs to take a prescription for 10 days for a urinary tract infection
    3. A client with long-standing asthma who has a prescription for a different inhaler
    4. A surgical client being discharged; the wound is healing without complications, and the sutures have been removed

38. You have planned to do a client's wound care at 10 AM. Your schedule is busy, and you know the client will probably be discharged tomorrow. When you enter the room, you find that the client's son has just arrived from out of state. You would:
    1. know that psychosocial needs are important, and delay the wound care.
    2. ask the son to leave the room, and hurriedly do the wound care without teaching.
    3. ask the client if the son can stay and include him in the teaching.
    4. tell the son he will have to come back later.

MANAGING CLIENT CARE

PURPOSE

This chapter introduces you to nursing management and the roles of a nurse-manager at different levels in an organization. It describes how these roles involve managing quality, budgets, people, change, and risk.

MATCHING

1. _____ accountability
2. _____ authority
3. _____ change-of-shift report
4. _____ concurrent audit
5. _____ continuous quality improvement (CQI)
6. _____ delegation
7. _____ for-profit
8. _____ leadership
9. _____ management
10. _____ non-profit
11. _____ not-for-profit
12. _____ nurse-manager
13. _____ peer review
14. _____ performance appraisal
15. _____ policy
16. _____ primary nursing
17. _____ procedure
18. _____ protocol
19. _____ quality assurance
20. _____ responsibility
21. _____ retrospective audit
22. _____ risk management
23. _____ Standards of Practice
24. _____ Standards of Professional Performance
25. _____ team nursing
26. _____ total client care
27. _____ transactional leadership
28. _____ transformational leadership

a. being held answerable for personal actions or the actions of others
b. the obligation to provide an accounting or rationale for personal actions or the actions of others
c. a nurses role in organizational management that shares the goal of providing quality services to meet client needs

d. the process of identifying, evaluating, and reducing or financing the cost of predictable losses
e. the ability or legitimate power to make decisions, implement strategies, and elicit work from others
f. involves assigning responsibility for certain tasks to other people, thereby allowing the manager to concentrate on higher level activities
g. involves showing others the way, directing others in a course of action, going before others, or going with and inspiring others
h. the implementation of strategies that promote effective and efficient use of resources to achieve organizational goals
i. refers to the process of achieving an optimal degree of excellence in the services rendered to every client
j. a combination of nursing personnel who work together and share responsibility for the care of a group of clients
k. enhances comprehensive care by assigning each client to a nurse at the bedside who is responsible for the client's care over a 24-hour period
l. an oral report given by an off-going nurse to an on-coming nurse who will assume responsibility for the care of a client
m. a hospital or agency that exists to make a profit
n. a hospital or agency that may make a profit that is returned to the institution to maintain or upgrade equipment; but does not exist for that purpose
o. a hospital or agency that does not make a profit and may be supported by charitable donations or taxes
p. a detailed description of a specific method of accomplishing a task or performing nursing care
q. a set of rules and regulations that govern nursing practice and nursing care
r. detailed guidelines for nursing care for clients with specific conditions or medical treatments
s. a competent level of nursing care as demonstrated by the critical thinking model known as the nursing process
t. a style that seeks to motivate others through a cost-benefit, economic exchange in which followers' material and psychic needs are met in return for services rendered

u. authoritative statements that describe a competent level of behavior in the professional role.

v. a style that seeks to motivate others by inspiration, arousing and satisfying higher needs and engaging the full person

w. an evaluation method that inspects the nursing staff's compliance with predetermined standards and criteria while care is being provided

x. an evaluation method that inspects the medical record for documentation of care in compliance with the applicable standards after the fact

y. a systematic approach to control and improve quality from the perspective of both professionals and clients

z. an organized, uniform method of evaluation of a nurse's job contribution, quality of work, and potential for advancement made by the nurse's supervisor

aa. an evaluation of the performance of one staff member by another staff member to judge the quality of care provided

bb. one nurse being assigned to provide comprehensive care to a small group of clients based on the nurse's expertise and the client's needs

TRUE OR FALSE

29. _____ Nurse-managers have become consensus builders who facilitate client care rather than acting as control systems.

30. _____ A nurse-manager who wanted to hire a new nurse could use information gained as part of fiscal management to justify the need.

31. _____ The overall definition of the business of health care for each institution is written in the form of a policy.

32. _____ A mission statement is used to identify institutional goals.

33. _____ Organizational goals are translated into specific objectives to guide the day-to-day operation of work units.

34. _____ Cost containment remains a major goal in health care today and affects all health care practitioners.

35. _____ An institution must be accredited by the JCAHO to be certified or licensed, or to receive reimbursement for services.

36. _____ A nurse who is verifying information for properly submitting a vacation request form would consult the nursing procedure manual.

FILL IN THE BLANKS

37. A nurse orientee who requests that the designated mentor nurse observe her while she performs a wound irrigation is engaged in the _____ audit method.

38. An assumption of a continuous quality improvement program is that quality can always be _____.

39. Because the position of nurse-manager involves inspiring others to work, all nurse-managers should be _____.

40. Managing _____ means accentuating positive outcomes as well as avoiding negative outcomes.

41. Nurse-managers evaluate how well policies and procedures facilitate the attainment of goals by measuring _____.

42. _____ and _____ are rules and outlined processes that define the steps taken to meet objectives.

43. Nurse-managers strive to ensure the highest quality care at the lowest possible _____.

EXERCISING YOUR CLINICAL JUDGMENT

Kristen Williams is a nurse-manager on a 40-bed surgical unit in a local hospital. She arrived at work at 7 AM and is developing her plan for the day after reviewing her scheduled appointments and meetings. She must attend a 9 AM meeting of the Policy and Procedure Committee, followed by a budget meeting at 10 AM. In the afternoon, she has a staff meeting planned to explore with staff how they can achieve more timely client discharges on the unit before new admissions arrive from the postanesthesia care unit. As she gathers the materials needed for the morning meetings, she realizes that in her role today she will be managing quality, people, budget, and change. She glances at her watch and determines that she has plenty of time to talk to the charge nurse and nursing staff about concerns on the unit before her planned schedule begins.

44. As Kristen enters the nurses' station, the charge nurse reports that there has been a sick call already for the evening shift. Which of the following actions would represent the best use of Kristen's time and skills and those of other staff?
    1. Delegate to the charge nurse the responsibility for calling part-time off-duty nurses to see if they can work
    2. Call the vice president for nursing to complain about how short-staffed the unit always is
    3. Make a mental note to bring this problem up at the budget meeting, and try to use it to demand more staff
    4. Tell the staff at 3 PM that they will have to work short and "make do."

45. At the Policy and Procedure Committee meeting, the first item on the agenda is a review of the effectiveness of a new policy and procedure for blood transfusion intended to reduce turn-around time from receipt of an order in the blood bank to the start time for infusion into the client.
    The committee determines that based on data available, 20 minutes have been eliminated in the process. The new policy and procedure are determined to be effective in improving which of the following?
    1. Communication
    2. Quality
    3. Cost
    4. Goals

TEST YOURSELF

46. Which of the following members of the hospital staff would not be part of a multidisciplinary team working with a client?
    1. Social worker
    2. Billing clerk
    3. Pastoral care provider
    4. Client's family

47. Which of the following activities undertaken as part of a planned change correlates with the analysis phase of the nursing process?
    1. Identify the need for change
    2. Identify potential action plans
    3. Identify the potential cause of a problem
    4. Incorporate new behaviors into structures or processes

48. Which of the following time management tips would be least useful and productive for a nurse-manager?
    1. Write down identified tasks, obligations, and activities
    2. Work on the most important task first
    3. Do not accept assignments that you are not capable of completing
    4. Adopt a strategy of needing to be perfect

49. The nurse-managers of an institution are meeting to determine how well they are complying with regulations of the Joint Commission on Accreditation of Healthcare Organizations. The group is motivated to be in compliance because this is necessary for:
    1. praise from the chief executive officer.
    2. national recognition.
    3. accreditation.
    4. high profit margins.

50. A client expresses satisfaction with the nursing care received on the clinical unit, and completes a patient satisfaction survey describing it as caring, thoughtful, and respectful. The nurse-manager documents this anecdote from the client, knowing that this information is an example of which of the following?
    1. Quality indicator
    2. Internal standard
    3. External standard
    4. Compliance with federal regulation

51. The nurse who is practicing nursing within the standards of a specialty nursing organization knows that these standards most often are derived from those of which of the following?
    1. Employer
    2. Joint Commission on Accreditation of Healthcare Organizations
    3. Department of Health and Human Services
    4. American Nurses Association

52. A nurse working on the cardiac telemetry unit has a set of standing physician's orders for treating chest pain. The nurse implementing these orders is working with which of the following?
    1. Policy
    2. Procedure
    3. Protocol
    4. Parameter

PURPOSE

The purpose of this chapter is to provide introductory information about nursing research and its methodology to assist you in understanding research studies.

MATCHING

1. _____ abstract
2. _____ data
3. _____ data collection
4. _____ dependent variable
5. _____ experimental research
6. _____ hypothesis
7. _____ independent variable
8. _____ informed consent
9. _____ institutional review board (IRB)
10. _____ instruments
11. _____ nonexperimental research
12. _____ operational definition
13. _____ qualitative research
14. _____ quantitative research
15. _____ quasi-experimental research
16. _____ research design
17. _____ research problem
18. _____ sampling
19. _____ theoretical framework

a. a short summary that contains brief information about the purpose of a study, the number of subjects, the methodology used to select subjects, the type of study being conducted, and the major results from the study

b. the process by which a researcher collects the information necessary to answer the research question

c. a type of research study in which a researcher manipulates a treatment or intervention, randomly assigns subjects to either a control or experimental group, and has control over the research situation

d. a tentative prediction of the relationship between two or more variables being studied

e. the variable in a research design that may show variation, but the variation is expected to remain constant in the study, although it influences or even causes change in another variable

f. the tools a researcher uses to conduct a study

g. the variable in a research design that is hypothesized to change with the treatment (i.e., has been caused by an independent variable)

h. used to designate the information the researcher is interested in collecting

i. a type of study in which the researcher collects data without the introduction of a treatment or intervention

j. a type of study that uses ideas that are analyzed as words

k. a type of study in which the researcher manipulates a treatment or intervention, but is unable to randomize subjects into groups or lacks a control group

l. a committee whose duties include ensuring that the proposed research meets the federal requirements for ethical research; the federal government mandates the committee if the institution is receiving federal funds for research

m. means that the subjects have been provided with sufficient information regarding the research to enable them to consent voluntarily to participate or decline to participate.

n. a type of study that uses variables that are analyzed as numbers

o. the meaning of the concept precisely as it is being used in the study, defined in a manner that specifies how the concepts will be measured

p. a researcher's strategy for testing a hypothesis

q. the process of selecting subjects from the population being studied

r. an observation, situation, occurrence, or even a hunch that an investigator chooses to research

s. a logical but abstract structure that suggests the relationship among the variables for a research study

TRUE OR FALSE

20. _____ One of the ANA priorities for nursing research is to analyze home health care services and data on elders at home and in long-term care facilities.

21. _____ One of the priorities for the National Center for Nursing Research is to test interventions for coping with chronic illness.

22. _____ Informed consent for research includes a clear statement that the subject is free to discontinue participation at any time the subject wishes.

23. _____ In the absence of a requirement for institutional review, researchers are free to skip some ethical guidelines.

24. _____ Research should not be performed on human subjects unless there is a clear possibility of benefit to society or individuals.

25. _____ When a research study shows a good correlation between two variables, causation can be inferred.

26. _____ Reading an abstract is sufficient to evaluate a study.

27. _____ The results of a study are a factual presentation of what is found.

28. _____ In the discussion that follows the results, the researcher tells what the findings mean in his or her opinion.

29. _____ Not all problems are amenable to research methods.

30. _____ The *Index Medicus* does not contain nursing journals.

31. _____ As a user of research, the operational definition can help you know if the information applies in a specific client situation.

32. _____ A research study is not worthwhile unless it proves the hypothesis.

33. _____ Research begins with a problem or a question that arises in the clinical practice setting.

34. _____ When you are reading a research study, always ask, "What else could have caused this effect?"

35. _____ The goal of using research findings is to improve the quality of care in the clinical setting.

FILL IN THE BLANKS

36. _____ _____ is the method used to develop or search for knowledge about issues important to nurses and nursing practice.

37. Because nursing research often involves _____ _____, ethical standards are especially important.

38. A _____ _____ is a type of research that involves the detailed investigation of an individual, group, or institution to understand which variables are important to the subjects—history, care, or development.

39. The concepts under investigation in a study are called _____.

40. In a _____ (random, nonrandom) sample, each member of the population has an equal chance of being selected as part of the sample.

41. In qualitative research, the data are analyzed by _____ of large volumes of narrative data into categories that can be identified as the concepts present in the situation.

42. Controlling _____ variables controls research bias.

43. When you ask if the passage of time has affected the results, you are asking a question about the validity classification of _____.

TEST YOURSELF

44. Select the statement that is true about the case study method of research.
    1. Case studies increase knowledge of clients with similar conditions.
    2. Case studies are not a valid method of research.
    3. Case studies focus on the psychosocial needs of clients.
    4. Case studies rule out the need to consider multiple variables.

45. Before you use the findings of a research study to make decisions in the clinical setting, you should make which of the following determinations?
    1. Whether the elements of the situation are precisely like those of the study
    2. Whether you have the qualifications to make decisions using research
    3. Whether your hospital is a research hospital
    4. Whether the elements of the situation are sufficiently similar to the conditions of study to make it likely that the intervention will work in this situation

46. Which of the following items would be consistent with one of the ANA priorities for nursing research?
    1. Finding a cure for AIDS
    2. Testing lifestyle management strategies for preventing AIDS
    3. Developing a vaccine against AIDS
    4. Describing the mutation mechanisms of the HIV virus

47. Select the most important criterion for deciding if a problem is worth studying.
    1. The solution can be expected to improve the quality of life for a number of clients.
    2. The solution to the problem will make the researcher famous.
    3. The problem is unusual and therefore interesting to study.
    4. Enough is known about the problem to make a solution feasible.

48. A nurse wants to study a technique for reducing infection rates in premature infants. Select the behavior that would be within ethical guidelines for research.
    1. Not informing the parents of the control group because nothing will change for their child
    2. Not informing the parents of the experimental group because their participation is not necessary
    3. Selecting the babies with greater weights for the experimental group to prevent causing harm
    4. Fully informing and seeking consent from parents of all infants

49. At which of the following times is the review of a research protocol by an institutional review board required?
    1. When federal support is sought to conduct the study
    2. Only when invasive procedures are used in the study
    3. Only when the subject is of a sensitive nature
    4. Only when the methods are known to cause harm

50. When considering the issue of informed consent for research, a vulnerable population is one that has which of the following characteristics?
    1. Is unable to give informed consent
    2. Is more likely to be harmed by the intervention
    3. Is at greater risk for complications
    4. Is unlikely to want to participate in the study

51. The population being studied refers to which of the following groups?
    1. Both the research subjects and the control group
    2. The group with the characteristics of the people who are selected as subjects
    3. The clients on the nursing unit where the study is being conducted
    4. Everybody living in a given geographical area

INFANCY THROUGH SCHOOL-AGE DEVELOPMENT

PURPOSE

This chapter explores concepts and principles of growth and development and factors that affect children from infancy through school age. It introduces you to the use of the nursing process for health maintenance and risk reduction in these client populations.

MATCHING

1. _____ attachment
2. _____ cephalocaudal
3. _____ concrete operations
4. _____ conservation
5. _____ critical periods
6. _____ development
7. _____ differentiated development
8. _____ growth
9. _____ object permanence
10. _____ proximodistal
11. _____ sensory stimulation
12. _____ symbolic play

a. the physiological development of a living being and the quantitative change seen in the body
b. development that starts with a generalized response and progresses to a skilled specific response
c. a progression of behavioral changes that involve the acquisition of appropriate cognitive, linguistic, and psychosocial skills
d. the stage of cognitive development at which children begin to project the self into other people's situations and realize that their own way of thinking isn't the only way
e. the awareness that unseen objects do not disappear; evidenced by the infant searching for an object that has been moved out of sight
f. pretend or imaginative play that enables preschool children to recreate experiences and to try out roles
g. periods of time when a person has an increased vulnerability to physical, chemical, psychological, or environmental influences

h. a pattern of neuromuscular growth and development that starts at the head and moves toward the feet
i. a pattern of skill development that starts at the midline of the body and moves outward
j. the development of strong ties of affection by an infant with a significant other
k. a child's ability to understand that changing the shape of a substance does not change its volume
l. the activation and exhilaration of the senses

TRUE OR FALSE

13. _____ Each stage of development depends on adequate completion of the previous one and forms the foundation for development of new skills.
14. _____ Jean Piaget described cognitive development as involving the increasing ability to think and reason in a logical manner.
15. _____ The list of developmental tasks is the same for all cultures.
16. _____ Crying is the primary means by which newborns make their needs and wants known.
17. _____ During parallel play, toddlers play beside, but not with, their friends.
18. _____ Socioeconomic factors, such as income, educational level, and single parenthood, influence the growth and development of children.
19. _____ The preschool years are a time of rapid weight gain for a toddler.
20. _____ It is normal for preschool children to create imaginary companions that they talk to and play with, and who become a regular part of their daily routines.

21. _____ Children between the ages of 6 and 11 have few fears, such as fear of darkness, animals, and high places.

22. _____ Children cannot be trusted to handle a gun safely, even though they have the mechanical skill and strength to fire one.

FILL IN THE BLANKS

23. A newborn's length is measured from _____ to _____.

24. Eyes begin to focus and fixate at _____ months.

25. An infant who cries when separated from parents or approached by strangers is having _____ _____.

26. Human milk is the most desirable form of milk for the first _____ months of life.

27. During the preschool years, a toddler's future body type becomes apparent. Body types include _____ (lanky build), mesomorphic (medium muscular build), and _____ (large build).

28. The vivid imagination of the _____- _____ child can turn a stuffed toy by day into a threatening monster in the dark.

29. Deaths from bicycling injuries usually result from _____ injuries.

30. Children under the age of _____ should not use skateboards or in-line skates because they are not developmentally prepared to protect themselves from injury.

EXERCISING YOUR CLINICAL JUDGMENT

Yung Hi, the 33-month-old Korean client from the chapter's case study, has undergone orthopedic surgery to reduce a fractured femur and is in skeletal traction. She has a nursing diagnosis of delayed growth and development related to prescribed dependence (traction) and separation from her parents at night. You are assigned to work with Yung on the evening shift, and are thus able to work with her while her mother is present, and on a one-on-one basis after her parents have gone home for the evening.

31. Which of the following age-appropriate toys would you recommend be brought to the hospital for Yung to play with during her recuperation?
    1. Mobile
    2. Rattle
    3. Toys that float in water
    4. Nontoxic crayons

32. You are trying to encourage continued physical growth during the period of recuperation. Which of the following strategies would be most useful?
    1. Try to have Yung eat the same amount of food every day.
    2. Keep foods separated from each other on the tray, and use her favorite cup at each meal.
    3. Use food as a reward for good behavior.
    4. Encourage Yung to eat every bit of food on her plate.

33. You would plan age-appropriate care by allowing time for Yung to have a 1- to 2-hour nap each day at:
    1. 9 AM.
    2. 10 AM.
    3. 1 PM.
    4. 4 PM.

TEST YOURSELF

34. Bringing toys and games to the bedside of an immobilized child would be primarily useful interventions for which of the following nursing diagnoses?
    1. Ineffective health maintenance
    2. Delayed growth and development
    3. Diversional activity deficit
    4. Health-seeking behaviors

35. The nurse would bring rattles that make noise and vinyl or cloth books to the bedside of a client who is how old?
    1. 1 to 2 months
    2. 2 to 3 months
    3. 4 to 7 months
    4. 1 to 2 years

36. The nurse providing immunizations to children would teach the parents to report to the health care provider which of the following adverse effects of an immunization?
    1. High fever
    2. Mild discomfort at the site
    3. Rash at the site
    4. Soreness in the area

37. The home health nurse would provide parent education after noting which of the following behaviors when visiting the home of a pediatric client?
    1. All crib rails raised
    2. Mother left toddler in tub to answer door
    3. Safety handles on all cabinet doors
    4. Gate positioned at the head of stairs

38. The nurse would avoid giving toys with small removable parts to a client younger than the age of:
    1. 6
    2. 4
    3. 3
    4. 5

39. Your client is upset because his mother left the room. She told him that she was returning in 2 hours. Fear of abandonment is a common concern for which of the following age-groups?
    1. 4- to 6-year-olds
    2. Teenagers
    3. School-age children
    4. Preschoolers

40. Establishing guidelines for behavior is representative of which of the following?
    1. Developing morality
    2. Discipline
    3. Limit-setting
    4. Parenting skills

41. The recommended screening for tuberculosis (TB) during childhood is at which of the following times?
    1. Twice during childhood
    2. Four times during childhood: 1, 4, 8, and 12 years old
    3. Three times during childhood: 12 to 15 months, before entering kindergarten, and at 14 to 16 years of age
    4. At entrance to school, unless otherwise indicated

42. Advice you can give working parents of latchkey children is to:
    1. not leave their children unsupervised.
    2. use the community resources available to latchkey children
    3. encourage them have their children remain at school until they can pick them up.
    4. consider working in jobs that allow them to be at home when their children are home.

PURPOSE

This chapter discusses the development tasks of the adolescent and young adult. It identifies factors that affect adolescent and young adult development and describes the assessment of this age-group. Nursing diagnoses interventions, and outcomes appropriate for adolescents and young adults are also included.

MATCHING

1. _____ adolescence
2. _____ constitutional delay of puberty
3. _____ egocentrism
4. _____ formal operations
5. _____ gynecomastia
6. _____ menarche
7. _____ nocturnal emission
8. _____ young adulthood

a. the ability to reason abstractly
b. a benign increase in breast tissue in adolescent boys associated with puberty
c. the period of life from age 20 to 34
d. an absence of early signs of puberty
e. refers to the tendency to spend so much time thinking about and focusing on your own thoughts and changes in your own body that you come to believe that others are focused on them as well
f. a progression of behavioral changes that involve the acquisition of appropriate cognitive, linguistic, and psychosocial skills
g. a discharge of semen during sleep
h. the time of the first menstrual period
i. a benign increase in breast tissue associated with puberty
j. a period of transition between childhood and adulthood; ages 12 to 21

TRUE OR FALSE

9. _____ Adolescents who are abused and neglected are at high risk for *Delayed growth and development*.

10. _____ Girls are affected by a constitutional delay of puberty more often than boys are.
11. _____ Most cases of short stature result from underlying disease.
12. _____ The number of adolescents living with chronic illness has increased, not because the incidence of disease has changed but because more children with chronic conditions are surviving.
13. _____ Alcohol is a factor in the most common causes of deaths and injuries among adolescents.
14. _____ Ninety percent of adolescents who suffer from anorexia nervosa are girls.
15. _____ Adults develop in a manner that is fairly consistent with others of their age-group with little if no effect from genetic or ethnic factors.
16. _____ Young adults are expected to perform many roles.
17. _____ Adults ages 18 to 24 are likely to have health insurance, with more than 75% covered by group health insurance.

FILL IN THE BLANKS

18. The chief developmental task of adolescence is the development of _____ versus _____.

19. Adolescents who live in poverty typically have poor nutrition, substandard housing, and limited access to _____ _____.

20. Adolescents must establish their own sets of _____ and _____ in order to gain autonomy from adults.

21. The leading causes of death for adults younger than 25 are _____ , _____ , and _____.

22. Most studies agree that at almost _____ of adolescents in the United States engage in intercourse during their high school years.

23. When performing the health assessment of an adolescent, it is important for you to remain _____.

24. Adolescents with a chronic illness may engage in risk taking by failing to _____ with their treatment program.

25. Erickson's young adult phase focuses on _____ versus _____.

26. Each plan of care must be _____ to a client's needs, age, and culture.

27. When educating a client regarding lifestyle changes, suggest _____ _____ rather than _____ ones.

28. An appropriate exercise program for adolescent and young adult clients should take into consideration their current level of _____.

29. Health-care planning for the well young adult is centered on the goals of maintaining _____ and preventing _____.

EXERCISING YOUR CLINICAL JUDGMENT

30. Jamie King, the 19-year-old client from the case study is experiencing weakness, lethargy, and high street levels since she moved into the dorm at college 10 weeks ago. Her dietary and exercise routines have changed since she moved out of her parents home. Jamie is experiencing which stage of psychosocial development?
    1. Identify versus identity diffusion
    2. Intimacy versus isolation
    3. Integrity versus despair
    4. Generativity versus stagnation

31. While Jamie lived at home, her mother prepated all of her meals. She is now visiting the cafeteria several times a week and eating quick food between classes. To help Jamie better manage her diabetes a realistic goal would be for her to:
    1. Schedule an appointment with her doctor for a complete physical examination
    2. Stop eating in the cafeteria and begin preparing well-balanced meals at the dorm
    3. Describe the connection between her change in diet and her blood sugar levels
    4. Eliminate all quick foods from her diet within 30 days

32. Jamie experienced a significant lifestyle change when she moved into the college dorm form her parent's home. An adolescent who is unable to cope successfully with this change may experience:
    1. Poor job performance
    2. High levels of stress
    3. A situation crisis
    4. Poor family relationship

TEST YOURSELF

33. You are discussing preventive health issues with an adolescent client. The response you get is, "Other people may have to worry about that, but I don't have to worry about it." This is an example of which hallmark of adolescent cognitive development?
    1. Egocentrism
    2. Elitism
    3. Fantasy world
    4. Concrete thinking

34. Which of the following statements is true for constitutional delay of puberty?
    1. It affects more girls than boys and is more likely to arise in a family in which the pubertal development of the same-sex parent was delayed.
    2. It is more likely to arise in a family in which the pubertal development of the same-sex parent was delayed.
    3. It affects more boys than girls and is more likely to arise in a family in which the pubertal development of the same-sex parent was delayed.
    4. It affects males and females equally and is related to heredity.

35. Your adolescent client was involved in a homicide. Which of the following statements is the most accurate?
    1. Homicide is a serious public health problem in the United States, and a leading cause of deaths among young adults.
    2. Homicide-related deaths are among the top three causes of death among adolescents.
    3. Homicide deaths occur among adolescents, but are not among the primary causes of deaths among adolescents.
    4. Homicide is a serious problem because of alcohol abuse among teenagers.

36. One of the most effective ways for parents to help prevent their teenagers from becoming pregnant is to:
    1. use the "just say no" approach.
    2. buy them condoms.
    3. condone their behaviors, so they feel comfortable coming to their parents when they want advice.
    4. talk with their teenagers about sex in a nonjudgmental and informative manner.

37. Your client, a high school student, earns straight A's and is very active in school activities. She is thin and appears underdeveloped for her age. Her weight is 98 lb. and height is 5 ft 8 in. She confides in you that she feels fat. Which of the following nursing diagnoses would be most appropriate?
    1. *Ineffective health maintenance*
    2. *Ineffective individual coping*
    3. *Disturbed body image*
    4. *Delayed growth and development*

38. You should do which of the following diagnostic screening tests with young adult clients?
    1. TB, vision, Papanicolaou smear, breast examination
    2. TB, prostate-specific antigen test, cholesterol
    3. BP, breast examination, prostate-specific antigen test
    4. TB, sigmoidoscopy, vision

39. Your assessment of a 20-year-old client reveals that she has had several unwanted pregnancies, and that she abuses alcohol. Which nursing diagnosis would be most appropriate?
    1. *Ineffective health maintenance*
    2. *Knowledge deficit*
    3. *Ineffective management of therapeutic regimen*
    4. *Delayed growth and development*

Chapter 18

THE MIDDLE, AND OLDER ADULT

PURPOSE

This chapter discusses key concepts related to the developmental tasks of middle and older adulthood. It identifies the various factors that affect adult development. It also differentiates among the variety of diagnoses appropriate for the adult seeking knowledge or health care related to growth and development. It discusses nursing interventions to maintain health and reduce risk factors.

MATCHING

1. _____ ageism
2. _____ geriatric nursing
3. _____ gerontology
4. _____ menopause
5. _____ middle adulthood
6. _____ midlife crisis
7. _____ older adult
8. _____ retirement
9. _____ sandwich generation

a. a stereotype, prejudice, or discrimination against people, particularly older adults, based on their age
b. caught between the needs of adjacent generations; caring for ill or frail parents while handling the competing demands of children and employment
c. any person age 65 years and older
d. the period from ages 35 to 64
e. a stressful life period during middle adulthood precipitated by the review and reevaluation of one's past, including goals, priorities, and life accomplishments, during which the person experiences inner turmoil, self-doubt, and major restructuring of personality
f. the stage in the female climacteric during which hormone production is reduced, the ovaries stop producing eggs, and menstruation ceases
g. the permanent withdrawal from one's job
h. a comprehensive study of aging and the problems of older adults
i. a branch of nursing that deals with the problems and diseases of old age and aging people

TRUE OR FALSE

10. _____ A person's growth and development always represent the interaction of genetic makeup and environment.
11. _____ Gerontology is the comprehensive study of aging and the problems of the aged
12. _____ Erickson's theory of psychosocial development identifies the older adult stage as generativity versus stagnation.
13. _____ Regular exercise promotes appetite, mental health and balance, and stress reduction.
14. _____ Alcohol abuse in the older adult is often very easy to determine.
15. _____ The Centers for Disease Control and Prevention (CDC) report that at least 1 in 10 deaths in North America is related to cigarette smoking.
16. _____ Stress is the most common cause of illness in our society.
17. _____ A key to wellness for the adult is appropriate screening, especially for clients in high-risk groups.
18. _____ Chronic diseases account for 70% of all deaths in the United States.

FILL IN THE BLANKS

19. Erickson's seventh stage of psychosocial development, _____ versus _____ is reached during middle adulthood.

20. Levinson conceived of development as a sequence of qualitatively distinct eras or _____, each of which has its own time and brings certain psychological challenges to the forefront of a person's life.

21. Chronic drug users are particularly susceptible to _____ _____ and are considered high-risk transmitters.

22. _____ is a stereotype, prejudice, or discrimination against people, especially older adults, based on their age.

23. Clients who are _____ experience a great deal of functional impairment, resulting in lost work time, decreased job performance, and decreased family and social functioning.

24. _____ is associated with limited access to health care, poor nutrition, substandard housing, and inadequate prenatal care.

25. The leading causes of death for adults are cancer, _____, _____ _____ _____, influenza, and _____.

26. Working older adults are discovering that more of their after-tax dollars are spent on _____ _____.

27. Urinary _____ is not a normal age-related change in the older adult.

EXERCISING YOUR CLINICAL JUDGMENT

28. Mr. Cognomi, the 70-year-old client from the chapter's case study, states that he feels his life is without meaning. He has become self-absorbed and distant from his family. Mr. Cognomi may be experiencing which psychosocial stage of development?
    1. Intimacy versus isolation
    2. Industry versus inferiority
    3. Integrity versus despair
    4. Generativity versus stagnation

29. Mr. Cognomi has been gradually withdrawing from social roles and has little interest in pursuing acitivities with friends or family members. He is most likely experiencing:
    1. poor job performance.
    2. a situational crisis.
    3. disengagement.
    4. poor family relationships.

30. To help persuade Mr. Cognomi to change his high-risk behaviors, you will need to:
    1. give Mr. Cognomi both oral and written health education material.
    2. have Mr. Cognomi join a support group made up of men his age.
    3. identify Mr. Cognomi's beliefs relevant to his high-risk behaviors, and provide him information based on this foundation.
    4. give Mr. Cognomi your recommendations regarding his most serious high-risk behavior so he may begin working on modifying it.

TEST YOURSELF

31. Middle adulthood is the period from ages 35 to 64 when mature adults are concerned with:

1. developing philosophies of life and personal lifestyles.
2. balancing a career with raising small children.
3. establishing a significant relationship with a partner.
4. establishing and guiding the next generation in their roles as parents, teachers, mentors, guardians of the culture, etc.

32. Your client has a child in high school and is caring for his elderly parent. As a group, clients in this situation are often commonly called the:
    1. midlevel generation.
    2. x-generation.
    3. sandwich generation.
    4. midlife transition generation.

33. You are admitting a client to your health care facility. What is the most important thing you need to do to ensure that you obtain a thorough and accurate history of the client's problems?
    1. Read the admission record prior to your assessment.
    2. Develop a trusting relationship with the client.
    3. Obtain biographical data, history, and chief complaint.
    4. Obtain family history and chief complaint.

34. You should do which of the following diagnostic screening tests with your middle-aged adult female clients?
    1. BP, Papanicolaou smear, cholesterol
    2. TB, colonoscopy, hemoglobin and hematocrit
    3. HIV, BP, cholesterol
    4. CBC, cervical culture, breast exam

35. Your assessment of a 75-year-old client reveals that he has poor personal hygiene and has missed several scheduled health care visits. Which nursing diagnosis would be most appropriate?
    1. *Ineffective health maintenance*
    2. *Knowledge deficit*
    3. *Ineffective management of therapeutic regimen*
    4. *Delayed growth and development*

36. Your client is involved in an adult day care program. This type of long-term-care service offers which of the following?
    1. Temporary respite for family caregivers by allowing a resident to live in assisted living community or nursing home
    2. Inpatient care designed for adults who have an acute illness, injury, or exacerbation of disease process
    3. Community-based group programs designed to meet the needs of functionally impaired adults through individualized plans of care
    4. Twenty-four-hour nursing care for residents available from licensed nurses

PURPOSE

This chapter discusses key concepts that relate to the nursing diagnosis *Health-seeking behaviors*. It provides you with definitions of health and describes the perception of health for individuals, families, and communities. In addition, this chapter identifies health goals and expected outcomes when planning care for individuals, families, and communities. It also discusses factors affecting health and interventions you can use to promote health.

MATCHING

1. _____ disease
2. _____ etiology
3. _____ health goals
4. _____ health-illness continuum
5. _____ health perception
6. _____ health promotion
7. _____ health within illness
8. _____ illness
9. _____ population health
10. _____ preventive health care
11. _____ primary health care
12. _____ primary prevention
13. _____ secondary prevention
14. _____ tertiary prevention
15. _____ well-being
16. _____ wellness

a. knowledge and experience of one's state of wellness and well-being

b. refers to the personal experience of feeling unhealthy, caused by changes in a person's state of well-being and social function

c. an event that can expand human potential by providing an opportunity for personal growth and well-being despite having an illness

d. the advancement of health through the encouragement of activities that enhance the wellness of individuals, families, and communities

e. a subjective perception of a good and satisfactory existence in which the individual has a positive experience of personal abilities, harmony, and vitality

f. considers health problems encountered as a result of being a part of a group, and focuses intervention on the population rather than on the individual

g. a specific disorder characterized by a recognizable set of signs and symptoms and attributable to heredity, infection, diet, or environment

h. consists of actions that are considered true prevention because they precede disease or dysfunction and are applied to clients considered physically and emotionally healthy to protect them from health problems

i. outlines broadly what needs to be done to achieve health for individuals, families, and communities

j. the cause of the disease

k. ranges from high-level wellness—an optimal state of mental and physical well-being—to premature death

l. consists of actions that focus on the early diagnosis and prompt treatment of people with health problems or illnesses and who are at risk for developing complications or worsening conditions

m. all care necessary to people's lives and health, including health education, nutrition, sanitation, maternal and child health care, immunizations, and prevention and control of endemic disease

n. recognition of the risk for disease and actions taken to reduce that risk

o. a state of optimal health or optimal physical and social functioning

p. involves minimizing the effects of a permanent irreversible disease or disability through interventions directed at preventing complication and deterioration

TRUE OR FALSE

17. _____ Health perception is the knowledge and experience of one's state of wellness and well-being.

18. _____ Countries around the world are seeking to establish and attain health goals for their citizens.

19. _____ The World Health Organization (WHO) has declared that it is unrealistic to believe that health is a fundamental right of all people.

20. _____ All diseases can be cured by removing their etiology.

21. _____ Every person exists at some point on the health-illness continuum and may move back and forth between the two extremes.

22. _____ Population health is primarily concerned with public policies and interventions.

23. _____ The key element of *Health-seeking behaviors* is choice.

24. _____ Society at large is responsible for the health of its members.

FILL IN THE BLANKS

25. The _____ _____ _____ has defined health as a state of complete physical, mental, and social well-being, and not merely the absence of illness.

26. The goal of *Healthy People 2010* is increasing the _____ and _____ of healthy life.

27. Wellness is a _____ that cannot be _____ achieved.

28. Health care is the _____ and treatment of disease based on a specific disorder and its etiology.

29. The _____ _____ _____ recognizes that more than one factor is necessary to determine a person's state of health.

30. Health in a community is defined by the parameters of _____ health.

31. A statement of health goals flows from the _____ of health.

32. Primary _____ care refers to care provided at the point at which a client first enters the health care system.

TEST YOURSELF

33. You are organizing a public forum to identify health goals for the local teen center. Your plan is to have teens actively seek ways to alter detrimental personal health habits so they can move toward a higher level of health. You are doing your health care planning based on the goals of *Healthy People 2010*. The goals of *Healthy People 2010* include which of the following?
    1. To help individuals of all ages increase life expectancy and improve their quality of life and to eliminate health disparities among different segments of the population
    2. Essential health services must be available to all persons without regard to age, risk category, present health status, or ability to pay.
    3. Essential health services should be planned, funded, and supervised on a nonprofit basis by public authorities.
    4. Essential health services should be available to those eligible when they are away from home.

34. When planning your assessment of the teen center, which broad social issues might you consider assessing?
    1. Whether or not it is a safe environment, and whether or not it offers cost-effective health services
    2. Whether or not the teens have good relationships with their peers
    3. Whether or not the teens have good coping skills
    4. Whether or not the teens have the capacity to make healthy lifestyle decisions

35. You are concerned about the high levels of depression in the teen population. You organize and screen the teens for depression. This type of prevention is:
    1. primary.
    2. secondary.
    3. tertiary.
    4. evaluation.

36. The WHO has defined health as:
    1. the absence of disease.
    2. a state of complete physical, mental, and social well-being.
    3. knowledge and experience of one's state of wellness and well-being.
    4. a state of complete physical, mental, and social well-being, and not merely the absence of disease.

37. When assessing community health, your nursing care plan may include which of the following broad social issues of community health?
    1. Positive, supportive interpersonal family relationships, safety and security issues, affordable housing
    2. Community design, joint action for minority and cultural health, social services, and public policy
    3. A safe environment, preventive health services, and consequences of lower-status occupations
    4. Access to and appropriate use of health care services, affordable housing, and a safe environment

38. Immunization programs are an example of which level of preventive care?
    1. Primary prevention
    2. Secondary prevention
    3. Tertiary prevention
    4. Disease prevention

HEALTH MAINTENANCE: LIFESTYLE MANAGEMENT

PURPOSE

This chapter introduces you to worldviews of health, health care, and behavior change that affect one's decisions about lifestyle changes as part of a therapeutic regimen. It helps you to use the nursing process when working with clients seeking to make these lifestyle changes to enhance health and well-being.

MATCHING

1. _____ action stage
2. _____ contemplation stage
3. _____ counseling
4. _____ emic dimension
5. _____ etic dimension
6. _____ lifestyle
7. _____ maintenance stage
8. _____ perceived barriers
9. _____ perceived benefits
10. _____ perceived severity
11. _____ perceived susceptibility
12. _____ precontemplation stage
13. _____ preparation stage
14. _____ referral
15. _____ self-efficacy
16. _____ social support
17. _____ termination stage

a. client's subjective perception of the risk of contracting a health condition.
b. the client does not intend to change a high-risk behavior in the foreseeable future (the next 6 months), primarily because he or she is unaware of the long-term consequences of the behavior
c. perceived negative aspects of a health action or the perceived impediments to undertaking the recommended behaviors
d. the client changes risky behaviors and the context of the behavior (environment, experience), and makes significant efforts to reach goals
e. the perceived seriousness of contracting an illness or leaving it untreated
f. the client intends to change the behavior within the next 6 months
g. the conviction that one can successfully execute the behavior required to produce the outcomes

h. takes place during the 6 months after the client changes the high-risk behavior
i. refers to an individual's or social group's subjective perceptions and experiences related to health
j. the subjective feeling of belonging, or being accepted, loved, esteemed, valued, and needed for oneself, not for what one can do for others
k. a behavior or group of behaviors chosen by the person that may have a positive or a negative influence on health
l. a process designed to provide the client with access to health care and supportive services that are not available form the sending institution
m. refers to the objective interpretation of health by a scientifically trained practitioner
n. the client is no longer tempted to engage in old behavior
o. a method of communication that actively involves the client in the recognition of personal risk factors and management of necessary behavior changes
p. the client's perceptions and beliefs about the effectiveness of the recommended actions in preventing the health threat
q. the client intends to take action in the very near future, usually within the next month

TRUE OR FALSE

18. _____ To effectively help others, health care professionals must first understand the health and quality of life perspective of the client.
19. _____ According to the health belief model, clients will take action to control ill health if the anticipated barriers to taking the action are outweighed by the benefits.
20. _____ Impaired verbal skills or language differences do not interfere with the ability of a client to effectively express health needs to health care professionals.
21. _____ Clients with health insurance are more likely to seek health care at the onset of symptoms than those who do not have insurance.

22. _____ A client's spiritual values and beliefs always coincide with recommended interventions to promote, maintain, or restore health.

23. _____ The nursing diagnosis *Noncompliance* is used when a client desires to comply but factors are present that deter adherence to health-related advice given by health care professionals.

24. _____ Counseling is different from education in that counseling involves guiding the client through decision making rather than merely providing the information needed to make a decision.

25. _____ A nurse should anticipate problems in managing the therapeutic regimen if the client has poor eyesight, decreased mobility, or reduced manual dexterity.

26. _____ The nurse is solely responsible for the discharge planning process.

27. _____ If no noticeable change occurs in unhealthy behaviors within a reasonable time, the client should be reassessed to determine what prevented progress.

FILL IN THE BLANKS

28. The theory of _____ _____ is a human behavior framework designed to explain a client's intention to perform a behavior.

29. Health practices and behaviors that have potential negative effects on health are known as _____ _____.

30. A health-risk appraisal provides clients with essential information about health threats from hereditary factors, _____, and _____ history.

31. A client with a nursing diagnosis of *Health-seeking behaviors* does not necessarily have a _____ diagnosis.

32. A nurse who provides specific information to a client about a health problem in order to motivate health behavior is striving to increase the client's _____ level.

33. _____ _____ is a self-discovery process that may be helpful in assisting a client to make health-related choices when faced with one or more alternatives.

34. Building rewards into effective management of the health care regimen is a method of providing _____ or _____ factors.

35. A client who is in _____ is not likely to see the need for or benefit of health care services that are provided through referral.

36. _____ planning begins at the time of admission, but should be finalized with a specific plan before the client leaves an institution.

37. The assistance of family and friends in facilitating health-related behavioral change is considered a type of _____ support.

EXERCISING YOUR CLINICAL JUDGMENT

Mr. Kitchen, the African-American client from the chapter's case study, has a nursing diagnosis of *Ineffective therapeutic regimen management*. His identified health problem is heart failure, and he was prescribed digoxin (a cardiac glycoside) and Lasix (a loop diuretic) at his first clinic visit. Mr. Kitchen did not return to the clinic when he was scheduled for a follow-up appointment, but came in today after experiencing a return of shortness of breath. He had stopped taking his medication because he felt better, and because he disliked having to go to the bathroom so frequently. Recall that he is a widower with no family nearby, and he does not carefully plan meals or attend to his health. He also is a smoker who is not motivated as yet to stop smoking. You have been asked by the clinic nurse to provide teaching to Mr. Kitchen to enhance his ability to manage his health problems at home.

38. If Mr. Kitchen does not yet perceive that there are health benefits from smoking cessation, you would determine that he is in which of the following stages in the transtheoretical model of behavioral change?
    1. Precontemplation
    2. Contemplation
    3. Preparation
    4. Action

39. Which of the following factors is most likely to be responsible for Mr. Kitchen's lack of adherence to the medical regimen?
    1. Complexity of the therapeutic regimen
    2. Side effects of therapy
    3. Financial cost of the regimen
    4. Complexity of the health care delivery system

40. The most effective strategy to use when providing information to Mr. Kitchen about his health problem would be to:
    1. explain that he will have a steady downhill course if he does not adhere to the treatment plan.
    2. share with him the results of research studies that show the cost of treating other noncompliant clients who have similar health problems.
    3. increase his awareness that unhealthy lifestyle habits are related to the development of his symptoms.
    4. encourage him to hire a companion to cook his meals and make sure he takes his medication.

41. You realize that Mr. Kitchen needs supportive care in order to achieve and maintain lifestyle changes. Given this client's particular situation, you would select which of the following as the most important intervention for this client?
    1. Make referrals to all available services that are provided within the clinic setting.
    2. Contact other outside agencies to give follow-up care.
    3. Ask him to renew his relationships with family that lives out of town.
    4. Establish a trusting therapeutic relationship with him.

TEST YOURSELF

42. To improve overall health, the nurse would place highest priority on assisting the client to make lifestyle changes for which of the following habits?
    1. Drinking a six-pack of beer each day
    2. Eating an occasional chocolate bar
    3. Exercising twice a week
    4. Using relaxation exercises to deal with stress

43. A nurse who is assessing the health-related physical fitness of a client as part of a health assessment would focus on which of the following aspects of the assessment?
    1. Agility
    2. Speed
    3. Body composition
    4. Power

44. A nurse would interpret that which of the following clients is most likely to have a reduced ability to acquire knowledge about a newly prescribed diet and medication regimen due to cognitive perceptual impairment?
    1. One who has a slight decrease in hearing acuity
    2. One who has chronic confusion
    3. One who wears corrective lenses
    4. One who is 48 years old

45. A client with a newly diagnosed health problem has the choice of using either of two acceptable treatments for the problem. If the client has difficulty choosing between the two, the nurse would consider which of the following nursing diagnoses as most appropriate?
    1. *Health-seeking behaviors*
    2. *Knowledge deficit*
    3. *Ineffective health maintenance*
    4. *Decisional conflict*

46. A nurse is trying to motivate a client toward more effective management of a therapeutic regimen. Which of the following actions by the nurse is most likely to be effective in increasing the client's motivation?
    1. Determine whether the client has any family or friends living nearby.
    2. Develop a lengthy discharge plan and review it carefully with the client.
    3. Teach the client about the disorder at the client's level of understanding.
    4. Make a referral to an area agency for client follow-up.

HEALTH MAINTENANCE: MEDICATION MANAGEMENT

PURPOSE

This chapter describes concepts of medication management and a wide variety of factors that can influence the effectiveness of medication therapy. It provides specific guidelines and information related to nursing process that can assist you to effectively deliver medication therapy to clients.

MATCHING

1. ____ adverse effect
2. ____ anaphylaxis
3. ____ antagonistic effect
4. ____ bioavailability
5. ____ biotransformation
6. ____ chemical name
7. ____ controlled substance
8. ____ generic name
9. ____ hypersensitivity reaction
10. ____ idiosyncratic response
11. ____ intradermal (ID) route
12. ____ intramuscular (IM) route
13. ____ intravenous (IV) route
14. ____ loading dose
15. ____ official name
16. ____ parenteral route
17. ____ pharmacokinetics
18. ____ prescription
19. ____ side effect
20. ____ subcutaneous (subcut) route
21. ____ synergistic effect
22. ____ target organ
23. ____ teratogenic potential
24. ____ therapeutic effect
25. ____ topical route
26. ____ toxic effect

a. the amount of an administered drug that is available for activity in the target tissue
b. a mild allergic reaction to a drug
c. involves injection into the subcutaneous tissue just under the dermis
d. a medication side effect that is potentially harmful to a client
e. involves injection of a medication into a vein

f. the likelihood that a medication will harm a developing fetus
g. refers to a drug's activity from the time it enters the body until it leaves
h. a serious adverse effect of a medication that may even threaten life
i. an effect that occurs when one drug enhances or increases the effect of another drug
j. a body tissue or organ that is specifically affected by a drug
k. an unexplained and unpredictable response to a medication
l. the name assigned to a drug when it is first manufactured; also known as the nonproprietary name
m. involves injection into muscle tissue, specifically the body of a muscle
n. an effect of a medication that is not intended or planned but may occur as a result of use
o. drug that affects the mind or behavior, may be habit forming, and has a high potential for abuse
p. an effect that occurs when one drug reduces or negates the effect of another
q. an initial medication dose that exceeds the maintenance or therapeutic dose
r. the intended effect or action of a medication
s. used to deliver medication directly into a body site, such as skin, eyes, or ears
t. the name assigned by the Food and Drug Administration (FDA) after it approves a drug; often the same name as the generic name
u. involves injection into the dermis
v. an order for a medication that contains the client's name, medication name, dose, route, frequency, amount of medication to be dispensed, number of refills allowed, and prescriber's signature
w. the name that precisely describes the chemical and molecular structure of a medication; often long and complex
x. a drug route that is outside the GI tract
y. the process of inactivating and breaking down a medication
z. a life-threatening allergic reaction to a drug that requires immediate intervention to prevent possible death

TRUE OR FALSE

27. _____ In some states, revised Nurse Practice Acts have allowed selected groups of advanced practice nurses to write prescriptions.

28. _____ The blood-brain barrier permits transport of lipid-bound medications while preventing transport of many water-soluble drugs.

29. _____ No drug reaches the liver until it has passed through all body tissues.

30. _____ The peak serum concentration of a medication usually occurs just as the last bit of the most recently administered dose is being absorbed.

31. _____ There is a national standard recognized throughout all states that regulates how and when telephone and verbal medication orders should be given.

32. _____ The most common medication system in use today is the unit-dose system.

33. _____ A client's overall nutritional status can either positively or negatively affect medication actions in the body.

34. _____ Dehydration has no effect on drug transport because the dosage is unchanged.

35. _____ A client who subscribes to Western beliefs about health and illness typically expects to receive medication as part of a treatment plan.

FILL IN THE BLANKS

36. In the United States the _____ _____ Agency is empowered to enforce narcotic laws.

37. _____ _____ refers to the diminishing therapeutic effect of the same dosage of a drug over time, requiring increased dosing to achieve the same therapeutic effect.

38. _____-_____ drugs are coated to prevent them from dissolving until they reach the alkaline environment of the small intestine.

39. A drug that should be avoided during pregnancy because the risks outweigh any benefits is labeled as belonging to FDA Pregnancy Risk Category _____.

40. Drug dosages for infants and children are calculated according to either body surface area or _____ _____.

41. Nursing diagnoses that could apply due to the gastrointestinal side effects of medications include _____ and _____.

42. A client who develops signs such as oral lesions, diarrhea, or vaginal itching while taking antibiotic therapy could be developing _____.

43. In many agencies, a medication should be administered within _____ minutes before or after its scheduled time.

EXERCISING YOUR CLINICAL JUDGMENT

Mr. Connell, the 62-year-old Irish-American client from the chapter's case study, has high blood pressure. However, he stopped taking his prescribed medications because he "felt better." He has been treated in the local hospital emergency department for chest pain, and is now diagnosed with angina pectoris. You must teach Mr. Connell about the medications that are being resumed.

44. Which of the following items would you include in a discussion with Mr. Connell about general principles of medication self-administration?
   1. If a prescription runs out, use that of a relative or friend until it can be refilled.
   2. Change brand names depending on cost to motivate compliance with therapy.
   3. Develop and use a reminder system if forgetting medications is a problem.
   4. Put all types of medications into a single large container to make storage easier.

45. You are teaching Mr. Connell strategies to prevent dizziness, a common side effect of antihypertensive medications. Which of the following would you recommend?
   1. Use alcohol at will because it adds to the antihypertensive effect.
   2. Sit or stand up slowly when getting out of a bed or chair.
   3. Go out for long walks in hot weather for additive medication effects.
   4. Take the medication upon arising in the morning if dizziness is a chronic problem.

46. Which of the following directions would you give Mr. Connell about taking nitroglycerin because it is a sublingual medication?
   1. Chew the tablet thoroughly
   2. Swallow it whole
   3. Place it between the cheek and the gum
   4. Let it dissolve under the tongue

47. You would be careful to teach Mr. Connell about adverse medication effects knowing that he has an increased likelihood of experiencing these because of which of the following personal factors?
    1. Age
    2. Work history
    3. Medical diagnosis
    4. Cultural background

TEST YOURSELF

48. A client is exhibiting a toxic effect from a medication. Which of the following actions by the nurse is most appropriate?
    1. Withhold the dose and report the signs and symptoms to the prescriber.
    2. Administer half the dose for the next 3 days.
    3. Withhold the dose for 24 hours, then resume.
    4. Administer the next dose, but keep an antidote nearby

49. An adult client has an order for an intramuscular injection. The nurse selects an appropriate size syringe with which of the following needle lengths?
    1. ½ to ⅝ inch
    2. ⅝ to 1 inch
    3. 1 to 1½ inches
    4. 1½ to 2 inches

50. A client has a new order for a transdermal patch. Which of the following would the nurse teach the client about maintaining safety with this type of medication?
    1. Apply the patch on a hairy site to prolong absorption.
    2. Use firm pressure, especially around the edges to ensure good skin contact.
    3. If a patch falls off, leave it off until the next day.
    4. Trim the patch so it fits under clothing without being visible.

51. A client is due for a dose of a scheduled eyedrop. Which of the following would the nurse do to safely administer this medication?
    1. Have the client lower the chin.
    2. Ask the client to look down at the floor.
    3. Tell the client to squint or squeeze the eye shut after administration.
    4. Pull downward on the bony orbit to expose the lower conjunctival sac.

52. A client has an order to take 5 mL of a medication at each dose. The home health nurse tells the client that this amount is equal to which of the following household measurements?
    1. ½ teaspoon
    2. 1 teaspoon
    3. 2 teaspoons
    4. 1 tablespoon

PRIORITIZATION QUESTIONS

53. In which order should the following medications be administered?
    1. PO antibiotics for Mr. Lee, who is receiving them to treat his pneumonia
    2. IM pain medication for Mrs. Feeny, who had abdominal surgery yesterday
    3. Sublingual nitroglycerine for Mr. Henderson, who is complaining of chest pain
    4. Topical hydrocortisone for Miss Zender, who has a rash on her upper arms

54. Place the following steps required when mixing insulins in a single syringe in the correct order.
    1. If the insulin is in suspension, roll the vial between he palms of your hands
    2. Add air to the vial of regular insulin
    3. Add air to the vial of NPH insulin
    4. Invert the vial of regular insulin, and withdraw the correct dose

55. Prioritize the following nursing actions used when applying a topical medication to the skin.
    1. Apply the medication using long smooth strokes moving in the direction of hair growth.
    2. Cleanse the application site with soap and water unless contraindicated
    3. Use a tongue depressor or swab to remove creams, pastes, or ointments from the original container.
    4. Assess the condition of the client's skin.

PURPOSE

This chapter introduces you to the health problem of infection and the importance of infection control as it relates to nursing practice. It uses the nursing process as a framework in describing how to assess, diagnose, plan, implement, and evaluate strategies used to either prevent or treat infection.

MATCHING

1. _____ antibacterial
2. _____ antibiotic
3. _____ antibody
4. _____ antimicrobial
5. _____ bacterium
6. _____ differential cell count
7. _____ Gram stain
8. _____ iatrogenic infection
9. _____ immunization
10. _____ immunocompromised
11. _____ immunosuppression
12. _____ infection
13. _____ infection control
14. _____ inflammatory response
15. _____ isolation
16. _____ medical asepsis
17. _____ nosocomial infection
18. _____ pathogen
19. _____ quarantine
20. _____ septicemia
21. _____ standard precautions
22. _____ surgical asepsis
23. _____ virulence
24. _____ virus

a. a small, single-celled organism that can reproduce outside cells
b. a clinical syndrome caused by the invasion and multiplication of a pathogen
c. a set of actions, including performing hand hygiene and the use of barriers, designed to reduce transmission of infectious organisms
d. consists of practices designed to reduce the numbers of pathogenic microorganisms in the client's environment

e. having the ability to limit the spread of microorganisms
f. a tiny microorganism, much smaller than a bacterium, which can only replicate inside the cell of a host such as a human
g. infection in the bloodstream
h. a circulating protein that recognizes and destroys foreign invaders or immunoglobulins
i. a drug that kills bacteria
j. an infection acquired from a reservoir in the hospital that may also be resistant to several antibiotics
k. breaks down the number of white blood cells into their types
l. a disease-producing microorganism
m. a localized reaction to injury that is activated when there is tissue damage
n. a specific microscopic test used to obtain rapid results on a culture sent to the laboratory
o. identification of a client who has an infection, and implementation of precautions to prevent the spread of that infection
p. a medication administered to activate an immune response before exposure to the disease agent
q. suppression of the body's immune system
r. the power of an organism to cause disease
s. the protection of the client against infection before, during, and after surgery using sterile technique
t. a client whose body has a limited ability to fight infection
u. infections that are the direct results of treatments such as invasive procedures
v. management of infectious and communicable diseases, including preventing the spread of infection, monitoring clients with infections, and prompt treatment of infections to prevent spreading it to others
w. a substance that kills bacteria or inhibits their growth and reproduction
x. to isolate

TRUE OR FALSE

25. _____ The incubation period of an infection extends from the time of a client's first exposure to the organism to the appearance of the first symptoms.

26. _____ Virulence is a measure of the aggressiveness of an organism in causing a disease.

27. _____ Chickenpox is an example of an infection that is carried by a vector.

28. _____ An individual's level of immunity is age-related.

29. _____ People with dementia are at increased risk of infection due to impaired protective responses.

30. _____ The presence of an increased number of immature neutrophils, which can indicate infection, is sometimes called a *right shift.*

31. _____ A Gram stain tests the nature of bacterial cell walls by determining whether they take up a stain.

32. _____ A person's state of anxiety has no effect on one's protection against infection.

33. _____ Contact precautions involve use of standard precautions plus the use of barrier items such as gloves and gowns.

34. _____ Minor cuts and bruises should be washed with mild soap and water and patted dry.

FILL IN THE BLANKS

35. The period of _____ is the time following the height of the acute symptoms to the time the person experiences a return to normal health.

36. A place where an infectious agent can survive and possibly multiply until it can invade a susceptible host is called a _____ .

37. _____ infections are those that result from organisms that do not ordinarily cause disease.

38. An _____ factor that contributes to increased risk of infection is overcrowded living conditions.

39. Redness, swelling, pain, and heat are signs that accompany a _____ infection.

40. The sink and bathroom of a hospital room are generally considered to be _____ areas.

41. Gloves should never be used as a substitute for good _____ .

42. The _____ sterilization method kills microorganisms that are sensitive to heat and moisture.

43. _____ precautions refer to precautions used for organisms that can be spread through the air but are unable to remain in the air for distances greater than 3 feet.

EXERCISING YOUR CLINICAL JUDGMENT

Colleen Brown, the 8-month-old client from the chapter's case study, is admitted with dehydration secondary to possible infection. Colleen had been living with her parents and two siblings in an evacuation center in Louisiana where they spent 2 weeks. Mr. Brown is no longer employed due to the flooding and destruction in New Orleans. Colleen and her two older siblings have been complaining of stomach cramps, fever, and diarrhea that began 2 days after the family left the shelter in Louisiana. You are assigned to care for Colleen while she is hospitalized.

44. You would expect to note which of the following signs of systemic infection while caring for Colleen?
   1. Malaise
   2. Redness
   3. Swelling
   4. Pain

45. When considering what to teach Colleen's parents about reducing the risk of further infection, you would begin with which of the following health practices?
   1. Food storage
   2. Food preparation
   3. Performing hand hygiene
   4. Bathing

46. If Colleen had been found to have a viral infection, such as influenza, as the basis for her symptoms, which of the following types of isolation would be important to implement in her care?
   1. Airborne
   2. Droplet
   3. Contact
   4. Strict

47. Colleen is started on antibiotic therapy to treat her infection. If she still had general malaise and fever after 7 days of therapy, the nurse would evaluate that which of the following would be the most likely follow-up?
   1. Increase her fluid intake.
   2. Change the antibiotic to an antiviral agent.
   3. Send her home because hospitalization didn't help.
   4. Reculture her stool.

TEST YOURSELF

48. A nurse who is reviewing the medical record of a client would expect that the client has some type of infection if the results of the white blood cell count differential showed which of the following?
    1. Increased immature neutrophils
    2. Decreased monocytes
    3. Increased eosinophils
    4. Decreased basophils

49. The nurse is performing hand hygiene as part of medical asepsis. Which of the following nursing actions for rinsing the hands represents correct practice?
    1. Hands lower than elbows, water washing down hands to fingertips
    2. Hands lower than elbows, water washing from fingertips to wrists
    3. Hands higher than elbows, water washing down hands to fingertips
    4. Hands higher than elbows, water washing from fingertips to wrists

50. A client admitted with tuberculosis should be placed in isolation in which of the following rooms on the nursing unit?
    1. A two-bed room
    2. A four-bed room
    3. A private room with windows that open
    4. A private room with negative pressure

51. A home health nurse would provide client teaching about how to prevent infection in the home after noting which of the following?
    1. Sink and bathroom are clean
    2. Leftover cooked food is stored on countertop
    3. Individuals perform hand hygiene before touching food
    4. Individuals use tissues when sneezing

52. A nurse has an order to change a dressing using sterile technique. After opening a package of sterile gloves, the nurse would do which of the following first to put them on correctly?
    1. Grasp the glove from the inside edge
    2. Grasp the glove from the outside edge
    3. Grasp the folded edge of the cuff
    4. Grasp it anywhere desired

PRIORITIZATION

53. Mr. Benson had an appendectomy 3 days ago. After being discharged home, his surgical incision became erythematous with large amounts of purulent foul smelling drainage. He has just been admitted to your division with a diagnosis of postoperative wound infection, probable MRSA. Prioritize the following nursing actions:
    1. Initiate isolation as ordered.
    2. Observe for signs and symptoms of further infection.
    3. Administer IV antibiotics.
    4. Teach the client how to prevent infections at home.

54. You have completed giving care to a client in isolation. In what order should you remove your protective equipment?
    1. Mask
    2. Goggles
    3. Gloves
    4. Gown

55. Prioritize the following things you can do to prevent the spread of infection:
    1. Teach all clients the basics of infection control.
    2. Assess all clients entering the health care facility for *Risks for infection.*
    3. Be aware of infections that are currently present in the hospital.
    4. Perform hand hygiene properly before and after contact with each client.

56. When performing hand hygiene, place the following actions in the correct order:
    1. Apply soap to the hands.
    2. Wet the hands under running water.
    3. Turn off the faucet.
    4. Dry the hands with a paper towel.

Chapter 23

HEALTH PROTECTION: RISK FOR INJURY

PURPOSE

This chapter introduces you to concepts of injury and internal and external factors that are associated with increased risk. It uses nursing process as a framework to help you identify nursing actions that can help prevent injury and those that can minimize risk of further injury.

MATCHING

1. _____ asphyxiation
2. _____ aspiration
3. _____ burns
4. _____ choking
5. _____ injury
6. _____ poisoning
7. _____ restraint
8. _____ strangulation
9. _____ trauma

a. an internal obstruction of the airway by food or a foreign body
b. an interruption in breathing that results from a severe lack of oxygen (asphyxia) where there is no source of air, an inadequate supply of oxygen in the air, or a condition in which the air cannot be inhaled
c. a physical injury or wound caused by a forceful, disruptive, or violent action
d. constriction of the airway from an external cause
e. any injury caused by excessive exposure to electricity, chemicals, gases, radioactivity, or thermal agents
f. the inspiration of foreign material into the airway
g. a device intended for medical purposes that limits movement to the extent necessary for treatment, examination, or protection of the client
h. trauma or damage to some part of the body
i. an adverse condition or physical state resulting from the administration of a toxic substance

TRUE OR FALSE

10. _____ Injury can result from physical, mechanical, biological, or chemical agents.

11. _____ The biggest concern when an older adult falls is the threat of a hip fracture.

12. _____ Faulty electrical equipment is the leading cause of fatal residential fires.

13. _____ Older adults are at increased risk of fire death because they are more vulnerable to smoke inhalation and burns and are less likely to recover.

14. _____ A single, stressful lifting event is the cause of most back injuries.

15. _____ A person's lifestyle can raise the risk of injury.

16. _____ Potential hazards in the home are inadequate lighting, missing or broken steps or handrails, or the presence of throw rugs.

17. _____ A person's cognitive and perceptual abilities are crucial to promoting safety.

18. _____ All child car seats should be bought based on the child's weight and height.

19. _____ Substance abuse can reduce a person's judgment and coordination and the ability to complete typical tasks.

FILL IN THE BLANKS

20. Accidents that most commonly result in death include motor vehicle accidents and _____.

21. Clients who are unconscious from drugs or alcohol, or who have a cerebrovascular accident or cardiac arrest are at risk for _____ and _____.

22. _____ can enter the body through ingestion, inhalation, injection, application, or absorption of the noxious material.

23. Motor vehicle accidents are the leading cause of _____ deaths in the United States.

24. Potential _____ hazards to safety may result from noise, dust, air pollution, working with dangerous machinery, or being exposed to toxic substances.

25. A frequently cited reason for ignoring safety is a lack of _____ _____.

26. Clients at the developmental levels of _____ and _____ are particularly vulnerable to accidents and injuries because of their limited awareness of potential dangers.

27. When planning care for a client with an increased risk for injury, the nurse should focus primarily on _____.

28. The nurse can help prevent electrical shock by using equipment that is electrically _____.

29. The acronym RACE used in fire safety stands for _____, _____, _____, and _____.

EXERCISING YOUR CLINICAL JUDGMENT

Juanita Soto, a 75-year-old widow with rheumatoid arthritis who lives alone, is being followed by a home health nurse due to declining mobility and partial loss of vision. She recently fell and required a brief hospitalization.

30. Which of the following factors in Mrs. Soto's physical environment places her at risk for further falls?
    1. Intact stairs with treads
    2. Throw rugs on tile floors
    3. Night light in hallway
    4. Grab bars in bathroom

31. The home health nurse would reinforce to Mrs. Soto that she should do which of the following to prevent becoming burned in the home setting?
    1. Leave electrical outlets uncovered for ease of use.
    2. Keep pot handles facing the back of the stove.
    3. Use an open-flame heater for added warmth in cold weather.
    4. Use extension cords to maximize the ability to use electric plugs.

32. The nurse assesses Mrs. Soto for physiological risk factors for falls. The nurse would conclude that she is at no further risk if which of the following were discovered?
    1. History of dizziness
    2. Need for wheelchair due to reduced mobility
    3. Weakness and fatigue noted when climbing stairs
    4. Intact recent and remote memory

33. The nurse notes that Mrs. Soto has no fire extinguisher in the home. Which of the following types of fire extinguishers should be recommended?
    1. Water pump extinguisher (type A)
    2. Foam extinguisher (type B)
    3. Multipurpose extinguisher (types A, B, C)
    4. Dry powder extinguisher (type D)

TEST YOURSELF

34. When a nurse is working with older adults in the hospital, the nurse should assess each client for risk for falls. If the nurse assesses the client as having medium risk for falling while hospitalized, which one of the following would be true about the client?
    1. Has periods of confusion; noncompliance with safety measures
    2. Ambulates with a steady gait, can perform self-care activities without assistance, cognitively intact
    3. Needs some assistance when performing certain daily activities, alert, cooperative; may have a chronic physical problem that could prevent her from calling for help
    4. Denies obvious problems of ambulation or mobility; may refuse to call for assistance

35. The nurse working with a population of clients of all ages would interpret that which of the following clients has the least risk of poisoning?
    1. Toddlers
    2. Young children
    3. Older adults with sensory impairment
    4. Young adults

36. After calling the Poison Control Center, an ambulatory care nurse prepares to induce vomiting in a client being seen with overdose. The nurse should select which of the following as the agent of choice?
    1. Activated charcoal
    2. Syrup of ipecac
    3. Hypertonic saline
    4. Any solution containing phosphate

PRIORITIZATION

37. A fire occurs at your health care institution. Place the following actions in the correct order.
    1. Call for help by activating the fire alarm or calling the switchboard operator.
    2. Remove all clients from immediate danger.
    3. Extinguish the fire using the proper type of extinguisher for the fire involved.
    4. Turn off oxygen and electrical equipment.

38. When caring for a toddler, how are the teaching needs for the parents prioritized?
    1. Teaching how to detect and prevent ingestion of lead in the home
    2. Teaching about types of fire extinguishers and indications for their use
    3. Teaching about the importance of wearing a helmet when riding a bicycle
    4. Teaching about proper storage of toxic household substances to prevent ingestion

39. Mrs. Henderson, a 65-year-old client, has just been admitted to the hospital. Prioritize the following nursing actions with a goal of preventing accidents or injury.
    1. Teach the client how to call for help using the call light at the bedside and the emergency light in the bathroom
    2. Apply a restraint to prevent the client from falling and sustaining an injury
    3. Evaluate the client's cognitive and perceptual abilities
    4. Triple-check all medications before administering them

PROMOTING HEALTHY NUTRITION

PURPOSE

This chapter discusses key concepts that relate to normal nutrition. It provides an overview of how you will use the nursing process to assist clients in maintaining and/or improving nutritional health.

MATCHING

1. ____ amino acids
2. ____ anthropometric measurements
3. ____ calorie
4. ____ carbohydrates
5. ____ disaccharides
6. ____ fiber
7. ____ glycogen
8. ____ metabolism
9. ____ minerals
10. ____ monosaccharides
11. ____ nutrient
12. ____ nutrition
13. ____ nutritional status
14. ____ polysaccharide
15. ____ proteins
16. ____ recommended dietary allowance (RDA)
17. ____ starch
18. ____ triglycerides
19. ____ vitamins

a. measurements of physical characteristics of the body (such as height and weight), as well as the amount of muscle tissue or fat tissue in the body
b. simple or complex compounds composed of carbon, oxygen, and hydrogen
c. the form in which carbohydrates are stored in humans and in meat
d. a measure of the energy content of food
e. a biochemical substance utilized by the body for growth, maintenance, and repair
f. the condition of the body resulting from the use of essential nutrients available to it
g. subunits of carbohydrates that are six-carbon sugars (glucose, fructose, and galactose are examples)
h. compounds containing polymers of amino acids, linked together in a chain to form polypeptide bonds

i. compounds composed of carbon, hydrogen, oxygen, and an amino group that are classified as essential or nonessential, depending on whether the body can manufacture them from other sources
j. the level of a nutrient that is adequate to meet the needs of almost all healthy people, as determined by the Food and Nutrition Board of the National Research Council
k. organic substances found in food that serve as coenzymes in enzymatic reactions
l. composed of three fatty acids and a glycol unit; the chief form of fat in the diet and the main form of fat transport in the blood
m. the process by which energy from nutrients can be used by the cells or stored for later use
n. inorganic elements that are present in small amounts in virtually all body fluids and tissues
o. a group of monosaccharides joined together in a chain; they can be converted back to monosaccharides through a process called acid hydrolysis
p. the form in which plants store glucose
q. the structure of which plants are composed; includes cellulose, hemicellulose, pectins, gums, and mucilages
r. the science of food and nutrients, and the processes by which an organism takes them in and uses them for energy to grow, maintain function, and renew itself
s. molecules that form when two monosaccharides condense and join together to form a double sugar

TRUE OR FALSE

20. _____ A woman who is pregnant has an increased need for iron, calcium, and other vitamins.
21. _____ Most enzymatic digestion and virtually all absorption occur in the large intestine.
22. _____ The chemical energy from food is converted by the body to electrical, thermal, or mechanical energy, depending on the needs of the body.

23. _____ A diet high in fiber contains foods such as cereals, meats, and poultry.
24. _____ When the body is storing protein, negative nitrogen balance and catabolism occur.
25. _____ When taking medications, it is important to note whether there are foods that can cause drug-nutrient reactions.
26. _____ During pregnancy, the need for both calorie and fluid intake increases.
27. _____ Taking in the RDA of a nutrient will meet the body's needs for that nutrient regardless of whether the client is well or ill.
28. _____ Body composition can be determined by measuring the triceps fat fold and midarm muscle circumference.
29. _____ Eating a diet high in calories and fat or eating late at night are likely characteristics of a client with the nursing diagnosis *Imbalanced nutrition: more than body requirements*.
30. _____ Antioxidants are found in yellow and red and green leafy vegetables.

FILL IN THE BLANKS

31. _____ is the process by which the body changes food into elemental nutrients that can be absorbed.
32. Cellulose, pectins, gums, and mucilages are examples of _____.
33. As energy sources, both protein and carbohydrates provide _____ calories per gram.
34. _____ are organic substances found in food that serve as coenzymes in enzymatic reactions.
35. Zinc, iron, copper, and selenium are examples of _____.
36. Analysis of the type and amount of food eaten by a client is done by taking a _____.
37. Teaching clients about the type and number of food servings to eat each day can be done using _____ _____.
38. Albumin and prealbumin levels are indicators of _____ intake.
39. As a health promotion measure, nurses should teach clients to read the _____ _____ _____ _____ that must appear on all manufactured food products.

40. The five food groups included in MyPyramid are _____, _____, _____, _____, and _____.
41. _____ are plant compounds found in foods such as red wine, tea, apples, and grapes, and may reduce the risk of heart disease and cancer.

EXERCISING YOUR CLINICAL JUDGEMENT

Joan, a 20-year-old client, is of "normal weight" at 115 pounds for her 60-inch frame. She is an office secretary and participates in many church activities, but engages in very little physical activity. Joan denies hospitalizations or serious illnesses, but her medical record indicates that her cholesterol was elevated at her physical exam last year. Joan tells the nurse practitioner that she skips breakfast but snacks on cookies, candy, rolls, cheese, potato chips, and other snack foods from around 11:00 AM until dinner time. Her dinner usually consists of fried foods, potatoes, bread, and dessert. She expresses a dislike for fruits and vegetables. Her clinical evaluation reveals no abnormalities or specific alterations, and her triceps skin fold is within normal limits. Joan's total cholesterol remains elevated, and she asks how she can reduce it.

42. What is the most popular and easiest method the nurse can use for obtaining immediate data about Joan's dietary intake?
   1. 24-hour recall
   2. Food diary
   3. Calorie count
   4. Body mass index
43. Based on the information provided in the case study, which food groups are missing from Joan's current diet?
   1. Grains
   2. Fruits and vegetables
   3. Meats
   4. Dairy
44. How do you think Joan's current lifestyle is contributing to her elevated cholesterol level?
   1. She snacks rather than eating three meals a day
   2. Her diet contains foods high in fat such as fried foods and potato chips
   3. She has a sedentary job
   4. She dislikes fruits and vegetables
45. In providing teaching to Joan about the elements of a healthy diet, the nurse would find which of the following to be the most helpful resource to use during the information session?
   1. Recommended Dietary Allowances chart
   2. Nutrition book
   3. Textbook on nutrition
   4. MyPyramid

TEST YOURSELF

46. A nurse who is teaching clients about lowering the risk of hypertension (high blood pressure) would emphasize limiting which of the following types of substances in the daily diet?
    1. Salt
    2. Sugar
    2. Fiber
    3. Seeds and nuts

47. Although fats should be used sparingly in the diet, the nurse would encourage the use of which of the following types of fats when fat is needed during food preparation?
    1. Monounsaturated
    2. Polyunsaturated
    3. Hydrogenated
    4. Saturated

48. A prepubescent child has an increased need for calcium in the diet. The school nurse would teach children of this age-group to increase intake of which of the following types of foods to obtain this nutrient?
    1. Meats
    3. Fish
    3. Raw fruits
    4. Dairy products

49. The nurse would encourage a client who is pregnant to take which of the following dietary supplements that may not be met sufficiently with proper daily diet?
    1. Vitamin C and the B vitamins
    2. Vitamins A and D
    3. Ferrous iron and folacin
    4. Iron and magnesium

50. The nurse teaching clients about intake of high-fiber foods to protect against colorectal cancer would encourage the use of which of the following types of foods in the meal plan?
    1. Cooked fruits
    2. Cruciferous vegetables
    3. Lean meats
    4. Products made with refined flour

51. A female client asks about foods to eat that will provide a good source of phytoestrogen. Which of the following foods would the nurse recommend?
    1. Soy products
    2. Red meat
    3. Yellow vegetables
    4. Citrus fruits

PRIORITIZATION

52. List the following steps of the digestive process in the correct order.
    1. Pepsin and hydrochloric acid break down proteins
    2. Amylase, trypsin, and lipase are secreted to break down carbohydrates, proteins, and fats
    3. Ptyalin begins the breakdown of starches into simpler sugars
    4. Water and electrolytes are absorbed

53. In which order should the following steps be taken when working with a client with a diagnosis of *Imbalanced nutrition*?
    1. Assess the client's lifestyle and dietary patterns for risk factors.
    2. Identify nutritional needs, and develop goals for maximizing the client's nutritional status.
    3. Utilize formal and informal tools to measure learning.
    4. Educate the client providing information regarding the types and amounts of foods to eat.

54. Prioritize the following areas of dietary education needed for a client who has just learned that she is 8 weeks pregnant.
    1. The infant who has doubled his birth weight can control head movements and sits up with support is ready to start solid food.
    2. At least six to eight glasses of water per day are required to provide a sufficient volume of milk during lactation.
    3. Adequate calories and appropriate weight gain are necessary throughout pregnancy.
    4. Smoking, alcohol, and caffeine are potentially harmful and should be avoided during pregnancy.

RESTORING NUTRITION

PURPOSE

This chapter introduces you to nutritional deficits such as malnutrition and starvation, and the factors that aid in their development. It guides you in the use of the nursing process to facilitate optimum nutrition for clients with a nutritional deficit.

MATCHING

1. _____ anorexia
2. _____ catabolism
3. _____ deglutition
4. _____ dysphagia
5. _____ enteral nutrition
6. _____ malnutrition
7. _____ parenteral nutrition

a. the reflex passage of food, fluids, or both from the mouth to the stomach
b. any disorder of nutrition caused by unbalanced, insufficient, or excessive diet or from impaired absorption or metabolism of nutrients
c. the provision of total nutrition through a central or peripheral intravenous catheter
d. loss of appetite
e. the breakdown of muscle and lean body mass when nutrient intake fails to meet energy expenditure
f. difficulty in swallowing
g. any form of nutrition delivered to the gastrointestinal tract, although commonly used to refer to tube feedings

TRUE OR FALSE

8. _____ Nutritional deprivation can occur with problems that raise energy needs, such as infection, trauma, stress, or surgery.
9. _____ If a client has been starving for a period of time, the urine will be negative for ketones and nitrogen balance will be positive.
10. _____ Kwashiorkor is a condition of starvation caused by decreased protein intake, and usually occurs in young children after weaning.

11. _____ Marasmus is a condition of starvation that results from deficient caloric intake over a very short period of time.
12. _____ Bleeding tendencies can be associated with a deficiency of vitamin K.
13. _____ Approximately half of clients age 65 and older wear dentures, which can affect nutritional intake.
14. _____ Changes in appetite include anorexia, early satiety, lack of interest in food, and loss of taste.
15. _____ A weight gain program is generally considered successful if the client gains at least 5 pounds per month.
16. _____ Food intake can be enhanced by serving meals in an attractive manner and making the environment as pleasant as possible.
17. _____ A client who is diabetic should be allowed small amounts of concentrated sweets.

FILL IN THE BLANKS

18. Involuntary control of swallowing is coordinated in the lower pons and the _____ of the brain.

19. Pernicious anemia results from a deficiency of vitamin _____.

20. Anemia is most commonly associated with reduced intake of _____.

21. Premature infants may require tube feedings because the suck-swallow reflex does not develop until _____ to _____ weeks of gestation.

22. Serum studies are often ordered to evaluate a client who has unintentionally lost _____% of his or her weight during the past 6 months.

23. The first phase of swallowing that is evaluated when the client has impaired swallowing is the _____ phase.

24. A 1 L bag of 5% dextrose in water IV solution contains only _____ kilocalories.

25. Ginger ale, apple juice, and plain gelatin are considered to be part of a _____ liquid diet.

26. A _____ gram sodium diet is common for clients with hypertension.

27. If a client has severe kidney disease, such as renal failure, protein is generally _____ in the diet.

EXERCISING YOUR CLINICAL JUDGMENT

Mrs. Goldman, the 54-year-old client from the chapter's case study, is receiving chemotherapy following surgery for breast cancer. Her nursing diagnosis is *Imbalanced nutrition: less than body requirements, related to adverse effects of chemotherapy*. Specifically, she has early satiety and anorexia and says that food does not have much taste. You are working with Mrs. Goldman in the clinic setting to increase her nutritional intake with a Kosher diet, especially during the 3 remaining months of chemotherapy.

28. To increase Mrs. Goldman's sense of taste, you would recommend that she take supplemental doses of which of the following minerals?
    1. Magnesium
    2. Calcium
    3. Zinc
    4. Iodine

29. You would encourage Mrs. Goldman to increase intake at which of the following times, when intake is usually best?
    1. Breakfast
    2. Lunch
    3. Dinner
    4. Bedtime

30. To reduce the discomfort of mouth sores (xerostomia) that can accompany chemotherapy, you would advise Mrs. Goldman to avoid foods that have which of the following characteristics?
    1. Low in fat
    2. Spicy or acidic
    3. High in carbohydrates
    4. High in liquid content

31. To determine whether Mrs. Goldman has effectively increased the amount of iron in her diet, you would review the results of which of the following laboratory studies drawn at the next clinic visit?
    1. Blood urea nitrogen (BUN)
    2. Total protein
    3. Albumin
    4. Hemoglobin

TEST YOURSELF

32. The nurse giving enteral nutrition and medications through a feeding tube uses which of the following methods to prevent the tube from becoming occluded?
    1. Adequate flushing with water
    2. Instillation of meat tenderizer
    3. Flushing with cola
    4. Flushing with cranberry juice

33. The nurse measures and documents gastric residual for a client receiving continuous enteral nutrition at which of the following time intervals?
    1. Hourly
    2. Every 2 hours
    3. Every 4 hours
    4. Every day

34. A client is receiving parenteral nutrition via a central venous catheter. The nurse monitors this client for fluid overload from hyperosmolar fluids most effectively by taking which of the following actions?
    1. Monitoring temperature
    2. Listening to lung sounds
    3. Checking results of serum osmolarity
    4. Watching the color of the urine

35. The nurse would interpret that a client has had a *mild* reaction to lipid emulsion infusion if the client experiences which of the following?
    1. Fever and chills
    2. Vomiting
    3. Pain in the back or chest
    4. Itchy skin rash

36. The nurse would best promote effective swallowing in a client at risk for aspiration by placing the client in which of the following positions?
    1. On the right side with the head elevated 45 degrees
    2. Upright with the neck flexed 45 degrees
    3. Supine and on the left side
    4. In a comfortable chair that promotes relaxation

PRIORITIZATION

37. List the metabolic changes seen in a client with malnutrition in the order in which they occur.
    1. The body converts glycogen stores in the liver to glucose.
    2. The body attempts to lower energy use by lowering voluntary activity and the basal metabolic rate (BMR).
    3. The body breaks down fat for energy through lipolysis.
    4. The body breaks down muscle and lean body mass in a phenomenon called catabolism.

38. What is the sequence most commonly seen when advancing the diet of client who was NPO after abdominal surgery?
    1. Clear liquids
    2. Full liquids
    3. Soft diet
    4. General/regular diet

39. Place the following steps of administering an enteral feeding in the correct order.
    1. Flush the tube with water.
    2. Make sure the enteral feeding formula is at room temperature and within its expiration date.
    3. Elevate the head of the bed 30 to 45 degrees.
    4. Confirm placement of the tube and check for residual volume.

Chapter 26

MAINTAINING FLUID AND ELECTROLYTE BALANCE

PURPOSE

The purpose of this chapter is to introduce the concepts of fluid balance and its relationship to electrolytes in the body. You will learn introductory skills in providing intravenous therapy using physician orders.

MATCHING

1. _____ active transport
2. _____ anion
3. _____ cation
4. _____ colloid
5. _____ colloid osmotic pressure
6. _____ diffusion
7. _____ electrolyte
8. _____ filtration
9. _____ hydrostatic pressure
10. _____ hypertonic
11. _____ hypotonic
12. _____ isotonic
13. _____ metabolic acidosis
14. _____ metabolic alkalosis
15. _____ milliequivalent
16. _____ milliosmole
17. _____ nonelectrolyte
18. _____ osmolality
19. _____ osmolarity
20. _____ osmosis
21 _____ respiratory acidosis
22. _____ respiratory alkalosis
23. _____ third spacing

a. a process in which molecules move from an area of lower concentration to an area of higher concentration through an expenditure of energy
b. a passive process by which molecules move through a cell membrane from an area of higher concentration to an area of lower concentration without an expenditure of energy
c. macromolecules that are too large to pass though a cell membrane and do not readily dissolve into a solution (e.g., protein)
d. the movement of water through a semipermeable membrane from an area containing a lesser concentration of particles to an area of greater concentration of particles

e. osmotic pressure exerted by large molecules such as protein
f. positively charged ion (e.g., sodium, potassium, calcium, magnesium, hydrogen)
g. the passage of water and certain smaller particles through a semipermeable membrane, assisted by hydrostatic or capillary pressure
h. substance that, when placed in a solvent such as water, breaks up into positively charged particles called ions; will conduct electricity
i. the number of milliosmoles per liter of solution
j. pressure exerted by a fluid within a compartment that results from the weight of the fluid; for practical purposes it can be thought of as the portion of the pressure exerted by the fluid itself
k. substance that does not ionize, thus does not carry an electrical charge (e.g., glucose)
l. the movement of fluid into an area in which the fluid is physiologically unavailable to the body (e.g., peritoneal space—ascites; pericardial space—pericardial effusion; pleural space— pleural effusion; vesicles—burn)
m. the number of milliosmoles per kilogram of water
n. a pathological condition caused by an increase in bicarbonate or a decrease in acid, or both, in the extracellular fluid
o. a pathological condition caused by an increase in noncarbonic acids or a decrease in bicarbonate, or both, in the extracellular fluid
p. the unit of force from the dissolved particles in a solution
q. having an osmotic pressure greater than that of the solution with which it is being compared
r. one thousandth of a chemical equivalent; the measurement used to express the chemical activity or combining power of an ion
s. having an osmotic pressure equal to that of the solution with which it is being compared
t. having an osmotic pressure less than that of the solution with which it is being compared
u. negatively charged ion (e.g., chloride, bicarbonate, phosphate, sulfate, proteinate)

v. the result of rapid or excess elimination of carbon dioxide with a resultant increase in pH

w. the result of retention of carbon dioxide with a resultant decrease in pH

TRUE OR FALSE

24. _____ Clients with hyponatremia should be observed for low urinary output.

25. _____ Clients with hypernatremia should be observed for fluid retention.

26. _____ The most characteristic manifestations of hypokalemia are muscle flaccidity and ECG changes.

27. _____ Hyperkalemia occurs in the presence of high-volume urinary output.

28. _____ A client with hypocalcemia should be observed for seizures.

29. _____ Hypercalcemia is associated with kidney stones.

30. _____ Insensible water loss should be measured as part of intake and output.

31. _____ Cardiac failure is associated with retention of potassium and water.

32. _____ Tube feedings are hypertonic, thus a client may be at risk for fluid volume deficit unless water is given as a supplement.

33. _____ 5% Dextrose in water is given primarily for its glucose content.

34. _____ 5% Dextrose in ½ normal saline (a 25% solution) given at 3000 mL/day does not add sodium to the body.

35. _____ Hyponatremia can result from administration of excess D_5W.

36. _____ Plasma is used as a volume expander when a client is bleeding and there is no time to type and cross-match blood.

37. _____ Caution should be used with IV therapy to prevent air from entering a client's veins.

FILL IN THE BLANKS

38. Glucocorticoids cause _____ (retention, excretion) of fluid.

39. To pass a nasogastric tube, you should use a _____-_____ lubricant.

40. Nasogastric suction is used for gastrointestinal _____ in the presence of a bowel _____.

41. In a burn client, fluid is lost by _____ _____.

42. To pass a nasogastric tube, a client should be in the _____ _____ position.

43. _____ _____ is the only acceptable irrigant for a nasogastric tube.

44. When selecting an IV site, you should start with the most _____ (distal, proximal) vein that would support an intravenous catheter.

45. A(n) _____ -gauge needle is used for a venipuncture if you have reason to believe the client may need blood.

46. To clean a site for venipuncture, start _____ _____ _____ and clean in a circular motion _____ _____ (toward, away from) the site.

47. When you make a venipuncture, you confirm that you are in the vein by observing _____ _____.

EXERCISING YOUR CLINICAL JUDGMENT

Mrs. Thompson, the client from the chapter's case study, has experienced two types of fluid imbalance within the past few weeks. She is currently admitted to the hospital with congestive heart failure resulting from excess fluid volume.

48. Which of the following signs of excess fluid volume would the admitting nurse expect to note in Mrs. Thompson at the time of hospital admission?
    1. A weak thready pulse
    2. Sluggish skin turgor
    3. Neck vein distention
    4. Postural hypotension

49. Which of the following electrolyte values could be expected to accompany Mrs. Thompson's fluid volume excess?
    1. Sodium 131 mEq/L
    2. Potassium 5.4 mEq/L
    3. Sodium 140 mEq/L
    4. Potassium 4.3 mEq/L

50. Which of the following basic nursing interventions focused on fluid volume excess should be included in a care plan for Mrs. Thompson?
    1. Assess breath sounds.
    2. Assess the diet for potassium content.
    3. Encourage increased fluid intake.
    4. Discourage use of salt substitutes.

51. Mrs. Thompson has an order for 500 mL 0.9% sodium chloride to run at a keep vein open rate of 20 mL/hr. An infusion pump is not available. After selecting a microdrip infusion set with a calibration of 60 drops/mL, you would adjust the IV to deliver how many drops per minute (gtt/min) of solution?
    1. 10
    2. 20
    3. 30
    4. 33

52. Which of the following assessments provides the best evaluative data that Mrs. Thompson's fluid balance is returning to normal?
    1. Heart rate is 100 beats/min
    2. Voided 500 mL the previous 8-hour shift
    3. Weight has returned to baseline
    4. Took in 360 mL with breakfast

TEST YOURSELF

53. Six hours postsurgery your client has signs of deficient fluid volume. The doctor orders a fluid challenge of 200 mL lactated Ringer's IV over 20 minutes stat. You should assess for a positive response to this treatment by observing for which of the following?
    1. Decrease in blood pressure
    2. Crackles in lower lung bases
    3. Increase in specific gravity
    4. Increase in renal output

54. Prior to administering a potassium supplement, it is most important that the nurse assess the function of which of the following body systems?
    1. Hepatic
    2. Cerebral
    3. Renal
    4. Vascular

55. You determine that your client has been taking his diuretic at home whenever he thinks he needs it. Which of the following would be a typical side effect of excess furosemide (Lasix) to monitor for during visits to the health center?
    1. Nephrosis
    2. Metabolic acidosis
    3. Hypokalemia
    4. Hypernatremia

56. The nursing care plan for hypovolemia should include which of the following?
    1. Increasing fluid intake to 2000 mL/day
    2. Placing the client in supine position
    3. Increasing protein in the client's diet
    4. Auscultating for adventitious breath sounds

57. The most accurate means of determining the amount of fluid retention in an individual is by which of the following means?
    1. Measuring edema with a millimeter tape
    2. Accurately measuring the client's intake
    3. Determining the amount of neck vein distention
    4. Classifying edema as 1+, 2+, 3+, or 4+

58. Which one of the following vitamins plays the most important role in calcium absorption in the presence of hypocalcemia?
    1. Vitamin A
    2. Vitamin D
    3. Vitamin B
    4. Vitamin E

59. A 45-year-old client has just returned to your unit after having major abdominal surgery. Based on the impact of antidiuretic hormone (ADH) released during the stress of surgery, select the most likely client response.
    1. Increased urinary output for the first 24 hours
    2. Decreased urinary output for the first 24 hours
    3. No change in output from the previous 24 hours
    4. Intake equal to output for the first 24 hours

60. Signs and symptoms of circulatory overload include which of the following?
    1. Cold, clammy skin; decreased BP; SOB; hacking cough
    2. Rales, moist cough, neck vein distention, increased BP
    3. Decreased venous pressure, cyanosis, SOB, orthopnea
    4. Decreased BP; pitting edema; cold, dry skin

61. While reviewing your patient's laboratory test, you note a seriously low serum calcium. Which of the following would be an appropriate nursing intervention to incorporate into your care?
    1. Force fluid to 12 glasses/day.
    2. Monitor intake and output.
    3. Provide a quiet nonstimulating environment.
    4. Encourage bananas and orange juice in the diet.

62. Your client is to receive an IV infusion of 1000 mL D_5W over 10 hours. Your drip chamber delivers 15 gtt/mL. How many drops per minute would you run the IV infusion?
    1. 33
    2. 25
    3. 20
    4. 16

PRIORITIZATION

63. Mrs. Felders and her three children have been admitted to the emergency department after being without water or electricity in their home for the last 3 days during extremely hot weather. None of the clients have preexisting health problems, but all are showing signs of dehydration. List the clients in the order in which they should be evaluated.
    1. Mrs. Felders, a 35-year-old female
    2. Angela Felders, a 13-year-old female
    3. Bobbie Felders, an 8-year-old male
    4. Melissa Felders, a 3-year-old female

64. You are caring for a client with a bowel obstruction. He had an NG tube placed to decompress the stomach yesterday. The NG tube has stopped draining. Prioritize the following nursing interventions.
    1. Irrigate the NG tube with 30 to 60 mL of normal saline.
    2. Assess the equipment for function errors.
    3. Check for gastric pH using a pH test strip.
    4. Verify placement of the tube by aspirating for gastric secretions.

65. List the following steps taken when preparing to initiate IV therapy in the correct order.
    1. Mark an IV strip, and place it on the IV bag.
    2. Gather all of the equipment needed to perform the procedure.
    3. Check for client allergies and incompatibility between solutions or IV medications.
    4. Prime the IV chamber and tubing.

PROMOTING WOUND HEALING

PURPOSE

This chapter discusses key concepts that relate to the nursing diagnoses *Risk for impaired skin integrity*, *Impaired skin integrity*, and *Impaired tissue integrity*. It describes the skin disruptions, wound health, and problems of wound healing.

MATCHING

1. ____ abrasion
2. ____ debridement
3. ____ dehiscence
4. ____ epithelialization
5. ____ eschar
6. ____ evisceration
7. ____ exudate
8. ____ fistula
9. ____ granulation tissue
10. ____ hematoma
11. ____ hemorrhage
12. ____ laceration
13. ____ maceration
14. ____ pressure ulcer
15. ____ primary lesion
16. ____ secondary lesion
17. ____ slough
18. ____ wound

a. a disruption of normal anatomic structure and function that results from bodily injury or a pathological process that may begin internally or externally to the involved organ or organs
b. thick, leathery, necrotic, devitalized tissue
c. refers to the fluid and cells that have escaped from blood vessels during the inflammatory response and are left in the surrounding tissues
d. an accumulation of bloody fluid beneath tissue
e. the first lesion to appear on the skin in response to a causative agent
f. a superficial injury caused by rubbing or scraping the skin against another surface
g. bleeding from the wound bed or site
h. an abnormal passage between two internal organs or between an organ and the external skin surface

i. refers to a partial or total separation of the wound edges
j. the protrusion of an internal organ (such as a bowel loop) through an incision
k. the removal of dirt, foreign matter, and dead or devitalized tissue from a wound
l. a process in which epithelial cells move to the wound bed
m. open wound with jagged edges
n. any lesion caused by unrelieved pressure that leads to damage of underlying tissues
o. a lesion that results when changes occur in a primary lesion
p. necrotic tissue that is moist, stringy, and yellow in color
q. excessive exposure to moisture causing the skin to appear white and waterlogged
r. bright red tissue formed by fibroblasts during the reconstruction phase of wound healing
s. skin damage that occurs due to pressure or rubbing against linens or medical devices such as oxygen tubing

TRUE OR FALSE

19. _____ Skin lesions are related to the client's medical condition.
20. _____ A black wound indicates that the wound is not yet ready to heal because it has fibrous slough or exudate that must be cleansed and removed.
21. _____ Most acute wounds and surgical wounds close by primary intention.
22. _____ Internal hemorrhage can occur with no external evidence of bleeding.
23. _____ Wounds can heal when infection is present.
24. _____ Yellow drainage from a wound means the wound is infected.
25. _____ Radiation is the least common mechanism of skin injury.

FILL IN THE BLANKS

26. _____ is the primary function of the skin.

27. The _____-_____-_____ (RYB) classification system is based on wound bed color.

28. Typically, a _____ _____ is located over a bony prominence or an area that sustains prolonged pressure.

29. Adequate _____ is essential for the client with *Impaired skin integrity*.

30. Use the concept of the face of a _____ to help define landmarks and areas of the wound or impaired skin area.

31. Surgical wounds and incisions are usually closed with _____ or stainless steel _____.

32. Interventions for a client with *Impaired skin integrity* are developed by the multidisciplinary team. A valuable resource to medical and nursing staff is the certified _____ therapist nurse.

EXERCISING YOUR CLINICAL JUDGMENT

33. Mrs. Jacan, the client from the chapter's case study, is bedridden after her hip surgery. She has developed a pressure ulcer that looks like a blister or shallow crater. Her pressure ulcer is most likely in which stage?
    1. Stage I
    2. Stage II
    3. Stage III
    4. Stage IV

34. Which one of the following diagnostic tests will help determine if Mrs. Jacan has inflammation, or infectious or necrotic processes?
    1. Complete blood count
    2. Erythrocyte sedimentation rate
    3. Prealbumin and albumin levels
    4. Blood panel

35. Mrs. Jacan had a reddened area on her sacrum and bilateral heels. Twenty-four hours after admission, you chart the following: Hydrocolloid dressing intact, no drainage (you had applied dressings to her sacrum and to her heels). Which of the following nursing diagnoses would be most appropriate for an evaluation of your client's care?
    1. *Impaired tissue integrity*
    2. *Disturbed body image*
    3. *Hopelessness*
    4. *Impaired skin integrity*

TEST YOURSELF

36. Your client was wounded by a knife. What type of wound is your client most likely suffering from?
    1. Closed and clean wound
    2. Abrasion and contusion
    3. Open, contaminated, penetrating
    4. Open, contaminated, abrasion

37. The area around your client's wound has edema, erythema, heat, and pain. His wound is 1 day old. This is an example of which phase of wound healing?
    1. Inflammatory
    2. Proliferative
    3. Reconstruction
    4. Maturation

38. If your client has an incision and dressing on the anterior part of the neck, you would check which of the following to determine if she was hemorrhaging externally?
    1. Bloody drainage on dressing, distention of the affected area, a change in the amount or type of drainage from a drain
    2. Distention of the affected area, a change in the amount or type of drainage from a drain, signs and symptoms of hypovolemic shock
    3. Bloody drainage on dressing, signs and symptoms of hypovolemic shock
    4. Bloody drainage on dressing and areas around the dressing, and posterior to the wound site

39. Your client is a single 38-year-old female on her third postoperative day. She is very concerned about the large abdominal incision created during her hysterectomy and worries how this will affect her relationship with men she dates. Which of the following nursing diagnoses would be most appropriate?
    1. *Impaired tissue integrity*
    2. *Disturbed body image*
    3. *Hopelessness*
    4. *Impaired skin integrity*

40. For a wound to heal, the wound must be clean and free of bacteria. To cleanse a wound, you will need a wound cleaning solution. Which of the following is the preferred cleansing agent for most wounds?
    1. Normal saline solution
    2. Dakin's solution
    3. Povidone-iodine
    4. Hydrogen peroxide

PRIORITIZATION

41. You are caring for a client with a wound that requires irrigation and dressing change every shift. List the following actions to be taken in the correct order:
    1. Remove the old dressing
    2. Irrigate the wound using the irrigant ordered by the physician
    3. Medicate the client for pain if discomfort is anticipated
    4. Perform hand hygiene, and put on clean gloves

42. Prioritize the following nursing actions that should be taken when caring for a client with a wound evisceration.
    1. Cover the protruding intestine with a sterile dressing moistened with sterile normal saline.
    2. Assist the client into a semi-Fowler's position with the knees slightly flexed.
    3. Establish intravenous access to provide fluids and prepare for surgery as ordered.
    4. Assess vital signs and pulse oximetry readings.

43. The following clients have a nursing diagnosis of impaired skin integrity. In what order would you assess them based on the severity of the wound?
    1. A geriatric client with a stage I pressure ulcer on her sacrum
    2. An adult surgical client with a wound dehiscence
    3. A teenage client with a deep puncture wound on his hand
    4. A young adult client who is 24 hours post appendectomy

PURPOSE

The purpose of this chapter is to introduce you to the concepts of thermoregulation and associated clinical problems.

MATCHING

1. _____ fever
2. _____ heat exhaustion
3. _____ heatstroke
4. _____ hyperthermia
5. _____ hypothermia
6. _____ malaise
7. _____ pyrogen
8. _____ set-point

a. a nonregulated elevation in body temperature related to an imbalance between heat gain and heat loss
b. the temperature that thermoregulatory mechanisms attempt to maintain
c. a body temperature that exceeds 40.6° C (105° F), resulting in altered central nervous system function and shock
d. a feeling of indisposition; thought to be an adaptive response that decreases most daily activities, thereby maintaining energy stores for fever generation
e. any agent that causes or stimulates a fever; the initial stimulus for fever is often exogenous pyrogen
f. a regulated rise in body temperature that is mediated by a rise in temperature set-point
g. the state in which body temperature is reduced below normal
h. a rise in body temperature that is usually related to inadequate fluid and electrolyte replacement during physical activity in intense heat or the inability to acclimatize to intense heat

TRUE OR FALSE

9. _____ Fever is caused only by infection.
10. _____ During the initiation phase of a fever, pyrogens act on the hypothalamus to reset the temperature set-point higher than body temperature.
11. _____ Resolution of a fever by lysis is a gradual return to normal over several hours.
12. _____ Determination of the cause of fever can be difficult because of the many possible etiologies.
13. _____ A common finding in hypothermic clients is the incidence of low alcohol or other drug intake.
14. _____ An immunosuppressed client is able to generate a fever.
15. _____ Fever may not develop as readily in the elderly as in the younger population.
16. _____ Treatment for arthritis may mask a fever.
17. _____ Blood cultures are only used to identify bacteria in the blood.
18. _____ Blood cultures are best drawn through a central line IV site.
19. _____ An elderly client is more prone to heatstroke than a young adult.
20. _____ Febrile convulsions in infants are associated with temperatures greater than 105° F.
21. _____ Vasoconstriction decreases heat loss by radiation, convection, and conduction.
22. _____ In some clients, fever may not be present during infection.
23. _____ Hyperthermia occurs when a person falls through the ice of a lake and loses heat rapidly in the cold water.
24. _____ The change in heart rate with hypothermia will depend on the degree of hypothermia.
25. _____ The height of a child's fever does not seem to trigger febrile convulsions as much as a sudden spike in body temperature.

FILL IN THE BLANKS

26. The three phases of a fever are _____, _____, and _____.

27. During fever, the metabolic rate increases by _____ for every degree of increase in temperature.

28. A client with a fever has a(n) _____ (increased, decreased) need for fluids.

29. The symptoms of heatstroke include _____ _____, _____, _____, _____, and _____.

30. Alcohol use contributes to hypothermia by providing a false sense of _____, inhibiting _____ and _____ of the skin.

31. _____ _____ or fever of unknown origin is defined as fever of 3 weeks' duration with evaluation by a medical team for 1 week.

32. Side effects of aspirin include _____ and _____.

33. Acetaminophen should not be used in the presence of _____ disease.

34. Cooling blankets promote _____ heat loss.

35. Fans promote _____ heat loss.

36. Physical cooling is the standard for _____ (hyperthermia, fever).

37. _____ is the resolution of a fever.

38. The temperature control center is in the _____.

39. The two classes of interventions used for treating fever include _____ and _____ _____.

40. To assess for tolerance before feeding a febrile client, you would assess for _____ _____, _____ _____, and _____.

EXERCISING YOUR CLINICAL JUDGMENT

41. Mr. Stephen is 24 hours post cardiac bypass surgical procedure. His temperature is 102° F. You find signs of postoperative atelectasis and encourage him to cough and deep breathe. How often should you recheck his temperature?
    1. q4h
    2. qid
    3. bid
    4. q8h

42. A physician has written an order for Mr. Stephen for acetaminophen for a temperature greater than 102° F. A rationale for not giving the antipyretic for a lower temperature is that:
    1. fever is a host defense response.
    2. normal temperature is variable.
    3. antipyretics only work on high temperatures.
    4. only a high fever produces a headache.

TEST YOURSELF

43. A mother of a 3-year-old client asks for your advice about which antipyretic to use for her child's fever. Your best response would be:
    1. "Use acetaminophen. It is the best antipyretic."
    2. "Pediatricians often recommend avoiding aspirin in young children."
    3. "Never give your child antipyretics without the advice of a physician."
    4. "Acetaminophen can cause Reye's syndrome in young children."

44. A mother calls the emergency room. Her 6-year-old child has a fever of 101° F. Which information that she provides would prompt you to refer her to a physician?
    1. The child has not been exposed to a contagious disease.
    2. The child is having difficulty breathing.
    3. The child has clear drainage from the nose.
    4. The child is constipated.

45. A client with osteoarthritis has a painful swollen knee joint. Her temperature is 99.6° F. Select the best interpretation of her fever.
    1. Her knee has become infected.
    2. Her temperature is normally high.
    3. Her temperature is caused by inflammation.
    4. She is having a reaction to her medication.

46. Heatstroke results from:
    1. failure of the temperature-regulating capacity of the body, caused by prolonged exposure to the sun.
    2. a rupture of a blood vessel in the brain from getting overheated.
    3. pyrogens building up in the bloodstream because of kidney failure.
    4. a bacterial infection that attacks the temperature control center of the brain.

PRIORITIZATION

47. Prioritize the following instructions regarding febrile seizures to be given to parents of pediatric clients.
    1. Febrile convulsions are associated with a fever of 38.9° C to 40° C (102° F to 104° F).
    2. Make sure to take a child with a high fever to the doctor.
    3. Febrile convulsions do not cause brain damage.
    4. If a febrile seizure occurs, remain calm and protect the child from injury.

48. Mr. Parker has presented to the clinic on a hot summer day with mild signs of hyperthermia. He is dressed in several layers of heavy clothing and complains of fatigue and a headache. He tells the staff that he does not have air conditioning in his home and is afraid to leave the windows open. List the following nursing actions in order of importance.
    1. Assist Mr. Parker to remove extra layers of clothing so that he is dressed lightly.
    2. Encourage Mr. Parker to drink cool fluids.
    3. Refer Mr. Parker to the social worker for assistance with obtaining an air conditioner or fan for his home.
    4. Instruct Mr. Parker on strategies to avoid hyperthermia.

49. Based on the factors that affect thermoregulation, rate the clients listed below from highest to lowest risk for developing hypothermia in the absence of chronic or acute disease.
    1. Roger, a frail 84-year-old male
    2. Betty, a 42-year-old thin female
    3. Bob, a 27-year-old slightly overweight male
    4. Jamie, a 2-day-old infant

MANAGING BOWEL ELIMINATION

PURPOSE

This chapter introduces you to alterations in bowel elimination such as constipation, diarrhea, and bowel incontinence. It describes a variety of factors that affect bowel function and discusses the nursing process as a framework to use when caring for a client with an alteration in bowel elimination.

MATCHING

1. _____ bowel incontinence
2. _____ cathartic
3. _____ colostomy
4. _____ constipation
5. _____ diarrhea
6. _____ fecal impaction
7. _____ feces
8. _____ flatulence
9. _____ flatus
10. _____ guaiac
11. _____ ileostomy
12. _____ laxative
13. _____ occult blood
14. _____ ostomy
15. _____ paralytic ileus
16. _____ peristalsis
17. _____ steatorrhea
18. _____ stoma

a. the rhythmic smooth muscle contractions of the intestinal wall that propel the intestinal contents forward

b. body waste discharged from the intestine

c. the presence of abnormal amounts of gas in the GI tract, causing abdominal distention and discomfort

d. an amount of blood that is too small to be seen without a microscope

e. an amount of gas that occurs normally in the GI tract

f. the inability to voluntarily control the passage of feces and gas

g. a surgical procedure involving the creation of an opening between the colon and the abdominal wall

h. medication used to induce emptying of the bowel; often used interchangeably with a laxative, although it has a stronger action

i. a condition in which feces are abnormally hard and dry and evacuation is abnormally infrequent

j. a gray stool mixed with observable fat and mucus, resulting from the malabsorption of fat

k. the opening between the abdominal wall and intestine through which fecal material passes

l. the surgical procedure used to create an opening through the abdominal wall and into the intestine

m. the absence of peristalsis for more than 3 days

n. a test to measure occult blood

o. a collection of puttylike or hardened feces in the rectum or sigmoid colon that prevents the passage of a normal stool and becomes more hardened as the colon continues to absorb water from it

p. medication used to induce emptying of the bowel; often used interchangeably with a cathartic

q. a surgical procedure involving the creation of an opening between the ileum and the abdominal wall

r. the rapid movement of fecal matter through the intestine, resulting in poor absorption of water, nutrients, and electrolytes, and producing abnormally frequent evacuation of watery stools

TRUE OR FALSE

19. _____ Constipation is a major complaint among the elderly.

20. _____ Some risks of straining at stool include angina attacks, hemorrhoid development, and rupture of abdominal suture lines.

21. _____ It is exceptionally difficult to train the bowel to evacuate at a certain time.

22. _____ Spicy foods stimulate peristalsis by local reflex stimulation.

23. _____ Exercise has no effect on bowel elimination.

24. _____ Bowel elimination is usually not a problem for the adolescent unless there is a health problem.

25. _____ Motor or sensory disturbances, such as with spinal cord injury or neurological disease, can lead to diarrhea.

26. _____ A medication that is given to prevent constipation can cause diarrhea in some clients.
27. _____ The further down the bowel a colostomy is created, the greater the chance for being able to regulate the bowel.
28. _____ Mental depression plays no role in the development of constipation.

FILL IN THE BLANKS

29. A diet that is high in _____ tends to prevent the occurrence of constipation.

30. Chocolate, coffee, and prune juice are foods that can _____ the stool.

31. _____ is an out-pouching of the intestinal wall that can occur after age 40.

32. Impaired dentition in the older adult impairs _____, allowing food to enter the GI tract inadequately chewed.

33. A client is more at risk for cancer of the colon if the diet is high in _____ and low in _____.

34. The consistency of ileostomy drainage is _____.

35. As part of colon cancer screening, an annual digital rectal examination should be done every year after age _____.

36. Beans, beer, and cucumbers are examples of foods that can cause _____.

37. How the GI tract reacts to a particular food depends on the individual _____.

38. The overuse of laxatives can lead to physical and psychological _____.

EXERCISING YOUR CLINICAL JUDGMENT

Dr. Daley, the 92-year-old retired neurosurgeon from the chapter's case study, has a nursing diagnosis of *Constipation*. He is living in a long-term care facility because he can no longer manage on his own with a diagnosis of bone cancer. He has begun limiting the use of his opioid analgesic, morphine, because it could worsen the constipation. The nurse from the previous shift reports having just assessed Dr. Daley's abdomen and suspects impaction. You are now taking over the care of the clients on this unit.

39. Dr. Daley has chosen to use Milk of Magnesia as his laxative. You recall that this medication belongs to which of the following categories of laxatives?
   1. Bulk-forming
   2. Lubricant
   3. Saline
   4. Stimulant

40. The medication given to Dr. Daley has not worked, so you obtain an order for an oil retention enema. When administering it to Dr. Daley, you ask him to try to retain it in the bowel for at least how long?
   1. 5 minutes
   2. 15 minutes
   3. 30 minutes
   4. 1 hour

41. The enema is successful and you are exploring with Dr. Daley strategies that can be used to prevent a recurrence. You both agree that he should try to walk to the toilet at which of the following times, when stimulation of the gastrocolic reflex is strongest?
   1. Upon awakening
   2. After breakfast
   3. After lunch
   4. Before bedtime

42. You begin an intake and output record to keep track of Dr. Daley's fluid intake. You encourage him to drink at least how much fluid per day to minimize the risk of constipation recurrence?
   1. 1.5 liters
   2. 3 liters
   3. 4 liters
   4. 5 liters

TEST YOURSELF

43. The nurse caring for a client with an ostomy would do which of the following to maintain the skin integrity around the stoma?
   1. Use a skin barrier.
   2. Limit the use of skin paste.
   3. Wash peristomal skin but do not dry it.
   4. Try to have the pouch last about 2 weeks.

44. A client has abdominal pain related to flatulence. Which of the following items would the nurse suspect is contributing to the problem?
   1. Walking
   2. Eating slowly
   3. Eating cauliflower
   4. Drinking water

45. The BRATY diet is recommended for children and adults with nausea and vomiting associated with gastroenteritis for up to 24 hours. The nurse should offer this client which of the following products?
    1. Cheese
    2. Yogurt
    3. Skim milk
    4. Orange juice

46. An older adult with multiple health problems has a severe case of diarrhea. The nurse would assess this client for which of the following common complications of diarrhea in this client population?
    1. Thirst and ruddy skin color
    2. Diverticulitis
    3. Nausea and vomiting
    4. Fluid and electrolyte imbalances

PRIORITIZATION

47. The physician has ordered a large-volume enema the night prior to your client's abdominal surgery. List the following nursing actions in the correct order.
    1. Position the client on his left side and administer the solution as ordered.
    2. Prepare the enema solution ordered by the physician, and set up the equipment.
    3. Help the client to the toilet, or assist him with the bedpan or commode.
    4. Assess the client for risk factors associated with the receipt of an enema.

48. Prioritize the following actions necessary when initiating a bowel training program for a client with bowel incontinence.
    1. With the client, decide on a routine for bowel elimination.
    2. Assess and diagnose the factors causing the incontinence.
    3. Discuss with the client his previous bowel habits.
    4. Discuss bowel training with the client and significant others if the client desires.

49. Place the following steps for changing an ostomy bag or pouch in the correct order.
    1. Remove the old bag or pouch and stoma wafer and discard.
    2. Clean the stoma and skin with warm water and soap, rinse, and pat dry.
    3. Place an appropriately sized stoma wafer over adhesive around the stoma and press lightly.
    4. Snap the new ostomy bag or pouch onto the ring of the stoma wafer.

Chapter 30

Managing Urinary Elimination

PURPOSE

This chapter introduces you to basic nursing measures for clients with urinary problems. You will learn to recognize signs and symptoms of urinary problems and intervene to improve urinary function. Additionally, the chapter introduces procedures for collecting a urine specimen from a Foley catheter, using a condom catheter, and inserting a Foley catheter.

MATCHING

1. _____ anuria
2. _____ bacteriuria
3. _____ diuresis
4. _____ dysuria
5. _____ enuresis
6. _____ functional urinary incontinence
7. _____ hematuria
8. _____ Kegel exercises
9. _____ micturition
10. _____ nocturia
11. _____ oliguria
12. _____ polyuria
13. _____ reflex urinary incontinence
14. _____ residual urine
15. _____ stress urinary incontinence
16. _____ total urinary incontinence
17. _____ urge urinary incontinence
18. _____ urinalysis
19. _____ urinary frequency
20. _____ urinary hesitancy
21. _____ urinary incontinence
22. _____ urinary retention
23. _____ urinary urgency
24. _____ urination
25. _____ void

a. recurrent involuntary urination that occurs during sleep
b. the term used for nighttime urination
c. involuntary passage of urine
d. the person is unaware of cues to a full bladder and may be unaware of the incontinence; the incontinence is either continual or unpredictable
e. incontinence associated with neurological damage to the spinal cord above the level of the third sacral vertebrae
f. the inability to pass all or part of the urine that has accumulated in the bladder
g. incontinence reported or observed as dribbling with increased intra-abdominal pressure
h. the discharge of blood in the urine
i. incontinence reported or observed as a sudden desire to urinate and immediately seeking toileting facilities
j. the more commonly used term for the act of micturition; the term *void* is more common in clinical use
k. the increased secretion of urine
l. the symptom of difficulty with, or painful, urination; it may be accompanied by frequency, hesitancy, or urgency of urination
m. the absence of urine production
n. the amount of urine remaining in the bladder after voiding
o. sudden, forceful urge to urinate; further assessment is needed to determine the cause
p. a physical, chemical, and microscopic examination of the urine
q. urination that occurs at shorter-than-usual intervals without an increase in daily urine output
r. a diminished, scanty amount of urine
s. a large amount of urine usually associated with diabetes mellitus or diabetes insipidus
t. exercises to strengthen the floor of the pelvis
u. bacteria in the urine
v. the process of emptying the bladder
w. a delay in starting the urine stream, commonly with a decreased force of stream
x. synonymous with urination or micturition, emptying of the bladder
y. the inability of a usually continent person to reach the toilet in time to avoid unintentional loss of urine

TRUE OR FALSE

26. _____ The bladder is under the involuntary control of the sympathetic nervous system.

27. _____ Enuresis occurs in only about 7% of children by the age of 8.

28. _____ Urinary retention can be caused by obstruction or inability of the detrusor to contract.

29. _____ Urinary incontinence is an expected or normal part of aging.

30. _____ Six to eight glasses of water is equivalent to 1500 to 2000 mL.

31. _____ The external urinary sphincter is smooth muscle under control of the parasympathetic nervous system.

32. _____ A primary factor in incontinence for some elderly persons is urge incontinence in the presence of impaired mobility.

33. _____ Constipation can be a factor in incontinence of urine.

34. _____ Bilirubin is excreted in the urine when the biliary tract is obstructed.

35. _____ There is no reason to test the urine for blood unless the urine is red or cloudy.

36. _____ You need a minimum of 30 mL of urine to send for urinalysis.

37. _____ All clients need an antibiotic after a cystoscopy.

FILL IN THE BLANKS

38. The _____ valve is the connection between the ureters and the bladder.

39. The _____ is the primary muscle of the bladder.

40. The kidneys control the excretion of these waste products: _____, _____, _____ _____, _____, and _____ _____ _____.

41. Among other electrolytes, the kidneys control the excretion of the two primary electrolytes, _____ and _____.

42. Urine moves through the ureters by gravity and _____.

43. Dysuria is often related to _____, _____, or _____ of the lower urinary tract.

44. Voiding every hour would be described as _____.

45. The normal range for feeling the urge to urinate is _____ to _____ mL.

46. _____ _____ measures the function of the bladder and urethra by measuring the flow rate of urine passing through the urethra.

47. _____ (creatinine, BUN) is the more specific test for renal function.

48. _____ incontinence is associated with postmenopausal atrophy or the presence of a cystocele.

49. The Alzheimer's client who has progressed to the point of no neurological control over the bladder has _____ incontinence.

50. As a means to control incontinence, _____ _____ is recommended for clients who can learn to recognize some degree of bladder fullness or the need to void.

51. As a means to control incontinence, _____ _____ is recommended for clients for whom a natural pattern of voiding can be determined.

52. _____ _____ can help the client who has stress incontinence.

EXERCISING YOUR CLINICAL JUDGMENT

Mrs. Al-Kandari the client from this chapter's case study, is scheduled to have an indwelling urinary catheter removed this morning. It is now her second postoperative day following vaginal hysterectomy surgery. You have been assigned to Mrs. Al-Kandari's care for the day shift.

53. For what reason is it most important that Mrs. Al-Kandari's catheter be removed as early as possible in the course of recovery from surgery?
    1. Because of the high risk of infection
    2. Because she has a higher risk of retention with each passing day
    3. Because an indwelling catheter often provokes bladder spasms
    4. Because she will ambulate more easily without the catheter and drainage bag

54. To minimize discomfort during removal of the catheter, you should ask Mrs. Al-Kandari to do which of the following during catheter removal?
    1. Cough
    2. Take a deep breath
    3. Bear down as if to void
    4. Encourage her to squeeze your hand

55. The catheter was removed at 8:30 AM. On the report sheet to be used later in the day for intershift report, you note that Mrs. Al-Kandari is due to void *no later than* which of the following times?
    1. 10:30 AM
    2. 2:30 PM
    3. 4:30 PM
    4. 8:30 PM

56. Which of the following instructions would be best to give to Mrs. Al-Kandari to increase the likelihood that she will void successfully after catheter removal?
    1. Ambulate at least hourly.
    2. Take a diet of clear liquids only.
    3. Encourage her to keep a bedpan nearby.
    4. Encourage her to increase her fluid intake.

TEST YOURSELF

57. You are assessing a 57-year-old female client. She says she continues to have stress incontinence despite using Kegel exercises regularly for 6 months. Her doctor has talked about surgery, but she is reluctant. She asks you if she should keep trying the exercises. Which of the following is the best response?
    1. "If you haven't had success in 6 months, you should see your doctor about surgery."
    2. "I can review the technique with you if you like; sometimes it is difficult to contract the right muscle."
    3. "Kegel exercises only work for a small number of women."
    4. "It is always best to follow your doctor's advice."

58. Which of the following techniques is best to prevent the most serious complication of a condom catheter?
    1. To hold the catheter in place, use a soft flexible band that is snug but not tight.
    2. Inspect and clean the skin at least daily.
    3. Arrange the drainage tubing to ensure that urine drains from the condom.
    4. Tape the catheter collecting tubing to the leg, allowing slack in the catheter.

59. You are assigned a client who has urinary incontinence. You see a nursing order on the care plan for prompted voiding. To correctly assist with this intervention, you would take which of the following actions?
    1. Take the client to the bathroom every 4 hours, or offer the bedpan.
    2. Insist that the client go to the bathroom or use the bedpan every 2 hours.
    3. Admonish the client for wetness and insist that the client use the call light.
    4. Check the client for wetness every 2 hours, and offer assistance to the bathroom or bedside commode.

60. Which of the following clients is the best candidate for whom a Foley catheter may be used to prevent urinary retention?
    1. A client who has had bladder surgery where some bleeding is expected
    2. A client who has had surgery for a fractured hip
    3. A client who is in shock (blood pressure 88/50)
    4. A client with terminal cancer, who is expected to die within 24 hours

61. Your client is a 60-year-old male. He is 6 feet 4 inches tall and weighs 225 pounds. Select the catheter size that is most appropriate.
    1. 6 Fr
    2. 10 Fr
    3. 14 Fr
    4. 18 Fr

62. You are performing a Foley catheterization. You accidentally contaminate the connection tubing, but know the catheter is sterile. Which of the following actions would be most cost-effective and still be correct?
    1. Ask someone to bring you a new sterile catheter.
    2. Obtain a new tray and start over.
    3. Ask someone to bring you a new sterile bag and tubing.
    4. Continue with the catheterization, avoiding the connection tubing until you have inserted the catheter.

63. Which of the following is the best rationale for maintaining straight continuous gravity drainage from a Foley catheter?
    1. To be more aesthetically pleasing to the client
    2. To prevent the backflow of urine into the bladder
    3. To keep the bladder empty of urine
    4. To keep the catheter patent

64. Your client has had bladder surgery. The surgeon has ordered a three-way Foley catheter with continuous irrigation with normal saline. You enter the room and notice that the urine is dark red with only a small amount flowing through the drainage tubing. Which of the following is the best action to take?
    1. Call the surgeon immediately.
    2. Force fluids by mouth.
    3. Increase the flow of the irrigant until the urine clears.
    4. Turn the client in bed.

65. Your client has a urinary diversion that is well healed and has been functioning normally. She is currently admitted for pneumonia, is very weak, and needs assistance with caring for her elimination needs. You notice that urine is leaking under the stoma wafer applied to her skin. Which of the following is the best action to take?
    1. Use nonporous tape to secure the wafer.
    2. Remove the wafer, and apply a new one.
    3. Pad the site to collect the leakage.
    4. Remove the wafer, and insert a catheter to collect the urine.

66. Which of the following suggestions to acidify the urine would be best to make to a client?
    1. Take ascorbic acid bid.
    2. Drink four glasses of nonfat milk daily.
    3. Use 1 teaspoon sodium bicarbonate bid.
    4. Drink four glasses of orange juice daily.

PRIORITIZATION

67. List the steps of collecting urine from an indwelling (Foley) catheter in the correct order.
    1. Label the container with the client's name, date, and time of collection.
    2. Withdraw 10 mL of urine using a needle and a 10 mL syringe.
    3. Clean the collections port with an alcohol wipe.
    4. Inject the urine into a sterile specimen container.

68. Prioritize the following interventions used to manage urinary tract infections.
    1. Encourage clients to void when they feel the urge.
    2. Modify the diet by encourging cranberry juice to acidify the urine.
    3. Teach preventive measures to prevent future infections.
    4. Encourage clients to drink 6 to 8 glasses of fluid per day.

69. What is the correct sequence of steps for performing prompted voiding?
    1. Ask the client if he or she feels the need to use the toilet, and assist as needed.
    2. Give positive feedback if the client can correctly identify that he or she is dry.
    3. Elicit subjective data, and observe for evidence of wetness at scheduled times.
    4. Give positive feedback for appropriate toileting.

MANAGING SELF-CARE DEFICIT

PURPOSE

This chapter introduces you to key concepts that relate to the nursing diagnoses *Bathing/hygiene self-care deficit, Impaired skin integrity, Altered oral mucous membrane, Ineffective individual coping*, and *Powerlessness*. The chapter also outlines procedures related to assisting the client with self-care needs.

MATCHING

1. _____ alopecia
2. _____ caries
3. _____ cerumen
4. _____ dentures
5. _____ gingivitis
6. _____ perineum
7. _____ plaque
8. _____ tartar

a. a waxy secretion of the glands of the external acoustic meatus; commonly called *earwax*

b. a destructive process causing decalcification of the tooth enamel and leading to continued destruction of the enamel and dentin with resulting cavitation of the tooth

c. an inflammation of the gums usually manifested by the primary symptom of bleeding of the gums

d. a yellowish film of calcium phosphate, carbonate, food particles, and other organic matter deposited on the teeth by saliva

e. a complement of teeth, either natural or artificial, ordinarily used to designate an artificial replacement for the natural teeth

f. loss of hair and baldness

g. the pelvic floor and associated structures occupying pelvic outlet, bounded anteriorly by the symphysis pubis, laterally by the ischial tuberosities, and posteriorly by the coccyx

h. a soft, thin film of food debris, mucin, and dead epithelial cells that is deposited on the teeth and provides a medium for the growth of bacteria

TRUE OR FALSE

9. _____ The outer portion of the skin, the epidermis, is composed of stratified squamous epithelium that contains keratinocytes, which produce keratin, the substance that is responsible for the color of the skin.

10. _____ Hair grows faster at night than during the day and faster in warm weather than in cold.

11. _____ If your nails are thick and yellow, this may be indicative of bacterial infection.

12. _____ If you presuppose lack of ability when some ability may be present, it can further reinforce a client's sense of independence and helplessness.

13. _____ Total hygiene care consists of bathing, skin care, oral care, hair care, perineal care, back massage, shaving, changing the bed linens, and changing a client's gown or pajamas.

14. _____ Problems with nail and foot care may occur because of neglect or abuse.

15. _____ The benefits of bathing in a tub or shower (instead of a sponge bath) for the client are so significant that if the option is available, you should use it even if it may be difficult and time-consuming.

16. _____ Studies show that a client who needs to be fed will eat more food if the person doing the feeding switches from one food to another during the meal.

FILL IN THE BLANKS

17. _____-_____ is the ability to meet hygiene needs without the assistance of another person.

18. The skin helps screen out ultraviolet (UV) rays from the sun, but it also lets in some necessary UV rays that convert a chemical in the skin called 7-dehydrocholesterol into _____.

19. If the origin of a client's halitosis is _____, oral hygiene will not remove the odor.

20. Dental _____ is a disease of the calcified structure of the tooth.

21. Body lice suck _____ from the skin and live in clothing, making them hard to detect.

22. Skin _____ are prominent in aging skin.

23. Complete _____ _____ is giving a complete bath without any assistance from the client.

24. For clients with very curly hair, it is often useful to use a _____-_____ comb or a hair _____.

EXERCISING YOUR CLINICAL JUDGMENT

25. Joy Wilson, the 78-year-old African-American client from the chapter's case study, suffers from a stroke (cerebrovascular accident). She is unable to bathe herself. Which nursing diagnosis would be most appropriate?
    1. *Ineffective individual coping*
    2. *Bathing/hygiene self-care deficit*
    3. *Activity intolerance*
    4. *Impaired physical mobility*

26. Ms. Wilson's daughter gives her a hot-water bath. Which of the following best describes the purpose of this type of bath?
    1. Decrease pain and inflammation
    2. Relieve muscle spasm and muscle tension
    3. Relax and soothe
    4. Soothe skin irritation

27. Ms. Wilson's cognitive status is impaired because of her short-term memory loss. She has difficulty caring for her basic needs. Which nursing diagnosis would be most appropriate?
    1. *Ineffective individual coping*
    2. *Bathing/hygiene self-care deficit*
    3. *Activity intolerance*
    4. *Disturbed thought processes*

TEST YOURSELF

28. You advise the client to do regular oral care and that dental intervention may be necessary. Which problem of the oral cavity is your client most likely suffering from?
    1. Halitosis
    2. Gingivitis
    3. Periodontal disease
    4. Stomatitis

29. Your client is having difficulty following through on doing self-care. A careful assessment of the client's cognitive status is essential because although she appears to be well oriented and capable of self-care, a more careful assessment may reveal that she has which of the following?
    1. Short-term memory loss
    2. Long-term memory loss
    3. Difficulty coping with stressors
    4. Lack of full range of motion

30. Which of the following best describes the term *smegma*?
    1. Loss of hair and baldness
    2. Cheesy-like substance secreted by the sebaceous glands
    3. Oily substance secreted by the sebaceous glands
    4. The reaction of bacteria with perspiration

31. Your client is a 58-year-old poorly nourished woman who was diagnosed with Alzheimer's disease 3 years ago. She has shown rapid deterioration and now is unable to care for any of her basic hygiene. Which nursing diagnosis is most appropriate?
    1. *Disturbed thought processes*
    2. *Disturbed sensory perception*
    3. *Activity intolerance*
    4. *Impaired physical mobility*

32. Your client is a 43-year-old female who has had severe rheumatoid arthritis for 15 years. She has severe limitations of both her lower and upper extremities. She has difficulty grasping objects because of malformation of her hand and fingers. Which nursing diagnosis is most appropriate?
    1. *Disturbed thought processes*
    2. *Disturbed sensory perception*
    3. *Activity intolerance*
    4. *Impaired physical mobility*

PRIORITIZATION

33. List the correct order for bathing the following areas for a client who cannot assist with the procedure.
    1. Wash the client's chest and abdomen.
    2. Wash the client's arm, axilla, and hand.
    3. Wash the client's eyes, face, and neck.
    4. Wash the client's legs and feet.

34. Prioritize the following safety measures needed when assisting a client with a tub bath or shower.
    1. Assess the client's tolerance for activity, cognitive status, and musculoskeletal function.
    2. Assist the client into the tub or shower, and place all articles needed within reach.
    3. Prepare the bathroom by making sure the equipment is clean, placing a bath mat next to the tub or shower and adjusting the temperature of the room to a comfortable level to avoid chilling.
    4. Adjust the water to a comfortable temperature to avoid burns.

35. Place the following actions taken when assisting an adult client with eating in the proper order.
    1. Position the client appropriately, and assist the client to the degree necessary.
    2. Check the tray for the client's name, diet, and completeness of dietary items against the dietary order and the client's identification bracelet.
    3. Help the client to wash his hands and complete oral hygiene if desired.
    4. Assist the client with urinary or bowel elimination.

RESTORING PHYSICAL MOBILITY

PURPOSE

This chapter introduces key concepts that relate to the nursing diagnoses *Impaired physical mobility* and *Activity intolerance*. It describes the concepts of the structure and function of the musculoskeletal system pertaining to mobility and discusses factors affecting mobility.

MATCHING

1. _____ flaccid
2. _____ hemiparesis
3. _____ hemiplegia
4. _____ isometric exercise
5. _____ isotonic exercise
6. _____ kyphosis
7. _____ paraparesis
8. _____ paraplegia
9. _____ PQRST model
10. _____ proprioception
11. _____ quadriparesis
12. _____ quadriplegia
13. _____ range-of-motion (ROM) exercises
14. _____ spastic
15. _____ synovium

a. the inner layer of the articular capsule surrounding a freely movable joint
b. a sensation pertaining to stimuli originating from within the body regarding spatial position and muscular activity or to the sensory receptors that they activate
c. stands for: Provoking incidence, Quality, Region, Radiate, Relieve, Severity, and Timing of pain
d. an abnormal condition characterized by paralysis of the arms, legs, and trunk below the level of an associated injury to the spinal cord
e. a numbness or other abnormal or impaired sensation in all four limbs and the trunk
f. paralysis characterized by motor or sensory loss in the legs and trunk
g. paralysis of one side of the body
h. a numbness or other abnormal or impaired sensation experienced on only one side of the body that limits mobility and activities of daily living (ADLs)

i. an abnormal condition of the vertebral column characterized by increased convexity in the thoracic spine when viewed from the side
j. the state of being weak, soft, and flabby; lacking normal muscle tone; or having no ability to contract
k. contraction of skeletal muscles below the injury by reflex activity rather than by central nervous system control
l. a form of active exercise that increases muscle tension by applying pressure against stable resistance
m. a form of active exercise in which the muscle contracts and moves
n. any body action (active or passive) involving the muscles, joints, and natural directional movements, such as abduction, extension, flexion, pronation, and rotation
o. a numbness or other abnormal or impaired sensation in the legs and trunk

TRUE OR FALSE

16. _____ Widening your base of support by moving your feet apart helps you to maintain stability.
17. _____ Postmenopausal women's vertebral bone mass increases, and the thoracic spine becomes more convex, or curved.
18. _____ The most common congenital spinal deformity is scoliosis.
19. _____ Some medications have side effects that cause muscle atrophy.
20. _____ If a client can perform ADLs, a slight limitation of ROM is still unacceptable, especially for older adults.
21. _____ A client with *Impaired physical mobility* is at risk for injury from falls and fractures as a result of osteoporosis.
22. _____ For a postoperative client with a total knee replacement, a realistic intermediate outcome is that the client is expected to walk in the hospital room using a walker.

FILL IN THE BLANKS

23. At about the age of 35 years, _____ activity becomes greater than osteoblastic activity, which results in decreased bone that predisposes middle-aged and older adults to bone injury.

24. Muscle _____ causes weakness that can limit physical mobility.

25. An abnormal fixed position of the feet is _____ _____, or pigeon toe, a deformity that can worsen and delay physical development if not corrected.

26. The most common complaints associated with musculoskeletal health problems are pain, _____ _____, and inflammation.

27. _____ is a continuous grating sound caused by deterioration of a joint.

28. _____ and occupational therapists perform detailed assessments of muscle strength using various scales.

29. _____ nurses are specialists in helping clients return to or attain maximum function and a sense of well-being and independence.

EXERCISING YOUR CLINICAL JUDGMENT

30. Kristina Lasauskas, the client from the chapter's case study, had an open reduction and internal fixation to repair her fractured left hip. What nursing diagnosis would be most appropriate?
    1. *Impaired physical mobility*
    2. *Pain*
    3. *Activity intolerance*
    4. *Risk for injury*

31. Ms. Lasauskas needs help to learn how to increase her mobility skills after her surgery for a fractured left hip. Which one of the following discipline's primary role is improving clients' mobility skills?
    1. Rehabilitation nurse
    2. Physical therapist
    3. Occupational therapist
    4. Rehabilitation physician

32. Ms. Lasauskas will need ROM exercises while she is bedridden. What type of exercises are these?
    1. Isotonic
    2. Isokinetic
    3. Isometric
    4. Muscle toning

TEST YOURSELF

33. Pulling is usually easier than pushing, so pull clients toward you rather than push them. This can help do which one of the following?
    1. Reduce workload
    2. Decrease opposition from gravity
    3. Maintain stability
    4. Prevent muscle strain

34. Your client is having problems with her ankle. To assess her ankle's range of motion, which ROM exercises will you have her do?
    1. Flexion, extension, hyperextension
    2. Flexion, extension, abduction, adduction
    3. Plantar flexion, dorsiflexion, eversion, inversion
    4. External rotation, internal rotation

35. Your elderly client fell and fractured her hip and has degenerative arthritis in both knees. What nursing diagnosis would be most appropriate?
    1. *Impaired physical mobility*
    2. *Pain*
    3. *Activity intolerance*
    4. *Risk for injury*

36. Your teenage client has rheumatoid arthritis. She uses a walker to ambulate short distances, but relies on a wheelchair most of the time. She becomes very fatigued when walking. What nursing diagnosis would be most appropriate?
    1. *Impaired physical mobility*
    2. *Pain*
    3. *Activity intolerance*
    4. *Risk for injury*

37. Which one of the following discipline's primary role is improving clients' ADL abilities?
    1. Rehabilitation nurse
    2. Physical therapist
    3. Occupational therapist
    4. Rehabilitation physician

PRIORITIZATION

38. What is the correct order in which the following steps are taken when assisting a client to get out of bed without a transfer belt?
    1. Place the bed in its lowest position, and raise the head of the bed.
    2. Position a chair or wheelchair at a 45-degree angle to the bed on the client's stronger side.
    3. Help the client to rise to a standing position, and pivot toward the chair or wheelchair.
    4. Assist the client to a full sitting position, and support the client with his or her legs dangling over the side of the bed.

39. In what order should ROM exercises on the following areas of the body be performed?
    1. Wrist
    2. Elbow
    3. Shoulder
    4. Neck

40. In what order should the following actions be taken when preparing to move a client using a mechanical lift?
    1. Place the sling under the client.
    2. Practice using the lift.
    3. Make sure that the lift works correctly and safely.
    4. Lock the wheels on both the bed and the wheelchair.

PREVENTING DISUSE SYNDROME

PURPOSE

This chapter discusses key concepts that relate to the nursing diagnosis *Risk for disuse syndrome*. It describes the physiological concepts underlying the diagnosis and the factors that may lead to immobility and disuse.

MATCHING

1. _____ atrophy
2. _____ bedrest
3. _____ contracture
4. _____ deep vein thrombosis (DVT)
5. _____ disuse
6. _____ excoriation
7. _____ footdrop
8. _____ friction injury
9. _____ hypomotility
10. _____ hypostatic pneumonia
11. _____ immobility
12. _____ inactivity
13. _____ interface pressure
14. _____ maceration
15. _____ orthostatic hypotension
16. _____ orthostatic intolerance
17. _____ osteoporosis
18. _____ pressure ulcer
19. _____ pulmonary embolus
20. _____ renal calculi
21. _____ shear
22. _____ trochanter roll
23. _____ Valsalva maneuver
24. _____ wrist drop

a. the inability to move the whole body or a body part
b. a prescribed or self-imposed restriction to bed for therapeutic reasons
c. a decrease in the size or physiological activity of a normally developed tissue or organ as a result of inactivity or diminished function
d. the abnormal condition of joint flexion resulting from shortening of muscle fibers and associated connective tissue, with resistance to stretching and eventually to flexion and, finally in permanent fixation

e. a contracture deformity in which the muscles of the anterior foot lengthen
f. a condition in which there is a decreased mass per unit volume of normally mineralized bone, primarily from a loss of calcium that makes bones brittle and porous
g. any lesion caused by ischemia from unrelieved pressure that leads to damage of the skin and underlying tissues
h. pressure created in tissues that are compressed between the bones and a support surface by the weight of the body
i. a mechanical action in which an applied force exerted against the skin causes the tissue layers to slide in opposite but parallel directions, resulting in torn blood vessels
j. the epidermal layer of skin is rubbed off, possibly by a restraint, dressing, or tube
k. an injury to the epidermis caused by abrasion; scratching; a burn or chemicals, such as sweat; wound drainage; or feces or urine coming in contact with skin
l. a softening of the epidermis caused by prolonged contact with moisture, such as from a wet sheet or diaper
m. a drop in systolic blood pressure of 20 mm Hg or more and a drop in diastolic blood pressure of 10 mm Hg or more for 1 or 2 minutes after a client stands up
n. results when a piece of a deep vein thrombus breaks free, floats in the bloodstream to the pulmonary circulation, and lodges in a pulmonary blood vessel
o. the condition caused when a blood clot (thrombus) develops in the lumen of a deep leg vein, such as the tibial, popliteal, femoral, or iliac vein
p. an inflammation of the lungs, caused by stasis of secretions, that becomes a medium for bacterial growth
q. stones formed in the kidney when the excretion rate of calcium or other minerals is high, as when osteoclastic activity releases calcium from the bones during immobility
r. means to cease or decrease use of organs or body parts, to restrict activities, or to be immobile

s. a contracture of the wrist in the flexed position

t. an increase in abdominal pressure that results from forcing expiration against a closed glottis usually in preparation for work such as lifting or when having a bowel movement

u. a drop in the blood pressure that occurs when a client moves to a standing position, commonly resulting from immobility

v. decreased peristalsis from lack of stimulation of the gastrocolic reflex

w. a positioning device used to prevent external rotation of the hip joint

x. lack of performing or being used; usually related to an individual who is not active but sedentary or inert

TRUE OR FALSE

25. _____ Inactivity and immobility have a cyclic relationship with the development of complications.

26. _____ When muscles atrophy, they lose size and strength.

27. _____ Duration of immobilization of a client is not directly related to a higher risk of complications for the client of disuse.

28. _____ A pressure ulcer is a local defect or excavation of the surface of an organ or tissue that is produced by sloughing of necrotic inflammatory tissue creating impaired systemic circulation.

29. _____ Orthostatic intolerance is a rise in systolic blood pressure of 20 mm Hg or more and a drop in diastolic blood pressure of 10 mm Hg or more for 1 or 2 minutes after a client stands up.

30. _____ Clients who are at minimal *Risk for disuse syndrome* should be assessed every 4 to 6 hours.

31. _____ Constant contact with a bed made wet by perspiration causes maceration of the skin.

FILL IN THE BLANKS

32. _____ can affect a single body part or multiple interrelated body systems.

33. The _____ a client is immobile, the higher the risk of complication of disuse.

34. When a client is immobile, the body breaks down muscle mass to obtain _____.

35. Pressure _____ account for a large proportion of skin injuries that result from bed rest.

36. Low blood pressure and _____ _____ increase a client's risk of falling.

37. Stasis of the urine and infection increase the risk for _____ to form in the kidneys, renal pelvis, or urinary bladder.

38. You should assess and intervene every _____-_____ _____ with clients who have high *Risk for disuse syndrome.*

EXERCISING YOUR CLINICAL JUDGMENT

39. Mr. Jackson, the 58-year-old African-American client from the chapter's case study, has developed a friction injury. This type of injury results from which of the following factors?
    1. The epidermal layer of skin is rubbed off.
    2. The client is neither very young nor very old.
    3. There is a decrease in range of motion.
    4. There is maximal inactivity of long duration.

40. Mr. Jackson has moderate inactivity of maximal duration, is middle-aged, has normal to slight increased body weight, minimal discomfort, and low environmental risk. Your client is at moderate *Risk for disuse syndrome.* How often should you assess and intervene with this client?
    1. Every 4 to 6 hours
    2. Every 2 to 4 hours
    3. Every 1 to 2 hours
    4. Every shift

41. You encourage Mr. Jackson to exercise his right arm and leg against resistance three times daily. Which nursing diagnosis does Mr. Jackson have?
    1. *Ineffective role performance*
    2. *Disturbed sensory perception*
    3. *Risk for disuse syndrome*
    4. *Self-care deficit*

TEST YOURSELF

42. Your client has been immobile for several weeks. Once he begins ambulating, he is more susceptible to ambulation problems and injury caused by what?
    1. Footdrop
    2. Contracture
    3. Osteoporosis
    4. Falling

43. Your client has a deformity that involves flexion of the wrist and fingers and opposition of the thumb. You would state in the intershift report that the client has which of the following?
    1. Hand drop
    2. Wrist drop
    3. Osteoporosis
    4. Ankylosis

44. Your client has softening of the epidermis caused by prolonged contact with a wet sheet. What type of injury is this?
    1. Maceration
    2. Shear
    3. Friction injury
    4. Excoriation

45. There are two purposes that are unique to assessing the immobile client. One is to detect the risk of complication of immobility. The second purpose is to determine which of the following?
    1. The client's needs
    2. How much assistance the client will need to manage the activities of daily living and prevent complications
    3. The client's emotional well-being
    4. The client's level of understanding of his or her situation

46. To relieve pressure, how often do you turn the client to a new position?
    1. Every 1 to 2 hours
    2. Every hour
    3. Twice a shift
    4. Every 3 hours

PRIORITIZATION

47. What is the correct sequence for assisting a client who is in bed to turn onto his side?
    1. Lower the head of the bed and the knee gatch, and raise the bed to a comfortable working height
    2. Assess the client's condition and his ability to assist with the procedure
    3. Lock the wheels on the bed
    4. Cross the client's arms and legs
    5. Move the client to one side of the bed
    6. Roll the client toward you

48. When utilizing the Braden scale to predict pressure ulcer risk, rate the following client conditions from lowest to highest risk.
    1. The client makes major and frequent changes in position without assistance.
    2. The client is unable to make even slight changes in body or extremity position without assistance.
    3. The client makes frequent though slight changes in body or extremity position without assistance.
    4. The client makes occasional slight changes in position, but is unable to make frequent or significant changes without assistance.

49. Based on your understanding of *Risk for disuse syndrome*, rate the following clients from lowest to highest risk for developing complications of disuse.
    1. A 47-year-old client who had an abdominal hysterectomy under general anesthesia this morning
    2. A 66-year-old client with end-stage renal disease, incontinence, and malnutrition
    3. A 35-year-old client who had an uncomplicated vaginal delivery last night
    4. A 52-year-old client who had an arthroscopy on her shoulder yesterday afternoon

SUPPORTING RESPIRATORY FUNCTION

PURPOSE

The purpose of this chapter is to review anatomy and physiology of the respiratory system and to introduce you to basic respiratory nursing measures. You will learn to recognize the signs and symptoms of respiratory distress and intervene to improve respiratory function. Additionally, you will be introduced to some advanced procedures, such as managing a chest tube, suctioning the airway, and caring for a tracheostomy.

MATCHING

1. ____ bronchospasm
2. ____ chest percussion
3. ____ chest physiotherapy
4. ____ cough
5. ____ cyanosis
6. ____ diaphragmatic (abdominal) breathing
7. ____ dyspnea
8. ____ endotracheal tube
9. ____ hemoptysis
10. ____ hypercapnia
11. ____ hyperventilation
12. ____ hypoventilation
13. ____ hypoxemia
14. ____ hypoxia
15. ____ incentive spirometer
16. ____ postural drainage
17. ____ pulse oximetry
18. ____ pursed-lip breathing
19. ____ respiration
20. ____ sputum
21. ____ ventilation
22. ____ vibration

a. a bluish color to the skin that results from the concentration of deoxygenated hemoglobin close to the surface of the skin

b. spasm of the smooth muscles of the bronchi or the bronchioles that results in decreased airway diameter

c. using cupped hands to rhythmically clap on the chest wall over various segments of the lungs to mobilize secretions

d. a sudden audible, forceful expulsion of air from the lungs, usually an involuntary, reflexive action in response to an irritant

e. coughing and spitting up blood as a result of bleeding from any part of the lower respiratory tract

f. a catheter passed through the nose or mouth into the trachea for the purpose of establishing an airway

g. a high carbon dioxide level in the blood, usually resulting from failure of the lungs to remove carbon dioxide

h. breathing in which the majority of ventilatory work is accomplished by the diaphragm and abdominal muscles; deliberate use of the diaphragm and abdominal muscles to control breathing

i. an approach to mobilizing and draining secretions from gravity-dependent areas of the lung that uses a combination of postural drainage, chest percussion, and vibration

j. the subjective sensation of difficulty in breathing

k. increase in the rate and depth of breathing, clinically defined as $PaCO_2$ less than 35 mm Hg

l. a method of measuring the oxygen saturation of functional hemoglobin in the blood

m. a technique in which a client assumes one or more positions that will facilitate the drainage of secretions from the bronchial airways

n. a technique of mouth breathing that creates slight resistance to exhalation by contracting the lips to reduce the size of the opening, thus maintaining an even reduction of intrathoracic pressure during exhalation

o. deficient oxygenation of the blood

p. mucus secreted from the lungs, bronchi, and trachea; may include epithelial cells, bacteria, and debris

q. a device that provides a visual goal for and measurement of inspiration, thus encouraging the client to execute and sustain maximal inspiration

r. decrease in the rate and depth of breathing, clinically defined as $PaCO_2$ greater than 45 mm Hg

s. the process of exchanging air between the ambient air and the lungs; *pulmonary ventilation* refers to the total exchange of air, whereas *alveolar ventilation* refers to the effective ventilation of the alveoli

t. a technique of chest physiotherapy whereby the chest wall is set in motion by oscillating movements of the hands or a vibrator for the purpose of mobilizing secretions

u. the exchange of oxygen and carbon dioxide between the atmosphere and the cells of the body; a series of metabolic activities by which living cells break down carbohydrates, amino acids, and fats to produce energy in the form of ATP (adenosine triphosphate)

v. deficient oxygenation of body tissues

TRUE OR FALSE

23. _____ The accessory muscles of respiration become more active during forceful expiration.
24. _____ The work of breathing is directly related to the amount of airway resistance.
25. _____ Tidal volume is the amount of air inhaled with a deep inspiration.
26. _____ Oxygen and carbon dioxide are exchanged through the alveolar membrane by the passive process of diffusion.
27. _____ Fowler's position is the position of optimum ventilation/perfusion ratio.
28. _____ In the older adult, decreased compliance and elasticity increase the risk for respiratory complications during illness or surgery.
29. _____ Nicotine patches have a 50% success rate in helping people quit smoking.
30. _____ Fractured ribs are a type of obstructive respiratory disease.
31. _____ Asthma is more common when there is a history of asthma in the family.
32. _____ Ambulation is an efficient, noninvasive, inexpensive method of stimulating respiration.
33. _____ Endotracheal suctioning is a sterile procedure without regard to the client's condition or setting.
34. _____ Always ask if the client has COPD before beginning oxygen in amounts greater than 4 L/min.

FILL IN THE BLANKS

35. The primary muscle of respiration is the _____.
36. _____ _____ is the tendency of the lungs to return to a nonstretched state.
37. _____ is a lipoprotein secreted by the alveolar epithelium and acts like a detergent to reduce the surface tension and hold the alveoli open.

38. _____ stimulates the production of surfactant.
39. _____ _____ is any surface of the airways that contains air but does not participate in gas exchange.
40. The _____ is the opening at the top of the larynx between the resting vocal cords.
41. A _____ _____ _____ is the diagnostic test that provides information about the oxygen-carrying capacity of the blood.
42. The _____ _____ _____ is the volume of air forcefully (with maximum effort) exhaled after a maximum inhalation.
43. A saturation of _____% is the critical value for oxygenation to support life.
44. _____ describes the client rendered insensitive to painful stimuli by reducing the level of consciousness with a narcotic or anesthetic. This client has rapid shallow breathing.
45. _____, _____ sputum is difficult to cough out and may be associated with dehydration.
46. The client with pain from a high abdominal surgical incision is at risk for the nursing diagnosis of _____ _____ _____.
47. Cyanosis represents the presence of increased amounts of _____ _____ in the blood.
48. _____ is a medication used to reverse the action of narcotics, thus stimulating respiration.

EXERCISING YOUR CLINICAL JUDGMENT

Mrs. Wilheim, the client introduced in the chapter's case study, has been admitted to the hospital with a diagnosis of pneumonia. Her physician orders include antibiotic therapy and oxygen therapy.

49. Mrs. Wilheim is placed on oxygen via nasal cannula, a low-flow oxygen delivery system. Which of the following statements best describes this therapy?
    1. The wall-mounted oxygen flow meter delivers 35% to 45% oxygen to the nasal cannula.
    2. The client supplements the flow of oxygen with room air to maintain the minute ventilation.
    3. A low-flow system can only deliver 28% oxygen.
    4. 100% oxygen from the wall is mixed precisely with room air to deliver the ordered percentage of oxygen.

50. Mrs. Wilheim is hypoventilating because of her disease process. Which of the following pieces of client data best fits the definition of hypoventilation?
    1. Respiratory rate of 36, with visible chest wall movement in the upper third of the chest
    2. Measured tidal volume of 500 with a rate of 12
    3. Arterial carbon dioxide level of 43, oxygen saturation of 94%
    4. Respiratory rate of 10, no dyspnea, color good, skin warm and dry

51. Mrs. Wilheim is subsequently given medication via metered-dose inhaler to enhance her breathing. The nurse teaching her to correctly use a metered-dose inhaler would instruct her to do which of the following?
    1. Activate the inhaler, and then take a deep breath
    2. Take a deep breath, and then activate the inhaler
    3. Simultaneously activate the inhaler and take a deep breath
    4. Activate the inhaler, close the mouth, and take a deep breath

TEST YOURSELF

52. Your client had a thoracentesis 30 minutes ago. He is complaining of shortness of breath. You listen to his lungs. Which finding indicates the possibility of the complication of atelectasis?
    1. Bilateral crackles (rales) in the bases
    2. Diminished breath sounds on the side where the thoracentesis was performed
    3. Harsh sonorous sounds over the bifurcation of the bronchi
    4. Wet, bubbling sounds over the midsternum

53. Your client is having an asthma attack. You hear wheezes throughout the lung fields. You can attribute the sounds to which of the following?
    1. Mucus in the bronchioles
    2. Atelectasis
    3. Bronchospasms
    4. Inflammation of the pleura

54. A client who has a dry, hacking cough and wheezes throughout the lung fields would be given which of the following nursing diagnoses?
    1. *Ineffective airway clearance*
    2. *Ineffective breathing pattern*
    3. *Impaired gas exchange*
    4. *Obstructive airway disease*

55. Your postoperative client has an order for an incentive spirometer treatment q2h for the 72 hours following surgery. He asks you why he needs this treatment when his surgery was on his abdomen. Which of the following responses is best?
    1. "It will help you use all of your lungs when you breathe and prevent a respiratory infection."
    2. "It will help you maintain a maximal inspiration, thus preventing atelectasis."
    3. "It will increase the perfusion to your lungs for better arterial oxygen saturation."
    4. "It will increase the blood flow to your lungs so you can get more oxygen from the air that you breathe."

56. Your client with chronic obstructive pulmonary disease has chronic inflammation in her lungs. She is taking a corticosteroid by metered-dose inhaler. She asks why she can't just take a pill. Which of the following would be the most accurate response?
    1. "Your doctor prefers a metered-dose inhaler."
    2. "You can use the metered-dose inhaler anytime you need it."
    3. "The medication in a pill form won't reach your lungs."
    4. "You are less likely to have the complication of failure of your adrenal glands to produce corticosteroids."

57. You observe all of the following in your client with a chest tube. Select the finding that represents the most serious complication of a chest tube.
    1. 100 mL of serosanguineous drainage in an 8-hour period
    2. Itching under the pressure dressing around the chest tube
    3. Air from the pleural space bubbling in the water-sealed drainage system
    4. Sucking air into the pleural space through the chest tube

58. Which of the following would be the primary purpose of pursed-lip breathing?
    1. To increase the resistance to expiration to maintain functional residual volume
    2. To help the client focus on the respiration during times of stress
    3. To increase the inspiratory capacity thus improving exercise tolerance
    4. To produce the relaxation response during times of dyspnea

59. Which of the following would be the primary reason for a client to learn diaphragmatic breathing?
    1. To increase the strength and use of the diaphragm for exhalation
    2. To increase the strength and use of the diaphragm for inhalation
    3. To produce the relaxation response and reduce stress
    4. To reduce the strength and use of the accessory muscles of respiration

60. You are suctioning the client's airway through a tracheostomy. Which of the following actions represents a correct nursing action during this procedure?
    1. Apply suction continuously as you enter the airway.
    2. Apply suction intermittently as you enter the airway.
    3. Apply suction continuously as you exit the airway.
    4. Apply suction intermittently as you exit the airway.

61. For which of the following reasons is the Yankauer tip suction device used for safety in oral suctioning?
    1. The tip has multiple openings thus preventing damage to the oral mucosa.
    2. It can be attached only to low-suction devices.
    3. The hard plastic catheter cannot be swallowed by the client.
    4. The openings are not large enough to cause mucosal damage.

62. Which of the following represents the primary principle in assisting the client to clear the airway?
    1. To use the most aggressive procedure first to reduce the time needed for treatment
    2. To use the least invasive procedure necessary to produce the desired results
    3. To avoid invasive suctioning until the secretions are life-threatening
    4. To suction when the level of need is preventive

63. The most serious complication of suction is represented by which of the following data?
    1. Streaks of blood in the sputum
    2. Oxygen saturation of 88%
    3. Large amount of watery sputum
    4. Moderate amounts of yellow sputum

PRIORITIZATION

64. List the respiratory defense mechanisms in the order in which they assist in maintaining an internal environment essentially free of microorganisms and foreign matter.
    1. Lungs
    2. Glottis
    3. Pharynx
    4. Nose

65. Prioritize the following interventions that can be implemented with a client who has an ineffective breathing pattern
    1. Administering medications such as bronchodilators
    2. Encouraging use of an incentive spirometer
    3. Positioning the client for maximum ventilatory function
    4. Stimulating respiration through ambulation

66. The physician has ordered that the client receive oxygen at 3 L/min via nasal cannula. Prioritize the following actions the nurse should take when preparing to administer the oxygen.
    1. Check the function of the system after establishing oxygen flow; observe for bubbling in the water.
    2. Obtain a humidification device, and fill it with sterile water.
    3. Remove all smoking materials from the room, and post a "No Smoking" sign.
    4. Place the nasal cannula on the client, and adjust the tubing to avoid pressure.
    5. Attach the connecting tube and the delivery device.
    6. Set up the system, and insert the flowmeter into the oxygen source.

67. List the steps required to teach a client to use an incentive spirometer in the correct sequence.
    1. Assist the client to an upright (sitting) position.
    2. Explain the purpose of the incentive spirometer to the client, and assess his or her ability to understand the teaching.
    3. Assist the client to position the mouthpiece of the upright spirometer between his or her teeth, and instruct him to close the lips around the mouthpiece.
    4. Instruct the client to breathe out normally.
    5. Instruct the client to take a slow deep breath and hold it for 2 to 6 seconds after reaching his or her preset goal.
    6. Instruct the client to exhale slowly, and repeat the process 5 to 10 times per hour.

PURPOSE

This chapter discusses concepts of and factors affecting cardiovascular function. It uses the nursing process as a framework to discuss management of *Decreased tissue perfusion* as a result of common cardiovascular problems.

MATCHING

1. _____ afterload
2. _____ antidiuretic hormone (ADH)
3. _____ atherosclerosis
4. _____ baroreceptors
5. _____ bradycardia
6. _____ cardiac output
7. _____ claudication
8. _____ diastole
9. _____ dysrhythmia
10. _____ edema
11. _____ inotropic agent
12. _____ ischemia
13. _____ necrosis
14. _____ preload
15. _____ stroke volume
16. _____ systole
17. _____ tachycardia
18. _____ viscosity

a. specialized cells located in the aorta, carotid, and other large arteries that detect pressure changes in the vascular system
b. cramplike pains in the calves caused by poor circulation of blood to the leg muscles
c. a heart rate above 100 beats/min
d. a decreased supply of oxygenated blood to tissues
e. contraction of the ventricles
f. the pressure against which the left ventricle pumps
g. a hormonal compensatory mechanism that is also called vasopressin
h. the amount of blood in the left ventricle immediately before contraction
i. the amount of blood pumped by the ventricles in 1 minute
j. refers to the relaxation of the ventricles

k. the relative ability of a fluid to flow that results from the thickness of the fluid
l. abnormalities of heart rate or rhythm
m. an abnormal accumulation of fluid in the interstitial spaces of tissues, commonly known as swelling
n. localized death of tissues caused by disease, oxygen deficit, or injury
o. medication that increases the contractility of the heart muscle, thereby increasing cardiac output
p. a pathological condition in which fat and plaque form deposits on the intimal (inner) surface of the arteries
q. the amount of blood ejected from the heart with each contraction
r. a heart rate less than 60 beats/min

TRUE OR FALSE

19. _____ Highly viscous blood encounters more resistance while moving through blood vessels.
20. _____ Starling's law indicates that stronger recoil of cardiac muscle tissue produces weaker stroke volume.
21. _____ Elevated blood glucose is a modifiable risk factor for cardiovascular disease.
22. _____ Nicotine produces vasodilatation, which increases blood flow to tissues, and increases the oxygen-carrying capacity of hemoglobin.
23. _____ Women have an increased incidence of Raynaud's disease, whereas men are more likely to have Buerger's disease.
24. _____ Atherosclerotic plaque deposits create a rough spot on the normally smooth inner surface of the blood vessel.
25. _____ Bacterial and viral infections of the heart are minor problems that leave no permanent heart damage as a result.
26. _____ Stress increases the heart rate and blood pressure, which, in turn, raise the body's oxygen demands.
27. _____ Excessive intake of high-fat foods can lead to elevated serum cholesterol levels.

28. _____ Lack of circulation destroys nerves and impairs motor function in the involved extremity.

FILL IN THE BLANKS

29. The average cardiac output is _____ to _____ L/min.

30. _____ and _____ are stimulants that increase heart rate and oxygen demand.

31. The primary effect of aging as a developmental factor on the circulation is the development of _____.

32. Hypertension is a condition in which the blood pressure is persistently higher than _____ / _____ mm Hg.

33. A _____ _____ is the blockage of a blood vessel in the brain through thrombus, embolus, or hemorrhage, which results in ischemia or death of brain tissue distal to the insult.

34. Fluid in the lungs is a prominent symptom in _____-sided heart failure.

35. _____ is needed to manufacture oxygen-carrying hemoglobin molecules.

36. Clients who take _____ and warfarin have a dangerous risk of bleeding.

37. Antihistamines and appetite suppressants are contraindicated for clients with hypertension because they cause _____.

38. Lifestyle choices such as _____, _____, and _____ have a direct effect on circulation.

EXERCISING YOUR CLINICAL JUDGMENT

Mr. Yoder, the client from the chapter's case study, is a 74-year-old Amish male who has a medical diagnosis of angina pectoris and a nursing diagnosis of *Ineffective cardiopulmonary tissue perfusion.* He was admitted 2 days ago with chest pain and underwent cardiac catheterization yesterday. You are assigned to take care of Mr. Yoder today and must develop and implement a teaching plan before his discharge, which is planned for later this afternoon.

39. To help Mr. Yoder conserve energy in order to decrease oxygen demand, you should encourage him to do which of the following?
   1. Take rest breaks between daily activities such as eating, bathing, and walking.
   2. Do all of his chores early in the morning provided he has had a good night's sleep.
   3. Save chores for late in the day so endurance will be greater.
   4. Stop all exertional activities and turn over responsibility for them to his son.

40. You would encourage Mr. Yoder to limit which of the following food items that typically has a high salt content?
   1. Vegetables
   2. Freshwater fish
   3. Sauces
   4. Fruits

41. Knowing that Mr. Yoder is being discharged with a prescription for an antihypertensive medication, which of the following general teaching points would you include in a discussion with him?
   1. Take the medication when eating a heavy meal.
   2. Wear slippers or shoes at all times.
   3. Take the medication whenever chest pain occurs.
   4. Rise slowly out of a bed or chair.

42. In teaching Mr. Yoder to avoid the Valsalva maneuver, you would tell him to avoid which of the following activities?
   1. Drinking lots of fluids
   2. Bearing down hard when having a bowel movement
   3. Walking up and down stairs
   4. Lying flat in bed

TEST YOURSELF

43. To determine the presence of jugular vein distention, the nurse would take which of the following actions?
   1. Raise the head of the bed to 30 to 45 degrees.
   2. Turn the client onto the right side.
   3. Lay the client supine in bed.
   4. Turn the client onto the left side.

44. A client has had a cardiac catheterization using the right femoral artery as the access site. The nurse would report which of the following peripheral vascular findings in the client's right leg following the procedure?
   1. Strong palpable pedal pulse
   2. Pink skin
   3. Warmth
   4. Numbness and tingling

45. The nurse would assess for which of the following peripheral vascular manifestations in a client with venous disease of the lower extremities?
    1. Pale, cool skin
    2. Decreased pulses
    3. Edema
    4. Tingling and burning sensations

46. A nurse has signed out a unit of blood from the blood bank at 2:00 PM. The unit must be hung by which of the following times in order to prevent bacterial contamination of the unit?
    1. 6:00 PM
    2. 4:00 PM
    3. 3:30 PM
    4. 2:20 PM

47. A nurse who has administered care to a client in shock interprets that the shock state is resolving. The nurse bases this conclusion on which of the following pieces of client data?
    1. Urine output is 45 mL/hour.
    2. Pulse rate is 128 beats/min.
    3. Blood pressure is 92/48 mm Hg.
    4. Client is experiencing neurological confusion.

PRIORITIZATION

48. Prioritize the following nursing actions required prior to administering blood.
    1. Assess if the client is at risk for a transfusion reaction by asking if he has allergies or has had a previous transfusion reaction.
    2. Obtain and document a set of baseline vital signs.
    3. Compare the blood and crossmatch slip from the blood bank with another RN.
    4. Check the physician's order to verify the type of blood product and number of units to be administered.
    5. Verify and document the required client information, blood donor number, and expiration date.
    6. Assemble necessary equipment including obtaining the blood from the blood bank.

49. Upon entering the client's room, you observe that he is lying on the floor. After shaking the client and calling his name, you have determined that he is nonresponsive. Place the following nursing actions in the correct sequence.
    1. Call for help by activating the facility's emergency response system.
    2. Remove visible food or vomitus from the client's mouth.
    3. Look, listen, and feel for breathing.
    4. If adequate respirations are not detected within 10 seconds, give two breaths.
    5. Open the client's airway.

50. During the administration of blood, a client develops chills and complains of dyspnea. Place the following nursing actions in the correct sequence.
    1. Stay with the client, and obtain vital signs
    2. Maintain the client's IV line.
    3. Stop the blood transfusion.
    4. Notify the physician, or ask another RN to notify the physician if you cannot do so without leaving the client's room.

51. You are caring for a 23-year-old male client who was brought to the emergency department after sustaining a severe laceration resulting in significant blood loss. You have identified that the client is at risk of hypovolemic shock. In what order would you expect to see the following signs of impaired tissue perfusion?
    1. Hypotension
    2. Cold, clammy skin
    3. Tachycardia
    4. Decreased urine output
    5. Restlessness, agitation, or confusion
    6. Weakened peripheral pulses

MANAGING SLEEP AND REST

PURPOSE

This chapter introduces you to concepts central to normal sleep and rest, and the variations from normal that can occur. It describes how to use the nursing process to assist the client in meeting personal needs for sleep and rest.

MATCHING

1. _____ bruxism
2. _____ circadian rhythm
3. _____ dyssomnia
4. _____ hypnotic
5. _____ insomnia
6. _____ multiple sleep latency test
7. _____ narcolepsy
8. _____ nightmare disorder
9. _____ nocturnal enuresis
10. _____ non–rapid eye movement (NREM) sleep
11. _____ obstructive sleep apnea
12. _____ parasomnia
13. _____ polysomnography
14. _____ rapid eye movement (REM) sleep
15. _____ rest
16. _____ restless legs syndrome
17. _____ sleep
18. _____ sleep deprivation
19. _____ sleep terrors disorder
20. _____ sleepwalking disorder
21. _____ sundowning
22. _____ zeitgeber

a. a biorhythmic pattern that is regularly repeated at 24-hour intervals
b. the state that results from a person not getting enough sleep
c. difficulty initiating or maintaining sleep, sleeping too lightly, easily disrupted sleep with many spontaneous arousals or early-morning awakenings, and the subjective sense that sleep quality is poor and inadequate
d. repeated occurrence of sleep terrors—abrupt awakenings from sleep usually beginning with a panicky scream or cry.

e. a sleep disorder manifested by periodic cessation of airflow at the nose and mouth during inspiration, which arouses the person from sleep
f. the continuous measurement and recording of physiological activity during sleep by using electroencephalogram, electrooculogram, electrocardiogram, and electromyogram.
g. a state in which consciousness, activity of the skeletal muscles, and metabolism are depressed
h. a direct, objective measure of sleepiness used to evaluate excessive somnolence and daytime sleepiness.
i. a state of being physically and mentally relaxed while being awake and alert
j. is characterized by high-voltage EEG activity and a high arousal threshold, which can make it difficult to arouse the sleeper
k. violent, repetitive grinding of the teeth that occurs during the lighter stages of sleep or during partial arousals.
l. a slow-wave sleep parasomnia associated with stereotypical "sleepwalking" behaviors
m. primary sleep disorders initiating or maintaining sleep or excessive sleep
n. repeated voiding of urine during nighttime sleep
o. a sleep disruption involving the nocturnal exacerbation of disruptive behaviors and agitation associated with clients who have dementia
p. a sleeping period without rapid eye movement (REM)
q. pathological REM sleep, manifested as excessive daytime sleepiness, disturbed nighttime sleep, cataplexy, sleep paralysis, and hypnagogic hallucinations
r. abnormal behaviors or physical events
s. a drug that acts on the CNS to shorten sleep onset, reduce nighttime wakefulness, or decrease anxiety when insomnia is associated with increased anxiety
t. repeated occurrence of frightening dreams that lead to awakening from sleep that occurs primarily during REM sleep and may occur every 90 to 110 minutes

u. a drug that exerts a soothing, tranquilizing effect on the CNS, resulting in a shortened sleep onset and the alleviation of anxiety

v. a familial sleep disorder characterized by intense, abnormal, lower-extremity sensations and irresistible leg movements that delay sleep onset

w. the stage of sleep characterized by rapid saccadic movement of the eyes

x. adjusting the human body's internal clock to a 24-hour solar day

TRUE OR FALSE

23. _____ Wrist actigraphs are transducers worn on the wrist so that all wrist movements can be recorded during sleep.

24. _____ A client who is physically rested is therefore also mentally rested.

25. _____ An electroencephalogram (EEG) can be used to distinguish among coma, sleep, and wakefulness when other assessment results are inconclusive.

26. _____ Restless legs syndrome is a rare sleep disorder.

27. _____ The half-life of nicotine is 1 to 2 hours.

FILL IN THE BLANKS

28. A _____ is an environmental trigger or synchronizer that adjusts the body's internal clock to a 24-hour day.

29. _____ is the "hormone of darkness" that regulates the circadian phase of sleep.

30. A person should avoid excess coffee, tea, or chocolate near bedtime because they contain the stimulant _____.

31. ICU psychosis is an iatrogenic complication that is strongly correlated with _____ sleep deprivation in ICUs.

32. The sleep-wake cycle is fully developed by the age of _____.

33. A person with sleep apnea should avoid sleeping on the _____.

EXERCISING YOUR CLINICAL JUDGMENT

Ms. Weiss, the client from the chapter's case study, is experiencing transient situational insomnia that she attributes to a new job and enrollment in graduate school courses. Personal habits include drinking a glass of wine to help with sleep, and smoking cigarettes and drinking coffee throughout the day. The nurse practitioner has asked you to counsel Ms. Weiss about nonprescription treatments for her sleep disorder.

34. Knowing that caffeine has stimulant properties, you would encourage Ms. Weiss to refrain from drinking coffee after which of the following times?
    1. Noon
    2. 2 PM
    3. 4 PM
    4. 8 PM

35. To reduce the interference of nicotine with Ms. Weiss's sleep, you would advise her to continue to try to have the last cigarette no later than:
    1. Midmorning.
    2. Lunchtime.
    3. Dinnertime.
    4. 1 hour before bedtime.

36. When discussing the Bootzin technique with Ms. Weiss, you would include which of the following points?
    1. Adjust the alarm clock nightly to a time that allows for 8 hours of continuous sleep.
    2. If you cannot get to sleep after 30 minutes of trying, get up and go into another room until sleepy.
    3. Take a nap at midday to make up for sleep lost the previous night.
    4. Go to bed at the same time each night, regardless of whether or not you feel sleepy.

37. You are instructing Ms. Weiss about progressive relaxation techniques as a method to promote sleep onset. Which of the following points would you include?
    1. Practice the exercises for 45 to 60 minutes before going to bed.
    2. Only do the exercises at bedtime, not during the night if wakefulness occurs.
    3. Do not do the exercises in conjunction with deep-breathing exercises.
    4. Relaxation begins with voluntary muscles in the feet and progresses upward to the face.

TEST YOURSELF

38. A client reports an inability to fall asleep, which is followed by awakening at night and a sense of not feeling well-rested in the morning. The nurse interprets that these symptoms are defining characteristics of which of the following nursing diagnoses?
    1. *Fatigue*
    2. *Disturbed sleep pattern*
    3. *Anxiety*
    4. *Altered thought processes*

39. The nurse who is planning behavioral outcomes for a client who has a problem with interrupted sleep would include which of the following suggestions?
    1. Do not eat heavy or fat-filled foods just before bedtime.
    2. Do not drink milk before bedtime.
    3. Drink a glass of wine or beer just before bedtime.
    4. Keep a bedside lamp on during the night.

40. When teaching a client cognitive strategies to reduce insomnia, the nurse would encourage the client to spend 20 minutes reflecting on daytime activities and achievements:
    1. Just after getting home from work, such as around 4 PM.
    2. Just before going to bed.
    3. Just after getting into bed for the night.
    4. In the early evening after dinner.

41. The nurse would encourage the client who has an order for a prn sleep medication to take it:
    1. Just after dinner.
    2. Two hours before bedtime.
    3. Shortly before bedtime.
    4. 1 hour after bedtime if not successful falling asleep.

42. The nurse would evaluate that interventions to treat a *Disturbed sleep pattern* were most effective if the client states:
    1. Complied with the interventions prescribed.
    2. Felt well-rested after sleep.
    3. Obtained 4 hours of uninterrupted sleep per night.
    4. Used at least half of the methods suggested by the nurse.

PRIORITIZATION

43. Mr. Phillips is a healthy 48-year-old client who complains of difficulty sleeping and fatigue during a visit to his employer's wellness center. In what order should the nurse complete the following?
    1. Obtain a sleep history with information about his normal sleep-wake patterns, bedtime routines, and risk factors
    2. Ask Mr. Phillips to complete a weekly sleep diary.
    3. Complete a physical exam looking for behavioral manifestations of insufficient sleep, nystagmus, ptosis, thickened speech, dark under-eye circles, yawning, muscle tremors, lack of coordination, and activity intolerance.
    4. Refer Mr. Phillips to his physician for further evaluation.
    5. Assist Mr. Phillips to develop a plan that includes routine bedtimes; exercise; avoidance of alcohol, caffeine, and nicotine in the evening; and elimination of sleep disturbances in the home.

44. You are caring for an 86-year-old female client who has recently been admitted to the long-term care facility in which you are working. She is complaining of mild low back pain and difficulty sleeping. What actions should you taking prior to administering the hypnotic ordered for prn use?
    1. Premedicate with an analgesic 30 minutes before bedtime.
    2. Provide a therapeutic back massage to relax tense muscles and relieve muscle spasms.
    3. Assist the client to maintain her normal bedtime routine.
    4. Offer a light snack.
    5. Prepare the environment for sleep by dimming the lights and shutting the door to decrease noise.

45. When traveling cross country on vacation, you experience "jet lag." Prioritize the following actions to decrease the impact of travel on your circadian rhythm.
    1. Reset your wristwatch while on the plane.
    2. Eat lightly and avoid alcohol on the plane.
    3. Adapt to the destination's circadian clock upon arrival.
    4. Adapt to the destination's time zone a few days before the trip.

Chapter 37 — MANAGING PAIN

PURPOSE

This chapter discusses key concepts that relate to the nursing diagnoses *Chronic pain* and *Pain*. It describes the physiological concepts supporting pain-related nursing diagnoses. It also describes pathophysiological, cognitive, affective, sensory, cultural, environmental, and other variables that affect the pain experience.

MATCHING

1. _____ acute pain
2. _____ adjuvant analgesic
3. _____ agonist analgesic
4. _____ analgesia
5. _____ antagonist
6. _____ atypical analgesic
7. _____ breakthrough pain
8. _____ chronic pain
9. _____ endorphin
10. _____ epidural analgesia
11. _____ equianalgesia
12. _____ first pass effect
13. _____ gate-control theory
14. _____ intrathecal analgesia
15. _____ mixed agonist-antagonist analgesic
16. _____ modulation
17. _____ neuropathic pain
18. _____ nociception
19. _____ nociceptive pain
20. _____ nociceptor
21. _____ nonopioid analgesic
22. _____ opioid analgesic
23. _____ opioid naive
24. _____ opioid receptor
25. _____ pain
26. _____ pain behavior
27. _____ patient-controlled analgesia (PCA)
28. _____ physical dependence
29. _____ pseudoaddiction
30. _____ psychological dependence
31. _____ referred pain
32. _____ rescue dose
33. _____ somatic pain
34. _____ suffering
35. _____ tolerance
36. _____ visceral pain

a. an unpleasant sensory and emotional experience associated with actual and potential tissue damage
b. the process of transmitting a pain signal from a site of tissue damage to areas of the brain where perception occurs
c. pain transmitted from a site of injury to the higher brain centers along an intact nervous system
d. the transmission of a pain signal from the site of injury to the higher brain centers via a nervous system that has been temporarily or permanently damaged in some way
e. well-localized pain, usually bone or spinal metastases or from injury to cutaneous or deep tissues
f. poorly localized pain
g. pain experienced at a site distant from the injured tissue
h. an internal or external restraining of the nociceptive process that inhibits transmission of the pain signal at any place along the transmission pathway
i. a portion of a nerve cell to which an opioid or opiate-like substance can bind
j. morphine-like drug that attaches to an opioid receptor and produces analgesia by blocking substance P
k. a drug that provides analgesia at the peripheral level by a mechanism other than the opioid receptor sites
l. an opioid that stimulates activity at an opioid receptor to produce analgesia
m. blocks activity at *mu* and *kappa* opioid receptors by displacing opioid analgesics that are currently attached
n. formulations that attach to both the *kappa* and *mu* receptor sites
o. an involuntary physiological phenomenon that occurs after repeated exposure to an opioid analgesic; it involves a decreased-level pain relief despite a stable or escalating opioid dosage
p. an involuntary physiological phenomenon that occurs after repeated exposure to an opioid analgesic

114

q. a chronic disorder demonstrated by overwhelming involvement with obtaining and using a drug for its mind-altering effects

r. anything a person says or does that implies the presence of pain

s. short-term, self-limiting pain with a probable duration of less than 6 months

t. long-term, constant or recurring pain without an anticipated or predictable end and a duration of more than 6 months

u. drugs not primarily indicated for pain but used to treat specific types of pain

v. a catheter is placed in the subarachnoid space between the dura mater and the spinal cord to allow immediate drug diffusion into the cerebrospinal fluid

w. a catheter is placed between the spinal vertebrae and the dura mater to allow the diffusion of an analgesic drug across the dura mater into the cerebrospinal fluid

x. a drug-delivery approach that uses an external infusion pump to deliver an opioid dose on a "client-demand" basis

y. intermittent episodes of pain that occur despite continued use of an analgesic

z. an as-needed dose of an immediate-release analgesic in response to breakthrough pain and in addition to the scheduled analgesic dosage

aa. the dosage that provides the same amount of pain relief independent of the drug or the route

bb. the partial metabolism of opioid analgesics by the liver before they reach the systemic circulation, thereby resulting in a decrease in opioid bioavailability

cc. those who have had minimal or no exposure to opioid analgesics

dd. any medication that may increase analgesic efficacy, thus allowing for a smaller opioid dosage

ee. the primary afferent fibers that initiate the pain experience when stimulated by tissue damage

ff. a group of internally secreted opiate-like substances released by a signal from the cerebral cortex

gg. unpleasant emotional response to pain

hh. a reduction in the perception or experience of pain

ii. hypothesizes an alteration in the transmission of the ascending pain signal by a spinal gating mechanism located in the dorsal horn; the pain signal may be inhibited or facilitated by multiple variables

jj. a syndrome of abnormal behavior that develops as a direct consequence of inadequate pain management; manifested by behaviors that mimic dependence

TRUE OR FALSE

37. _____ Pain is primarily a protective mechanism, but it is also a complex biopsychosocial phenomenon.

38. _____ Visceral pain is well-localized pain, usually from bone or spinal metastases or from injury to cutaneous or deep tissues.

39. _____ A single disorder may have components of both nociceptive and neuropathic pain.

40. _____ Educating a client about what to expect during a painful procedure decreases the pain's intensity and controls pain behaviors.

41. _____ Pain is the actual physical sensation of discomfort, whereas suffering is the unpleasant emotional response.

42. _____ Pain is a normal part of aging.

43. _____ The administration schedule of analgesia should be based on the known half-life of the drug.

FILL IN THE BLANKS

44. Pain functions as a _____ tool, an assessment variable, and a measure of _____ interventions.

45. _____ pain is experienced at a site distant from the injured tissue.

46. Behavioral expressions of pain are _____ from others.

47. _____ pain can quickly deplete a person's physical and emotional resources, immobilize the person, and lead to physical disability and subsequent loss of employment.

48. Once you choose a _____ _____ _____ for a client, continue to use the same scale throughout your ongoing assessment to keep the responses as comparable as possible over time.

49. Clients with _____ pain commonly have trouble finding adequate words to describe the sensation.

50. Nonmalignant etiologies are more likely to produce _____ pain, which tends to be difficult to treat and, at times, more disabling than cancer pain.

EXERCISING YOUR CLINICAL JUDGMENT

51. Mr. Joseph Valdez, the client from the chapter's case study, was born in Mexico City. He has recurrent gastric carcinoma and he hurts most of the time. His brothers told him to be tough and that he could "beat this thing." They were encouraging him to remain stoic even in the presence of severe pain. This is an example of which of the following?
    1. Religious beliefs
    2. Psychosocial modifiers
    3. Cultural norms
    4. Aggravating and relieving variables

52. Mr. Valdez is being admitted to an oncology unit for epidural catheter placement. He is experiencing unrelieved and severe pain. Which of the following nursing diagnoses would be appropriate?
    1. *Ineffective individual coping*
    2. *Hopelessness*
    3. *Pain*
    4. *Chronic pain*

53. Mr. Valdez experiences breakthrough pain. Which of the following actions would you take to treat him with rescue dosing?
    1. Call his physician and request that he receive a more effective analgesic
    2. Give him a one-time extra dose of his analgesic
    3. Change the schedule of his analgesic to be more effective
    4. Give him as-needed doses of an immediate-release analgesic in addition to the scheduled analgesic dosage

TEST YOURSELF

54. Which type of pain is described as squeezing, pressure, cramping, distention, or deep stretching?
    1. Somatic
    2. Visceral
    3. Referred
    4. Neuropathic

55. Your client develops withdrawal symptoms if the opioid is abruptly withdrawn or an opioid antagonist is administered. This is considered which of the following?
    1. Tolerance
    2. Physical dependence
    3. Psychological dependence
    4. Pseudo-addiction

56. You use a pain rating scale that is a 10 cm horizontal line. At its left endpoint is written *No pain at all*. At its right endpoint is written *Worst pain imaginable*. What type of pain rating scale is this?
    1. Self-report rating scale
    2. Verbal descriptor scale
    3. Numerical rating scale
    4. Visual analog scale

57. In the frail elderly, the most sensitive indicator of pain may be which of the following?
    1. Crying out in pain
    2. Moaning
    3. An observed decrease in the client's usual level of functioning
    4. Facial grimacing

58. If your client is receiving an opioid analgesic for acute or chronic pain and her respiratory rate is significantly affected (fewer than 8 breaths/min), the appropriate intervention is which of the following?
    1. Stop the opioid analgesic until the respiratory rate returns to normal.
    2. Slowly push intravenously 0.2 to 0.4 mg of naloxone (Narcan) as ordered that has been diluted in normal saline to equal 10 ml until an adequate respiratory rate returns but pain relief remains intact.
    3. Quickly push intravenously 0.4 mg of naloxone (Narcan) that has been diluted in normal saline to equal 10 ml until an adequate respiratory rate returns but pain relief remains intact.
    4. Give an intramuscular (IM) injection of 0.4 mg of naloxone (Narcan) that has been diluted in normal saline to equal 10 ml.

PRIORITIZATION

59. List the steps of the nociceptive process in their correct order.
    1. The pain signal is sent to the dorsal horn of the spinal cord and relayed to the thalamus.
    2. Injured cells release chemicals that stimulate nociceptors to initiate the pain signal.
    3. Initial injury (stimulus) occurs.
    4. The thalamus relays the pain signal to areas of the cortex where perception occurs.

60. Prioritize the following pain management principles.
    1. Identify the appropriate route needed for optimal analgesic effect.
    2. Titrate the medication to provide sufficient pain relief.
    3. Choose an administration schedule on the basis of the drug's half-life.
    4. Select the analgesic that is effective for the type and level of pain.

61. Prioritize the following management principles used when caring for a client with chronic pain.
    1. Develop a therapeutic relationship with the client.
    2. Partner with the client and family.
    3. Involve a multidisciplinary team in developing a treatment plan.
    4. Use multiple modes of therapy including nonpharmacological approaches.

SUPPORTING SENSORY/PERCEPTUAL FUNCTION

PURPOSE

This chapter discusses key concepts that relate to the nursing diagnosis *Sensory/perceptual alteration* (visual, auditory, kinesthetic, gustatory, tactile, and olfactory). It describes the normal physiology of sensation and perception, and a variety of factors affecting sensory/perceptual function.

MATCHING

1. ____ auditory
2. ____ gustatory
3. ____ kinesthetic
4. ____ olfactory
5. ____ ototoxic
6. ____ perception
7. ____ presbycusis
8. ____ presbyopia
9. ____ reticular activating system (RAS)
10. ____ sensation
11. ____ sensory deprivation
12. ____ sensory overload
13. ____ tactile
14. ____ visual

a. the reception of stimulation through receptors of the nervous system
b. the conscious mental recognition or registration of a sensory stimulus, as, for example, when a person smells a sweet fragrance and gets a mental image of a cherry
c. having a damaging effect on cranial nerve VIII or the organs of hearing and balance
d. results from excessive environmental stimuli or a level of stimulus beyond the person's ability to absorb or comprehend it
e. located in the midbrain and thalamus; keeps the brain aroused
f. a decrease in the elasticity of the lens with age that impairs the ability to focus on near objects
g. a sensorineural hearing loss of high-frequency tones that occurs in the elderly and may lead to a loss of all hearing frequencies
h. pertaining to the sensation of sight
i. pertaining to the sensation of hearing

j. pertaining to the sensation of taste
k. pertaining to the sensation of touch
l. pertaining to the sensation of smell
m. pertaining to the sensation of body position
n. inadequate reception or perception of environmental stimuli

TRUE OR FALSE

15. _____ Nurses observe sensory deficits more commonly in infants because of age-related changes in their sense organs.
16. _____ The cerebral cortex must be alerted or aroused to perceive and produce a conscious act in response to stimuli.
17. _____ Taste sensations decline normally with age.
18. _____ Adolescents are at risk for hearing loss if they are exposed to chronic loud noise.
19. _____ The Weber and Rinne tests are auditory screening tests used to evaluate the client for high-frequency hearing loss.
20. _____ Ageusia is the complete loss of taste.
21. _____ A hearing aid will not be damaged by x-ray examinations.

FILL IN THE BLANKS

22. _____% of all information received from the environment is visual.

23. _____ is commonly called *crossed eyes* and occurs in about 5% of children under the age of 4 years.

24. A _____ loss results from a problem in the outer and middle ear that reduces sensitivity to tones received by air conduction.

25. The sensation of smell declines with _____, nerve damage, or the presence of other odors in the nasal passages.

26. The _____ alphabet chart is used most commonly and appropriately for adults and older children to test their visual acuity.

27. Corneal _____ is indicated for diagnosis of corneal trauma, foreign bodies, corneal abrasions, or corneal ulcers.

28. The client hospitalized in an intensive care unit following major trauma or surgery is at risk for sensory _____.

EXERCISING YOUR CLINICAL JUDGMENT

29. Mrs. Pfannenstiel, the client from the chapter's case study, was most likely having difficulty doing which of the following things if she was scheduled for cataract surgery?
    1. Driving at night
    2. Selecting clothes that matched
    3. Reading a book since letters appeared small
    4. Reading a book because she had double vision

30. Mrs. Pfannenstiel was scheduled for cataract surgery. Which nursing diagnosis would be most appropriate?
    1. *Social isolation*
    2. *High risk for injury*
    3. *Disturbed sensory perception: visual*
    4. *Self-care deficit*

31. You instructed Mrs. Pfannenstiel to wear glasses, tape the metal shield over her operated eye at night, and not do heavy work, such as moving her furniture. Which nursing diagnosis would be most appropriate?
    1. *Social isolation*
    2. *Risk for injury*
    3. *Disturbed sensory perception: visual*
    4. *Self-care deficit*

TEST YOURSELF

32. Your client has double vision, which is also called:
    1. Presbyopia.
    2. Emmetropia.
    3. Diplopia.
    4. Ametropia.

33. Your elderly client has a hearing loss of high-frequency tones that may lead to a loss of all hearing frequencies. What type of hearing loss is this?
    1. Presbycusis
    2. Partial deafness
    3. Conductive loss
    4. Sensorineural

34. During a general assessment of your client's sensory/perceptual status, you asked the client if she was experiencing any numbness or tingling. Which of the following areas were you assessing?
    1. Hearing
    2. Sensation
    3. Vision
    4. Taste

35. You assessed bone conduction by placing the base of a vibrating tuning fork on the client's mastoid process and noting how many seconds passed before he could no longer hear it. Which of the following tests were you performing?
    1. Weber
    2. Rinne
    3. Whisper
    4. Finger-rubbing

36. Your 80-year-old client has had a progressive hearing loss over the past 8 months, has refused to participate in activities at the skilled nursing facility, and has often been found alone in his room. Which nursing diagnosis would be most appropriate?
    1. *Social isolation*
    2. *Altered thought processes*
    3. *Disturbed sensory perception: auditory*
    4. *Self-care deficit*

PRIORITIZATION

37. Prioritize the following steps required when assisting a client to insert a hearing aid.
    1. Perform hand hygiene.
    2. Turn down the volume, and insert the ear mold into the ear canal.
    3. Check that the battery is operating by turning up the volume.
    4. Inspect the hearing aid for cracks or cerumen.
    5. Slowly turn up the volume while speaking in a normal tone of voice until the client indicates that the volume is comfortable.

38. What is the correct manner in which to perform an ear lavage/irrigation?
    1. Explain the procedure to the client, and instruct him to avoid sudden movements.
    2. Cover the client's shoulder with a towel, and ask him to tip his head to the side being irrigated while holding an emesis basin under the ear.
    3. Check the temperature of the irrigant, and select an irrigating device.
    4. Direct the irrigation fluid toward the posterior wall of the ear canal, and lavage with a steady flow of solution.
    5. Examine the ear with an otoscope, and assess for an intact tympanic membrane and signs of otitis media.

39. Prioritize the following problems associated with disturbed sensory perception.
    1. *Impaired nutrition*
    2. *Impaired communication*
    3. *Risk for injury*
    4. *Social isolation*
    5. *Self-care deficit*
    6. *Disturbed thought process*

SUPPORTING VERBAL COMMUNICATION

PURPOSE

This chapter introduces you to the physiological and behavioral concepts underlying *Impaired verbal communication*. The chapter explores factors that affect communication and uses the nursing process as a framework for working with a client who has impaired verbal communication.

MATCHING

1. _____ aphasia
2. _____ articulation
3. _____ Broca's area
4. _____ communication
5. _____ dysarthria
6. _____ dysphagia
7. _____ dysphonia
8. _____ neologism
9. _____ paraphasia
10. _____ phonation
11. _____ resonance
12. _____ telegraphic speech
13. _____ Wernicke's area

a. difficulty swallowing
b. a word substitution problem of the aphasic client who speaks fluently
c. area of the brain that helps control the content of speech and affects auditory and visual comprehension
d. the process of molding sounds into enunciated words and phrases
e. the production of sound by the vibration of the vocal cords
f. the forced vibration of a structure that is related to a source of sound and results in changes in the quality of the sound
g. a complex process in which information is exchanged between two or more people
h. difficulty producing vocal sounds
i. a language disorder that results from brain damage or disease that involves speech centers in the brain
j. the creation of words that are meaningless to the listener; a common language problem of the aphasic client

k. the center of motor speech control
l. impaired articulation
m. telegram-like speech that lacks grammatical elements such as articles, prepositions, and conjunctions

TRUE OR FALSE

14. _____ Vocal abuse, as from cheerleading, smoking, and alcohol abuse; can lead to laryngeal cancer, which may result in loss of the vocal folds and the ability to communicate verbally.
15. _____ Although verbal communication varies from culture to culture, nonverbal communication remains the same.
16. _____ A stimulating environment for a very young child aids in language acquisition.
17. _____ Communication is an important aspect of the nurse-client relationship.
18. _____ Self-concept plays a major role in communication patterns with other people.
19. _____ The use of a team approach is often necessary when working with a client who has impaired verbal communication.
20. _____ Active listening, when used with the client with impaired verbal communication, focuses on the feelings of the client as well as nonverbal cues.
21. _____ Psychiatric illnesses do not affect communication with others.
22. _____ Self-talk involves talking about the activity as it is performed.
23. _____ When either the nurse or the client can speak the other person's language, but not fluently, they each know they are not at risk for misunderstanding the other.

FILL IN THE BLANKS

24. Adult loss of language usually stems from _____ diseases.

25. _____ speech is telegram-like speech that lacks grammatical elements, such as articles, prepositions, and conjunctions.

26. When the client cannot comprehend spoken language and cannot articulate or write words, it is called _____ aphasia.

27. A disorder of voice volume, quality, or pitch, known as _____, can result from damage or disease of the larynx or vagus nerve.

28. A _____ is a temporary or permanent upper airway diversion that results in altered speech production.

29. The nurse should allow ample time for the client with _____ aphasia to respond verbally.

30. An alternative communication method for the client who has had a laryngectomy is the use of _____ speech, which involves eructation of swallowed air.

31. Limiting environmental stimuli and reducing distractions may increase comprehension in the client with _____ aphasia.

32. A client who is unable to communicate due to language barrier, and who has no one who can interpret is likely to have a nursing diagnosis of _____.

33. An endotracheal tube, tracheostomy, or tumor is considered a _____ barrier to communication.

EXERCISING YOUR CLINICAL JUDGMENT

Señor Martinez, the client from the chapter's case study, is a Mexican-American client who has tuberculosis, a communicable disease. You have been asked by the nurse who admitted this client to provide information needed to manage this health problem.

34. If you become concerned that Señor Martinez is responding "yes" to your questions without fully understanding them, you should:
    1. Look for incongruity between the responses and the client's facial expressions.
    2. Assume that he will answer the important questions correctly.
    3. Ask the same question of his wife after the client answers.
    4. Refrain from asking any further questions.

35. After obtaining an interpreter to assist with communication, you would direct your attention to which of the following individuals when obtaining information from Señor Martinez?
    1. The interpreter
    2. Señora Martinez
    3. Señor Martinez
    4. Attend equally to all three

36. If Señor Martinez speaks English to some extent, it would be most appropriate for you to communicate about which of the following before an interpreter becomes available?
    1. Reason for coming to the hospital
    2. Informed consent
    3. Reason for procedures
    4. Medication information

37. You would formulate which of the following expected outcomes for the nursing diagnosis of *Impaired verbal communication* for this client?
    1. Answers all questions correctly
    2. Expresses satisfaction with the communication process
    3. Provides the nurse with sufficient information
    4. Adheres to instructions given while in the hospital

TEST YOURSELF

38. A nurse would assess the client with a tentative diagnosis of laryngitis for speech that is:
    1. Hoarse or soft.
    2. Spoken in a monotone.
    3. Garbled.
    4. Hesitant or deliberate.

39. A client is scheduled to have a tracheostomy performed. The nurse should make alternate plans for communication with this client:
    1. Before the surgery is done.
    2. Just after the client returns from surgery.
    3. On the day following surgery.
    4. As part of the discharge planning process.

40. The home health nurse notes that a client with the nursing diagnoses of *Impaired verbal communication* is frustrated about her ineffective communication skills and does not interact with family and friends as frequently as before. The nurse would tentatively make which of the following additional nursing diagnoses for this client?
    1. *Anxiety*
    2. *Powerlessness*
    3. *Impaired social interaction*
    4. *Altered role performance*

41. The nurse is communicating with a client who has Broca's aphasia. It would be most appropriate to do which of the following to enhance the client's ability to speak?
    1. Give directions in concise, quick, and sharp tones.
    2. Ask the client several questions at once so he or she can formulate answers to all.
    3. Give lengthy, detailed explanations.
    4. Allow ample time for the client to respond to the nurse's communications.

42. The nurse is providing health teaching to adolescents about the risk of brain and spinal cord injuries, which often result in impaired verbal communication. The nurse would encourage these individuals to avoid using which of the following?
    1. Drugs and alcohol
    2. Seatbelts
    3. Helmets
    4. Protective sports equipment

PRIORITIZATION

43. You have been assigned to care for a client who is scheduled for a permanent tracheostomy the next day. Prioritize the following nursing actions to be complete prior to surgery.
    1. Develop an alternative method of communication with the client and significant other to decrease anxiety.
    2. Explain to the client and significant other that speaking ability will be lost after surgery.
    3. Demonstrate the chosen techniques for communication to the client and significant other.
    4. Make arrangements with the speech-language pathologist to meet with the client to discuss long-term methods of effective speech.

44. What is the correct sequence of nursing actions when caring for a client from a different culture?
    1. Utilize a trained medical interpreter to communicate information about tests and procedures.
    2. Assess for a language or cultural barrier.
    3. Observe the client's nonverbal communication.
    4. Use caution when using bilingual friends or family members.

45. When caring for a client with Broca's (expressive) aphasia, the nurse should:
    1. Delay communication if the client is tired or frustrated.
    2. Utilize repeated practice of verbalization.
    3. Begin with questions that require a yes/no answer or movement of the head.
    4. Allow ample time for the client to respond.

MANAGING CONFUSION

PURPOSE

This chapter explores factors that affect normal cognition and concepts that underlie acute and chronic confusion. It describes how to use the nursing process to work with the client experiencing either acute or chronic confusion.

MATCHING

1. _____ affect
2. _____ agnosia
3. _____ apraxia
4. _____ attention
5. _____ awareness
6. _____ cognition
7. _____ confusion
8. _____ consciousness
9. _____ delirium
10. _____ delusions
11. _____ dementia
12. _____ executive function
13. _____ hallucinations
14. _____ judgment
15. _____ memory
16. _____ neurotransmitter
17. _____ orientation
18. _____ pseudo-dementia
19. _____ sundown syndrome

a. the state of being awake and alert enough to react to stimuli; also called *awareness*
b. the retention or storage of information learned about the world
c. false personal beliefs
d. an awareness of person, place, and time
e. the observable expression of feelings or emotions; changes as chronic confusion progresses, as does the client's personality
f. the ability to focus on an object or activity
g. the failure to recognize and identify objects or persons, or know what the use of the object is, despite having knowledge of the characteristic of those objects or persons
h. a severe form of depression resulting from a progressive brain disorder in which cognitive changes mimic those of dementia

i. the state in which the individual experiences or is at risk of experiencing a disturbance in cognition, attention, memory, and orientation of an undetermined origin or onset
j. the process of knowing and interacting with the world; also called *thought*
k. involves multiple cognitive deficits including impairment of memory and judgment, and resulting in a progressive decline in intellectual functioning
l. the state of being awake and alert enough to react to stimuli; also called *consciousness*
m. sensory reactions in the absence of real stimuli
n. the inability to execute or carry out skilled movements and gestures despite the functional ability to perform them
o. a disturbance in consciousness or a change in cognition that develops over a short time
p. the ability to make rational decisions
q. a worsening of behavior that occurs as the sun goes down, especially after dark
r. a constellation of cognitive abilities that include the ability to plan, organize, and sequence tasks and manage multiple tasks simultaneously
s. a chemical messenger released from the synaptic terminal of a neuron at a chemical synapse that diffuses across the synaptic cleft and binds to and stimulates the postsynaptic membrane

TRUE OR FALSE

20. _____ Confusion is a condition that occurs only in the older adult.
21. _____ Acute confusion in the older adult usually develops over hours or days.
22. _____ Perceptual difficulties, such as illusions and hallucinations, may occur in acute confusion.
23. _____ Because cognitive changes occur more slowly with chronic confusion, the client does not lose the ability to judge his or her own safety.
24. _____ The loss of ability to perform activities of daily living occurs in the third stage of chronic confusion.

25. _____ Lack of an appropriate and complete mental status examination can be a barrier to identifying confusion.
26. _____ A child who develops a high fever is at risk for experiencing acute confusion.
27. _____ The nurse should not include attention span when conducting a mental status exam.
28. _____ Anxiety is a common client reaction in both acute and chronic confusion.
29. _____ The nurse should use pale, muted colors or symbols to identify the room of a client with chronic confusion.

FILL IN THE BLANKS

30. Pick's disease is characterized by the formation of Pick's cells in the _____ and _____ lobes of the brain.

31. Cerebral hypoxia due to a medical condition can cause _____ confusion.

32. Acute confusion in the older adult typically occurs at _____.

33. A disrupted _____ rhythm is a classic symptom of acute confusion.

34. Dementia of the _____ type is the most common in older adults.

35. A client who does not brush the hair due to lack of recall about the purpose of the hairbrush is said to have _____.

36. Often an older adult will exhibit a change in mental status with a serious infection instead of a _____.

37. A client who can recall people and events from 30 years ago is said to have an intact _____ memory.

38. A client who is unaware of environmental hazards due to confusion may have the nursing diagnosis *Risk for* _____.

EXERCISING YOUR CLINICAL JUDGMENT

Mr. Tellis, the client from the chapter's case study, has a nursing diagnosis of *Acute confusion* related to disturbances in cerebral metabolism secondary to urinary tract infection as evidenced by agitation, inattention, and fluctuating consciousness. You have been assigned to work with Mr. Tellis on the day after hospital admission.

39. One of the expected outcomes formulated for Mr. Tellis in relation to this nursing diagnosis is "client will experience no injury." Which of the following actions would be most helpful in achieving this outcome?
    1. Restrict visitors as much as possible.
    2. Assist him with ambulation and toileting as needed.
    3. Leave the bed's side rails lowered at all times.
    4. Encourage him to stay in bed by obstructing the path to the bathroom with chairs.

40. Which of the following approaches to communicating with Mr. Tellis will be helpful in minimizing confusion and maintaining the client's dignity?
    1. Divide his care among several staff members.
    2. Give directions quickly and with a firm tone of voice.
    3. Focus on his real message and concerns during conversation.
    4. Quiz him about orientation level with each encounter.

41. Mr. Tellis lost most of his last night's sleep with the events surrounding admission. Which of the following strategies should be used to help reestablish his sleep-wake pattern?
    1. Schedule medications and care to allow for at least one uninterrupted 4-hour block of sleep each night.
    2. Make sure all visitors go home by at least 8 PM.
    3. Keep the door to his room open with the hall lights on.
    4. Encourage frequent naps during the day in case there are unexpected interruptions to sleep at night.

42. Mr. Tellis requires intermittent reorientation to his environment. Which of the following environmental cues would be most helpful?
    1. Bright lighting 24 hours a day
    2. No lighting during nighttime hours
    3. The names of caregivers written on a small pad on the night table
    4. A clock and a calendar on the wall at the foot of the bed

TEST YOURSELF

43. A nurse is conducting a mental status examination for a client who has just immigrated to the United States. Which of the following questions, if asked by the nurse, would be least helpful in determining whether confusion is present?
    1. "What is your name?"
    2. "What did you eat for breakfast?"
    3. "Did any family members visit you today?"
    4. "Who was the first president of the United States?"

44. The nurse who is working with a client with chronic confusion would not assess which of the following factors?
    1. Impaired socialization
    2. A change in level of consciousness
    3. Long-standing cognitive impairment
    4. Altered response to stimuli

45. A client has been placed in a protective environment due to chronic confusion and irreversible dementia. The client has been disoriented to person, place, and time for at least 6 months. Which is the most precise nursing diagnosis for this client?
    1. *Acute confusion*
    2. *Chronic confusion*
    3. *Impaired environmental interpretation syndrome*
    4. *Altered thought processes*

46. A nurse is caring for a client who seems confused and lost a spouse 3 months ago. The nurse would determine that the client is experiencing feelings of depression more than confusion if the client:
    1. Is worse in the morning than any other time of day.
    2. Has visual hallucinations.
    3. Is not preoccupied by certain people or events.
    4. Does not exaggerate and is unaware of inabilities.

47. A confused client is hallucinating that someone is trying to steal his clothing in the closet. The nurse who is looking for a deeper meaning to this episode would pursue which of the following themes in conversation with this client?
    1. Money
    2. Safety
    3. Food
    4. Loneliness

PRIORITIZATION

48. Prioritize the following nursing actions that should be implemented to minimize catastrophic incidents in the chronically confused client.
    1. Identify stressors that trigger combative, compulsive, or violent behaviors.
    2. Provide consistent caregivers.
    3. Prevent fatigue, overstimulation, or changes in the client's routine or environment.
    4. Observe for further illnesses or signs of acute confusion.

49. How can the nurse help the spouse of a client who is chronically confused reduce stress when providing care in a home environment?
    1. Take into account the capabilities of the caregiver.
    2. Encourage ongoing education and input into future planning.
    3. Help the caregiver consider the need for additional resources to prevent exhaustion.
    4. Provide education, resources, support, and information for the caregiver.

50. You are assigned to care for the following clients. Prioritize them in the order in which you will perform your initial assessments.
    1. A 94-year-old client with Alzheimer's disease who is disoriented to place
    2. A 63-year-old client with depression and short-term memory loss
    3. A 57-year-old client with a sudden onset of acute confusion
    4. A 79-year-old client with agnosia who is trying to wash his face with a slice of bread

PROMOTING SELF-CONCEPT

PURPOSE

This chapter introduces you to self-concept, self-esteem, personal identity, role performance, and body image as they relate to clients. It provides direction in using the nursing process in caring for a client with an alteration in one or more of the components of self-concept.

MATCHING

1. ____ body image
2. ____ personal identity
3. ____ role
4. ____ role performance
5. ____ self-concept
6. ____ self-esteem

a. a relatively enduring set of attitudes and beliefs about both the physical self and the psychological self
b. includes the roles a person assumes or is given
c. the organizing principle of the personality that accounts for the unity, continuity, consistency, and uniqueness of a person
d. the degree to which a person has a positive evaluation of self based on perceptions of how one is viewed by others as well as view of the self
e. a person's perception of his or her body
f. a homogeneous set of behaviors, attitudes, beliefs, principles, and values that are normatively defined and expected of someone in a given social position or status in a group

TRUE OR FALSE

7. _____ Self-concept is not a static state but one that develops and changes over time.
8. _____ Low self-esteem can result in lack of confidence and inability to act in one's own best interest.
9. _____ According to Maslow, self-esteem develops after the need for belonging and being loved by others is met.
10. _____ Erikson describes the development of self-esteem in eight stages that correspond to a period in the life span.

11. _____ Research has demonstrated a negative correlation between positive self-esteem and positive health practices.
12. _____ An inability to perform role responsibilities can negatively affect other aspects of self-concept, especially self-esteem.
13. _____ Socioeconomic status has no relationship to self-concept.
14. _____ Loss of a spouse, good job, or previous good health can easily lower self-esteem.
15. _____ Fatigue, illness, and surgery are examples of physiological factors that can affect self-esteem.
16. _____ Nurses should conduct an in-depth assessment of self-concept with all clients.

FILL IN THE BLANKS

17. The four components of self-concept are self-esteem, personal identity, role performance, and _____ _____.

18. At the top of Maslow's hierarchy of needs is _____-_____.

19. According to Erikson's stages of development, adolescence involves development of _____.

20. The ability to influence and control others, according to Coopersmith, is termed _____/_____.

21. The components of personal identity are _____, _____, and _____ images.

22. Self-esteem in infants and preschoolers can be related to the type of _____ a child receives.

23. Behaviors such as smoking, overeating, substance abuse, school difficulties, and early sexual experimentation can be associated with low _____-_____.

24. A sense of powerlessness can result in the nursing diagnosis of _____ *low self-esteem.*

25. If a client has a major change in body structure or function, the nurse should assess the client for the presence of the nursing diagnosis _____ _____ _____.

EXERCISING YOUR CLINICAL JUDGMENT

Nancy Ward, the 43-year-old Navajo woman from the chapter's case study, has a disturbance in self-esteem due to a breast mass that requires biopsy. Recall that Nancy's husband, who died 6 months ago from complications of alcohol abuse, diabetes, and heart disease, abused her physically and emotionally during their marriage. You see Nancy in the clinic when she comes to receive the biopsy results.

26. If you were focusing on the influence of her husband's behavior on Nancy's self-concept, you might have selected which of the following alternate nursing diagnoses?
    1. *Situational low self-esteem*
    2. *Chronic low self-esteem*
    3. *Ineffective role performance*
    4. *Disturbed body image*

27. If you were to focus on how to promote Nancy's feelings of acceptance/worthiness as part of her self-esteem, you would include which of the following people in her care?
    1. Physician and nurse manager of the clinic
    2. Tribal medicine man (shaman) and friend that came to clinic with her
    3. Clinic social worker and billing clerk
    4. Radiologist and continuing care nurse from the affiliated hospital

28. Nancy is told by the physician that the breast mass is cancerous and that surgery will be needed. You would interact with Nancy, expecting that which of the following will be her first reaction?
    1. Shock and disbelief
    2. Anger
    3. Depression
    4. Acceptance

29. In trying to assist Nancy to adjust to the idea of the loss of a breast, you could inquire whether she is interested in talking to which of the following individuals?
    1. The surgeon who took the breast biopsy
    2. The pathologist who did the examination of the breast tissue
    3. Someone from a breast cancer support group who has lost a breast herself
    4. The staff that will be doing her preadmission testing before surgery

30. To foster a sense of power and control in Nancy about her upcoming surgery, you would use which of the following approaches?
    1. Remind Nancy that emotional healing is a matter of determination and courage
    2. Tell Nancy of the scheduled date for surgery as soon as it is known
    3. Give Nancy a list of instructions that must be followed before the surgery
    4. Allow Nancy to make as many decisions about the upcoming procedure as possible

TEST YOURSELF

31. The nurse who is teaching a client with a new colostomy about colostomy care and management is indirectly increasing the client's sense of which of the following?
    1. Competence/mastery
    2. Power/control
    3. Moral worth/virtue
    4. Acceptance/worthiness

32. To reduce the impact of a recent loss on the client's self-concept, the nurse would assist the client to focus on which of the following?
    1. Past religious habits
    2. Personal successful coping skills
    3. The importance of forgetting negative events
    4. The negative attributes of the object of the loss

33. The nurse would look for other evidence of low self-esteem in a client who does which of the following?
    1. Accepts compliments with grace and ease
    2. Takes negative feedback from others in stride
    3. Continually seeks acceptance from others
    4. Is proud of personal accomplishments, but not boastful

34. The nurse would determine that which of the following clients is most at risk for developing issues with self-concept?
    1. A client who must take medication for allergies
    2. A client who gets short of breath after walking up two flights of stairs
    3. A client who has a gallbladder that must be removed
    4. A client who has suffered facial burns

35. A postoperative client who is also the mother of four is overexerting herself with housework and child-care responsibilities. In working with this client, the nurse incorporates the understanding that this client is experiencing a values conflict in which of the following areas of self-esteem?
    1. Competence/mastery
    2. Power/control
    3. Moral worth/virtue
    4. Acceptance/worthiness

36. The nurse is evaluating effects of an intervention on a client's self-concept. If the nurse were interested in using a subjective approach to evaluation, that nurse would select which of the following methods as most appropriate?
    1. The client's self-report of progress
    2. A standardized questionnaire
    3. A rating scale
    4. Observation of the client's behavior

MANAGING ANXIETY

PURPOSE

This chapter introduces you to concepts of anxiety as they are manifested in the health care setting. It uses the nursing process as a framework for interacting with clients experiencing anxiety.

MATCHING

1. _____ adaptation
2. _____ anxiety
3. _____ anxiety disorder
4. _____ anxiolytics
5. _____ fear
6. _____ homeostasis
7. _____ panic
8. _____ vulnerability

a. a serious, chronic medical illness that fills the client's life with overwhelming anxiety and fear becoming progressively worse if not treated

b. medications that act on the central nervous system to reduce the feelings of anxiety and associated symptoms such as muscle tension and restlessness

c. a state of internal stability of physiology and emotions

d. described as a diffuse, highly uncomfortable, sometimes vague sense of apprehension or dread accompanied by one or more physical sensations

e. self-regulation of the whole person in relation to change

f. a vivid, acute state of overwhelming fear with intense physiological, psychological, and behavioral symptoms

g. a feeling of helplessness, lack of control, and inadequate resources when faced with a threat or danger

h. response to a perceived threat that is consciously recognized as danger

TRUE OR FALSE

9. _____ Anxiety is caused by interplay of factors that can be internal, external, or both.

10. _____ A person can actually create or worsen his or her own anxiety.

11. _____ When a client is in a state of panic, he or she may faint or freeze.

12. _____ Anxiety disorders are fairly uncommon in today's society due to the number of medications available.

13. _____ A phobia is a specific type of fear that is often exaggerated and incapacitating.

14. _____ A healthy lifestyle does not make us immune to stress, but may help us to weather it better.

15. _____ Learning theory suggests that anxiety is not a learned behavior.

16. _____ Cognitive characteristics of anxiety can include blocking of thoughts, forgetfulness, and impaired concentration or problem-solving ability.

17. _____ The nursing diagnosis of *Fear* is appropriate when the client has an intense feeling of dread related to an identifiable source that the client can verify.

18. _____ A panic attack is a gradual, discrete feeling of overpowering fright accompanied by physiological symptoms and thoughts of losing control, impending catastrophe, or death.

FILL IN THE BLANKS

19. Anxiety can be considered as falling into one of two primary categories, either a threat to _____ integrity or a threat to _____ integrity.

20. A core dynamic theme found at all levels of anxiety is a sense of _____.

21. In the level of anxiety that is _____, the person's perceptual field is completely distorted.

22. If anxiety impedes daily living and productivity, it is labeled as _____.

23. A client who has a persistent thought, image, or impulse that causes anxiety, and that the client cannot set aside, is said to have an _____.

24. Being admitted to a hospital can be considered to be an _____ factor that produces anxiety.

25. An _____-_____ disorder is marked by uncontrollable thoughts, images, or impulses and behavioral rituals that the client cannot dismiss.

26. Lack of access to health care services due to inadequate insurance is considered to be an _____ factor contributing to anxiety.

EXERCISING YOUR CLINICAL JUDGMENT

Ms. Adkins, the 42-year-old divorced client from the chapter's case study, has a history of cardiac disease and panic attacks. Her 16-year-old son told her before the onset of symptoms that he wishes to move in with his father. While she is being evaluated for a cardiac cause of chest pain, she is also given the nursing diagnosis *Anxiety* by the admitting nurse. You come on duty to relieve the admitting nurse and take over the care of Ms. Adkins.

27. Ms. Adkins tells you that she cannot convince her son to remain living in her home. She goes on to say that she feels that she has no control over her situation or life events. Based on these statements, you might also consider which of the following viable alternate nursing diagnoses for Ms. Adkins?
    1. *Sensory-perceptual alterations*
    2. *Powerlessness*
    3. *Fear*
    4. *Altered thought processes*

28. You identify a short-term goal with Ms. Adkins, which is to identify her own anxiety symptoms and participate in care planning. You determine that she has met the first expected outcome when she is able to:
    1. Verbally identify signs and symptoms of escalating anxiety.
    2. Sleep at least in 6-hour blocks.
    3. Demonstrate relaxation techniques.
    4. Use problem-solving skills.

29. While you are talking with Ms. Adkins, you try to "tune in" to the feelings behind her words. In this instance, you are using which of the following interventions to reduce anxiety?
    1. Communicating a sense of caring
    2. Giving permission
    3. Listening actively
    4. Modifying the environment

TEST YOURSELF

30. The nurse who is assessing for physiological evidence of anxiety in a client would look for:
    1. Bradycardia.
    2. Excessive salivation.
    3. Constricted pupils.
    4. Urinary frequency.

31. The nurse would formulate which of the following expected outcomes to measure whether or not a client has experienced a reduction in anxiety?
    1. Inability to use problem-solving skills
    2. Inability to identify stressors associated with anxiety
    3. Reduced tension, irritability, tremors, and sweating
    4. Lack of participation in decision making

32. The nurse who assesses energy fields and uses appropriate interventions to modulate and balance the energy field is using which of the following forms of complementary therapy?
    1. Relaxation
    2. Music therapy
    3. Spiritual support
    4. Touch therapy

MANAGING VULNERABILITY

PURPOSE

This chapter describes the domains of the Vulnerable Populations Conceptual Model. It identifies factors affecting vulnerability and describes the key components of assessing a vulnerable population. It also describes key interventions for the diagnoses of *Hopelessness* and *Powerlessness* in vulnerable populations.

MATCHING

1. _____ community
2. _____ community forum
3. _____ community health nursing
4. _____ environmental resources
5. _____ epidemiology
6. _____ focus group
7. _____ health status
8. _____ human capital
9. _____ key informant
10. _____ opinion survey
11. _____ parish nurse
12. _____ participant-observation
13. _____ population
14. _____ public health nursing
15. _____ relative risk
16. _____ resource availability
17. _____ social integration
18. _____ social status
19. _____ vulnerable populations
20. _____ windshield survey

a. ratio of the risk of poor health among populations who do not receive resources and are exposed to risk factors compared with those populations who do receive resources and are not exposed to these risk factors

b. the field of nursing that promotes and preserves the health of populations

c. the practice of promoting and protecting the health of populations

d. the position of an individual in relation to others in the society

e. refers to the availability of socioeconomic and environmental resources

f. includes age- and gender-specific morbidity and mortality

g. a method of community assessment that examines formal and informal social systems at work

h. a registered nurse who is employed by (or volunteers for) a religious or health care organization for the purpose of providing nursing care to members of a church congregation

i. includes access to health care and quality of health care

j. social groups who have limited resources and consequently are at high risk for myriad health-related problems

k. a method of data collection in which the researcher drives through a neighborhood to conduct a general assessment of that neighborhood through observation

l. the study of the cause and distribution of disease, disability, and death among groups of people

m. a method of data collection in which 6 to 12 people from a group or aggregate are brought together for discussion and guided when necessary by a skilled, nonjudgmental leader

n. having a harmonious relationship with society in which the person participates as a full member of the society

o. includes income, jobs, education, and housing. Poverty, social inequality, poor educational resources, and limited vocational resources are just a few of the socioeconomic constraints found in vulnerable populations

p. a community leader, professional, politician, or businessperson who possesses knowledge of the needs of the community and who can act as a useful source of data and a supporter of new programs

q. a method of data collection performed through telephone interviews, mailed questionnaires, door-to-door interviews, or at clinic sites

r. a group of people who share common characteristics, such as an environment and common needs

s. a geographic location, or an aggregate or population of individuals who have one or more personal or environmental characteristics in common

t. an open meeting in which members of a community or group may come to share opinion and concerns about a particular issue

TRUE OR FALSE

21. _____ Resource availability includes human capital, social integration, social status, and access to health care.

22. _____ For adolescent girls, the combination of high socioeconomic status, poor academic achievement, lack of available jobs, and the resultant feelings of low self-esteem may lead to pregnancy as the only reasonable alternative.

23. _____ For a person to have hope, there must be a desire and some expectation that the desire will be fulfilled.

24. _____ A client who has a perception of power seeks knowledge and takes action to affect the outcome of the illness or to manage health.

25. _____ Hope cannot be present when the client feels no ability to control a situation.

26. _____ Both hope and power have to do with a client's ability to achieve goals.

27. _____ Only clients can empower themselves.

FILL IN THE BLANKS

28. The Vulnerable Populations Conceptual Model provides a framework for understanding the relationships among the limited resource availability, the health-related _____ factors, and the _____ status of vulnerable populations.

29. Human capital includes income, jobs, education, and _____.

30. _____ _____ is reflected in power to control the political process and the distribution of resources.

31. _____ isolation is one of the well-known risks of elderly persons who live alone in the community.

32. Hope on the unconscious level is a life force that provides the _____ to drive the individual forward.

33. The primary distinction between *Hopelessness* and *Powerlessness* rests in the concept of _____.

34. To empower another individual, you need to respect the individual's capacity for _____-_____.

EXERCISING YOUR CLINICAL JUDGMENT

Brenda Carter, the client from the chapter's case study, is a single mother living alone with her 2-year-old child. She tells you, "I am just stuck here with this baby with no chance to do nothing." She is socially isolated and has been in abusive relationships.

35. During your nursing assessment, you asked Brenda about her safety in her neighborhood. This would be an example of which type of needs assessment?
   1. Physical
   2. Psychological
   3. General
   4. Social

36. Brenda has broken off relations with her parents. She tells you she misses them. A potential nursing intervention would be to:
   1. Acknowledge her parents' disappointment with her.
   2. Help her contact her parents.
   3. Encourage her to make a new life for herself and her baby.
   4. Have her attend group counseling for pregnant teenagers.

37. You have been working with Brenda to help her deal with her feelings of hopelessness due to her parents' refusal to allow her to return home. She says that they told her, "You wanted to be an adult, now act like one." Brenda was diagnosed as suffering from *Hopelessness*. A few weeks later, she tells you that she has accepted living at the local home for unwed mothers and no longer feels hopeless about her situation. Your evaluation of *Hopelessness* may mean that she:
   1. Needs to continue trying to win her parents back.
   2. Has achieved acceptance of her situation, which cannot be changed at this time.
   3. Should immediately be referred to mental health for counseling about her parents' rejection of her.
   4. Is unrealistic about her situation.

TEST YOURSELF

38. Vulnerable social groups include which of the following?
    1. People subjected to intolerance, the poor, and those associated with a stigma
    2. Teenagers and people living in rural areas
    3. Infants and clients older than 60 years of age
    4. Those with resources, as well as children and the elderly

39. Your client has been diagnosed with breast cancer. She believes that through her own actions, behaviors, or personal characteristics she can affect her outcome. She feels in control of her situation. This is an example of which concept?
    1. "Power over"
    2. Human capital
    3. Hope
    4. Personal control

40. At the health department's teen clinic, adolescent girls and teen mothers are routinely screened for symptoms of conflict with their parents and with their partners. This is an example of which type of assessment of vulnerability?
    1. Hopelessness
    2. Physical needs
    3. Social needs
    4. Psychological needs

41. As a nurse, you can offer a client hope by:
    1. Offering empathy or understanding of the client's feelings associated with being in a desolate situation.
    2. Calling the mental health center and getting the client an appointment.
    3. Referring the client to the public health department for follow-up care.
    4. Telling the client to improve his or her self-esteem.

42. Your client has been diagnosed with diabetes. You can empower the client by:
    1. Helping the client to develop, obtain, and use resources.
    2. Calling the American Diabetes Association to obtain information for the client.
    3. Referring the client to the outpatient diabetic program.
    4. Waiting until the client requests help.

PURPOSE

This chapter discusses key concepts related to rehabilitation, common conditions that require rehabilitative services, role changes following injury, and the roles of various members of the interdisciplinary team. It cites assessment tools that can be used for a person with a functional disability and major nursing diagnoses for a person with a spinal cord injury.

MATCHING

1. _____ activities of daily living (ADLs)
2. _____ chronic illness
3. _____ chronicity
4. _____ community reintegration
5. _____ functional limitations
6. _____ instrumental activities of daily living
7. _____ interdisciplinary team
8. _____ phychosocial adaptation
9. _____ rehabilitation
10. _____ rehabilitation nursing

a. the process of adaptation or recovery, through which an individual suffering from a disabling condition, whether temporary or irreversible, participates to regain or attempts to regain maximum function, independence, and restoration

b. difficulties people may experience in performing activities of daily living (ADLs) or instrumental activities of daily living (IADLs)

c. the basic activities usually performed in the course of a normal day in a person's life such as eating, toileting, dressing, bathing, or brushing the teeth

d. food preparation, housekeeping, laundry, transportation, using the telephone, shopping, and handling finances

e. a group of people working together with the client to achieve mutually established goals for rehabilitation

f. a process by which a person adjusts, copes, or responds to changes that occur as a result of living with a physical or mental limitation or chronic illness

g. all impairments or deviations from normal that have one or more of the following characteristics: are permanent; leave residual disability; are caused by a nonreversible pathological condition; require special training of the client for rehabilitation; or are expected to require a long period of supervision, observation, or care

h. a broad term that encompasses chronic illnesses as well as disease or congenital defects that permanently alter a person's previous health status

i. the return and acceptance of a disabled person as a participating member of the community

j. a specialty in which nurses specialize in caring for people with functional limitations or disabilities

TRUE OR FALSE

11. _____ *Ineffective role performance* is the nursing diagnosis that applies when there is an adverse change in the way a person perceives or enacts a role.

12. _____ It is estimated that about 19% of the U.S. population has some form of disability.

13. _____ The Association of Rehabilitation Nurses (ARN) is the specialty organization for rehabilitation nurses.

14. _____ A prosthetist helps fit braces, orthoses, and adaptive equipment to assist with normal movement and prevent secondary complications.

15. _____ Assisted living facilities provide interdisciplinary care to people who do not require hospitalization but whose needs for care exceed availability from informal community resources.

16. _____ Environmental factors that can affect the ability and disability of clients with functional limitations include the person's living situation, workplace, or time spent in leisure activities.

17. _____ For a client who has functional limitations, you have primary responsibility for documentation of the overall health status and functional assessment.

18. _____ The client with sensory neglect may have minor neglect or be experiencing a more severe form, in which a body part, most often a paralyzed arm, is not recognized.

FILL IN THE BLANKS

19. Disabilities can be a result of _____, chronic illness, congenital defect, or _____ _____.

20. Nurses who care for those with functional limitations become experts in _____ and psychosocial assessment, _____ and bladder management, _____ care, nutrition, behavior, teaching, and family participation.

21. Clients with long-term health alterations often use prayer as a _____ mechanism and look to God or another spiritual being as a source of comfort.

22. _____ living facilities combine shelter with other support services, such as meals, housekeeping, and personal care.

23. The _____ with _____ Act is a significant piece of legislation that advocates for those with disabilities.

24. The _____ _____ _____ (FIM) scale is one of the most reliable and valid tools for measuring functional status.

25. Goals in rehabilitation are aimed at _____ function and preventing _____.

EXERCISING YOUR CLINICAL JUDGMENT

26. Which type of health care professional would most likely assess the range of motion, mobility, strength, balance, and gait of Robert, the 18-year-old client from the chapter's case study, who has a complete C5-6 spinal cord injury?
    1. Recreational therapist
    2. Physical therapist
    3. Rehabilitation nurse
    4. Occupational therapist

27. Robert receives respite care. What type of service does this represent?
    1. Help with home maintenance
    2. Comprehensive services requiring medical care that can be managed at home
    3. Assistance with personal care
    4. Temporary service enabling informal caregivers to take a break from their caregiving responsibilities

28. Robert is unable to perform most of the basic self-care activities such as feeding, bathing, and toileting. What nursing diagnosis would be appropriate?
    1. *Self-care deficit*
    2. *Impaired physical mobility*
    3. *Activity intolerance*
    4. *Risk for injury*

TEST YOURSELF

29. Which term is appropriate to describe the difficulties that your clients who have functional disabilities face with their physical challenges in performing ADLs?
    1. Impairment
    2. Functional limitations
    3. Chronicity
    4. Handicap

30. Your client receives assistance from homemaker services. What type of help does she receive?
    1. Help with home maintenance
    2. Comprehensive services requiring medical care that can be managed at home
    3. Assistance with personal care
    4. Temporary service enabling informal caregivers to take a break from their caregiving responsibilities

31. When your client's family is evaluating a nursing home for their frail, elderly family member, they ask the staff what infection-control measures are enforced. This question helps to evaluate which area of a nursing home assessment?
    1. Social, educational, recreational, and religious activities
    2. Location
    3. Safety
    4. Living environment

32. Your client with hemiplegia as a result of a stroke has tactile impairments. Which nursing diagnosis would be most appropriate for the problems associated with tactile impairments?
    1. *Self-care deficit*
    2. *Impaired physical mobility*
    3. *Disturbed sensory perception*
    4. *Risk for injury*

33. Falls are a common problem among older adults with reduced functional capacity and a major factor contributing to dependence. Which nursing diagnosis would be appropriate?
    1. *Self-care deficit*
    2. *Impaired physical mobility*
    3. *Disturbed sensory perception*
    4. *Risk for injury*

MANAGING LOSS

PURPOSE

This chapter discusses key concepts that relate to the nursing diagnoses of *Anticipatory grieving, Dysfunctional grieving*, and *Imminent death*. It describes a focused assessment of a dying client. It also discusses interventions to help the client and family feel understood and facilitate grief work.

MATCHING

1. _____ anger
2. _____ anticipatory grief
3. _____ bereavement
4. _____ code status
5. _____ denial
6. _____ disenfranchised grief
7. _____ dysfunctional/complicated grief
8. _____ grief
9. _____ grief attack
10. _____ grief work
11. _____ hospice
12. _____ loss
13. _____ mourning
14. _____ normal grief
15. _____ palliative care
16. _____ searching
17. _____ selective attention
18. _____ sense of presence
19. _____ thanatology

a. to rob or have something of value removed; is traditionally defined as being deprived through death, such as a widow who is deprived by the death of her husband

b. discipline of study and research that deals with death and death-related topics

c. the act of choosing when and to whom a person will give attention regarding a loss and allow thoughts and feelings to enter the conscious mind

d. occurs as the denial and disbelief are replaced with the growing awareness of reality

e. an unexpected, involuntary resurgence of acute grief-related emotions and behaviors triggered by routine events and sometimes accompanied by uncontrollable crying or emotional display

f. a term used to identify the specific orders for a client regarding whether to begin resuscitative actions, and the extent of those actions, at the time of a cardiac or respiratory arrest

g. a nonthreatening, comforting perception by the bereaved of the deceased's presence

h. the effort by a grieving person to acknowledge the physical and psychological pain associated with bereavement and to integrate the loss into the future

i. encompasses a very diverse and unique set of emotions and responses

j. the extended, unsuccessful use of intellectual and emotional responses by which individuals, families, and communities attempt to work through the process of modifying self-concept based on the perception of loss

k. grief that lacks social acknowledgment, validation, and support for the bereaved

l. the term used to describe social and cultural acts and expressions used by a bereaved person to convey thoughts and feelings of sorrow

m. a philosophical concept of providing palliative or supportive care to dying persons in which the goal of care at or near the end of life is to accentuate living and enhance the quality of life

n. involves the intellectual and emotional responses and behaviors by which individuals, families, and communities attempt to work through the process of modifying self-concept based on the perception of potential loss

o. the removal, change, or reduction in value of something valued or held dear and the feelings that result

p. refers to conscious and unconscious efforts by the bereaved to negate the reality of the loss through finding the deceased alive and well

q. an intellectual process that does not alter reality but is used to help the person cope with the undesired reality

r. the active total care of patients whose disease is not responsive to curative treatment, where control of pain, of other symptoms, and of psychological distress and spiritual distress is paramount

s. emotional, physical, cognitive, and behavioral responses to bereavement, separation, or loss

TRUE OR FALSE

20. _____ Mourning honors the dead and helps manage emptiness after death.
21. _____ Normal grieving can lead to lifelong problems and breakdowns in psychological and physical health.
22. _____ The ultimate loss a person faces is his own death.
23. _____ Normal anticipatory grief includes making plans for living after an ill person dies.
24. _____ Until the reality of the loss has been acknowledged, further grief work is constrained.
25. _____ Seldom do people have feelings of relief or emancipation from burdens after a person's death.
26. _____ If you are comfortable facing the reality of your own death, you will find it difficult to provide support to others facing these same circumstances and issues.

FILL IN THE BLANKS

27. Acts of mourning include _____ rituals, expressions of _____, and _____ practices.

28. The loss of _____ is recognized as the ultimate loss.

29. Cultural and societal mores commonly govern the behavioral responses associated with the _____ phase of grieving.

30. During the _____ phase, the mind comes to clearly understand that the loss is irreversible and that life has changed irrevocably.

31. When planning care for a terminally ill client, you are really caring for two clients, the dying person and the immediate _____ unit.

32. The most important intervention during the recognition: shock and denial phase of grief may be simply your _____.

33. _____ by other nurses or health care team members about attachments and feelings for clients in your care is detrimental both to you and to team dynamics.

EXERCISING YOUR CLINICAL JUDGMENT

34. Mr. Hashimoto, the 54-year-old first-generation Japanese-American client from the chapter's case study, died with his family by his side. After his death, his wife became nauseated, had abdominal cramping, and vomited. She felt heart palpitations and had trouble swallowing. She was in which phase of the grieving process?
    1. Dysfunctional grieving
    2. Recognition: shock and denial
    3. Reflection: physical, emotional, and spiritual suffering
    4. Redirection: reorganization and moving forward

35. Mr. Hashimoto did not talk to staff about his loss because he felt that they were not receptive to his concerns. This is an example of which type of cognitive denial?
    1. Selective attention
    2. Deception
    3. True denial
    4. Anger

36. A year after Mr. Hashimoto's death, Mrs. Hashimoto continues to experience periods of acute grief-related emotions and behaviors triggered by routine events and sometimes accompanied by uncontrollable crying or emotional display. Which type of psychological response is she experiencing?
    1. Sense of presence
    2. Intrusive memories
    3. Grief attacks
    4. Dysfunctional grief

TEST YOURSELF

37. Nurses wore a black band on their nurses' caps at the time of Florence Nightingale's death. This is an example of:
    1. Bereavement
    2. Mourning
    3. Loss
    4. Grief

38. This phase of the grief reaction has been called the "listen now, hear later" phase because it grants the grieving person time to buffer the truth while mobilizing coping resources to face the truth of a loss.
    1. Reflection: physical, emotional, and spiritual suffering
    2. Anticipatory grieving
    3. Recognition: shock and denial
    4. Redirection: reorganization and moving ahead

39. Sometimes a person develops physical symptoms experienced earlier by the deceased person, especially pains or specific somatic symptoms associated with the death. This is an example of which type of dysfunctional grief?
    1. Chronic
    2. Delayed
    3. Exaggerated
    4. Masked

40. Meeting the client's physical needs promptly, scheduling pain medications so they are being delivered to the client at the exact administration times, and touching and talking to the dying person are interventions to promote healthy grieving during which phase?
    1. Reflection: physical, emotional, and spiritual suffering
    2. Anticipatory grieving
    3. Recognition: shock and denial
    4. Redirection: reorganization and moving ahead

MAINTAINING SEXUAL HEALTH

PURPOSE

This chapter discusses key concepts that relate to the nursing diagnoses *Ineffective sexuality patterns* and *Sexual dysfunction*. It discusses general concepts and the biological, psychological, social, and cultural influences on development of sexuality. It also describes issues in the health care of lesbian women and gay men.

MATCHING

1. ____ androgyny
2. ____ arousal
3. ____ bisexual
4. ____ gender
5. ____ gender identity
6. ____ gender role
7. ____ heterosexual
8. ____ homophobia
9. ____ homosexual
10. ____ libido
11. ____ orgasm
12. ____ sexual desire
13. ____ sexual dysfunction
14. ____ sexual identity
15. ____ sexual orientation
16. ____ sexual patterns
17. ____ sexual response cycle
18. ____ sexuality

a. the state or quality of being sexual, including the collective characteristics that distinguish male and female
b. refers to a person's sex, either male or female
c. may be referred to as sexual identity, which is the internal belief or sense that one is male or female
d. may be referred to as gender identity, which is the internal belief or sense that one is male or female
e. refers to the outward appearance, behaviors, attitudes, and feelings deemed appropriate for males and females
f. an anthropological term; means that a person may display both male and female characteristics and may relate to both a male and female gender identity and role

g. refers to a person's sexual attraction and feelings of erotic potential toward a partner or toward members of either sex
h. type of sexual orientation in which one is attracted to members of the opposite gender
i. type of sexual orientation in which one is attracted to members of the same gender
j. type of sexual orientation in which one may be attracted to members of either gender
k. person's chosen expressions of sexuality
l. a wish to participate in sexual intimacy that is activated by thoughts, fantasies, emotions, and psychological wants and needs
m. physical and emotional stimuli heighten desire and begin the physiological changes that mark the sexual response cycle
n. a highly pleasurable involuntary response in which the clitoris, vagina, and uterus of the female or the penis of the male undergoes repeated muscular contractions
o. the conscious or unconscious sex drive or desire to pleasure or satisfy
p. implies a change or disruption in sexual health or function that the affected person views as unrewarding or inadequate
q. a fear of becoming homosexual through contact with lesbians and gay men or of having close or intimate feelings toward someone of the same sex
r. the four phases of bodily responses that occur during sexual arousal as identified by Masters and Johnson

TRUE OR FALSE

19. _____ Puberty is a physiologically stressful time.
20. _____ Gender identity is an external belief that one is either male or female.
21. _____ Sexual patterns generally fit with the prevailing expectations of a particular culture or society.
22. _____ A characteristic of being sexually healthy includes a person's willingness to make adjustments in sexual functioning when limitations of illness, injury, unavailability of a partner, or other situations occur.

23. _____ Nurses routinely discuss their client's sexual health and concerns.

24. _____ Numerous health problems can have a biochemical effect on sexual energy and the ability to engage in sex.

25. _____ It is a myth that it is best for a man to be on the bottom during sex after a heart attack.

FILL IN THE BLANKS

26. A person's sexuality is a vital component of health and is influenced by _____, psychological, social, and _____ forces.

27. Awareness of sexual feelings usually does not occur until _____, at the onset of mature sexuality.

28. _____ is a highly pleasurable involuntary response in which the clitoris, vagina, and uterus of the female or the penis of the male undergoes repeated muscular contractions.

29. The World Health Organization describes sexual health as the integration of somatic, _____, intellectual, and social aspects of sexual being in ways that are enriching and that enhance personality, communication, and _____.

30. Your anxiety or _____ in discussing sexual concerns will be communicated to your client.

31. A vital part of your assessment of a client with altered sexuality patterns is to understand the client's _____ knowledge and attitudes.

32. You should encourage children to tell a parent, teacher, or other trusted adult when a _____ is uncomfortable for them.

EXERCISING YOUR CLINICAL JUDGMENT

33. Lisa Simonelli, the 46-year-old client from this chapter's case study who was diagnosed with breast cancer and had a mastectomy 5 years earlier, expresses general concern regarding her sexuality. Which of the following nursing diagnoses would be most appropriate?
    1. *Ineffective sexuality patterns*
    2. *Sexual dysfunction*
    3. *Ineffective individual coping*
    4. *Hopelessness*

34. Ms. Simonelli states that she is feeling unattractive and expresses concern about the results of her biopsy. In addition, she reports she has had no intercourse with her husband for the past 3 months. With this expanded database of information, which of the following nursing diagnoses might the nurse also consider?
    1. *Ineffective sexuality patterns*
    2. *Sexual dysfunction*
    3. *Ineffective individual coping*
    4. *Hopelessness*

35. Ms. Simonelli is fearful of disclosing her personal anxieties and beliefs about sex. You assure her that sometimes sharing personal information is necessary to provide the best possible health care. This is an example of which step of the PLISSIT model?
    1. Permission
    2. Limited information
    3. Specific suggestions
    4. Intensive therapy

TEST YOURSELF

36. Gender roles (e.g., whether a wife is encouraged to cut the wood for the fireplace) refer to which of the following?
    1. Outward appearance, behaviors, attitudes, and feelings deemed appropriate for males and females
    2. Internal belief that one is male or female
    3. Awareness and feelings of being male or female
    4. A person's chosen expressions of sexuality

37. During which phase of the sexual response cycle does a male experience the following: the head of the penis enlarges slightly, the scrotum thickens further and tenses, and two or three drops of preorgasmic fluid emerge from the head of the penis?
    1. Excitement
    2. Plateau
    3. Orgasm
    4. Resolution

38. Your client was raised to think that sexual intercourse is disgusting and dirty. This is an example of what kind of factor that affects sexuality?
    1. Developmental
    2. Psychological
    3. Physiological
    4. Psychiatric disorder

39. After your client had heart surgery, what advice would you give him about maintaining his sexual patterns?
    1. "It is best for you to be on the bottom during sex."
    2. "Impotence and lack of sex drive always occur after a heart attack."
    3. "If angina occurs during sex, you should permanently stop having sex."
    4. "You can safely resume sex within a few weeks or as soon as you feel ready."

40. Your client, a 12-year-old boy, masturbates. His minister says that masturbation is sinful. Your client is concerned that he is not normal. Which of the following nursing diagnoses would be most appropriate?
    1. *Ineffective sexuality patterns*
    2. *Sexual dysfunction*
    3. *Ineffective individual coping*
    4. *Hopelessness*

SUPPORTING STRESS TOLERANCE AND COPING

PURPOSE

This chapter introduces you to the concepts of physiological and psychological stress, and the factors affecting one's ability to cope with stress. It provides guidelines on using the nursing process to work effectively with clients who are experiencing stress in their lives.

MATCHING

1. _____ adaptation
2. _____ adaptive coping
3. _____ anxiety
4. _____ coping
5. _____ crisis
6. _____ defense mechanism
7. _____ developmental crisis
8. _____ homeostasis
9. _____ maladaptive coping
10. _____ psychoneuroimmunology
11. _____ resilience
12. _____ situational crisis
13. _____ stress
14. _____ stressor

a. the study of the interface between the brain and immunology
b. the tendency of biological systems to maintain relatively constant conditions in the internal environment, while continuously interacting with and adjusting to changes originating within or outside the system
c. mental processes used, without planning or even full awareness, to protect or defend one's (psychological) self from stress and maintain psychological homeostasis
d. an individual's ability to recover from or successfully cope with both internal and external stresses
e. a physiological response produced by the normal wear and tear of bodily processes and external and internal demands
f. a physically or psychologically hazardous situation that is not easily anticipated and for which a person is inadequately prepared

g. any effort directed toward management of dangerous, threatening, or challenging situations
h. the description of a stress-causing agent
i. an upset in a balanced or stable state for which the usual methods of adaptation and coping are not sufficient
j. occurs when a person is unable to complete the tasks needed for a particular developmental level
k. a vague uneasy feeling, the source of which is often nonspecific or unknown to the individual
l. process through which individuals accommodate changes in the internal or external environment to preserve functioning and pursue goals
m. feelings and behavior that decrease the quality of life and lead to unhealthy outcomes
n. a process that fosters problem solving, growth, and development, and the ability to perceive reality and respond in a way that supports emotional and physical well-being

TRUE OR FALSE

15. _____ Stress results from attempts to balance internal and external environmental demands.
16. _____ In the resistance stage of the physiological stress response, the body cannot function defensively against the stressor.
17. _____ Lack of unconditional love can precipitate a developmental crisis in an infant.
18. _____ Sublimation involves using an excuse to justify behavior while disguising an unconscious motive.
19. _____ When assessing for stress tolerance and coping, it is helpful to ask clients if they are worrying about anything.
20. _____ Stress can cause some diseases and exacerbate others.
21. _____ What is stressful for one person in almost all cases is also stressful for another.
22. _____ Compensation is acting toward a stranger as if he or she were a significant other.

23. _____ Although all people react uniquely to stress, some have more reserve or capacity to resist challenges to self-integrity.

FILL IN THE BLANKS

24. The first stage of the physiological stress response is the _____ _____ stage.

25. A person in _____ is faced with overwhelming adaptive tasks.

26. There are two major types of crises: _____ and _____.

27. A person who attributes unacceptable thoughts or feelings to others is using the defense mechanism of _____.

28. How a person tolerates and copes with stress is influenced by _____, lifestyle, culture, and _____ _____.

29. The _____ nervous system activity increases heart rate, cardiac output, respiratory rate, muscle tension, mental alertness, and glucose levels during a stressful event.

30. Both anxiety- and crisis-provoking situations challenge a person's _____ skills.

31. An inability to have children is generally considered a developmental crisis of _____.

32. At certain stages of coping, _____ is a useful and healthy defense mechanism that permits a client to retain hope and allows an individual to organize more effective ways of adapting to a stressful event.

EXERCISING YOUR CLINICAL JUDGMENT

Billy Osceola, the Native American client from the chapter's case study, is diabetic, drinks alcohol, and has developed signs of stump infection following a recent left below-knee amputation. He was using a special herbal concoction made by the shaman to treat the painful stump area. After resisting attempts by a home health nurse to work with him in his home, he is ultimately readmitted to the hospital for treatment of the infection. You are now assigned to Mr. Osceola's care.

33. Based on your knowledge of Mr. Osceola thus far, you would select which of the following nursing diagnoses as most appropriate for him at this time?
   1. *Altered thought processes*
   2. *Ineffective denial*
   3. *Ineffective family coping*
   4. *Anxiety*

34. As a first step to assisting Mr. Osceola work through the stress of the amputation and its consequences, you would try to:
   1. Confront his denial of the infection before admission.
   2. Get a consult with a psychiatrist.
   3. Establish a therapeutic relationship.
   4. Make him identify past coping strategies.

35. If you wish to help Mr. Osceola cope by helping him gain control through knowledge, you would focus on teaching him:
   1. Relaxation and deep-breathing techniques.
   2. The relationship of his diabetes and drinking to the surgery he just had.
   3. That the medicine man, or shaman, is not very helpful in matters such as these.
   4. How to prevent further infection, control diabetes, and increase mobility.

36. Mr. Osceola shares with you that he finds comfort in listening to tribal music, especially the beat of the drums. Using knowledge of various coping methods, you would teach and encourage him to use which of the following while listening to this music?
   1. Relaxation
   2. Adaptive thinking
   3. Self-suggestion
   4. Coping thoughts

TEST YOURSELF

37. A coping method that is not conducive to alleviating stress in a healthy way would be:
   1. Listening to music.
   2. Overeating.
   3. Talking to others about the stressor.
   4. Crying or singing as an emotional release.

38. When working with a client experiencing a major stressor, the nurse would protect the client's "vulnerable self" by doing which of the following?
    1. Immediately breaking down any denial.
    2. Enlisting the help of the client's social supports.
    3. Helping the client identify inner strengths that can be used in this situation.
    4. Telling the client about the negative physiological effects of stress.

39. The nurse who is teaching relaxation techniques to a client would most likely incorporate which of the following methods in discussions with the client?
    1. Deep breathing and guided imagery
    2. Self-suggestion and coping thoughts
    3. Coping thoughts and inner dialog
    4. Adaptive thinking and self-suggestion

40. A client under extreme stress has come to the emergency room expressing thoughts of suicide. The nurse should take which of the following most appropriate actions?
    1. Locate and obtain resources to help with the crisis.
    2. Document the findings and then discharge the client to home.
    3. Encourage the client to resume antidepressant medications.
    4. Leave the client alone in a room to provide opportunity for reflective thought.

SUPPORTING FAMILY COPING

PURPOSE

This chapter describes the concepts of family, family function, family relationships, and caregiving. Family assessment criteria are identified as well as factors affecting an individual's ability to provide care family coping. The chapter provides potential nursing diagnoses that may be appropriate for family coping and caregiving. It provides goal-directed interventions to prevent or correct family problems and *Caregiver role strain*.

MATCHING

1. _____ caregiver
2. _____ caregiver burden
3. _____ caregiver burnout
4. _____ caregiver stress
5. _____ caring
6. _____ closed system
7. _____ coping patterns
8. _____ dysfunctional families
9. _____ extended family
10. _____ family
11. _____ family-centered nursing
12. _____ family dynamics
13. _____ intergenerational family
14. _____ nuclear family
15. _____ objective caregiver burden
16. _____ open system
17. _____ role conflict
18. _____ role stress
19. _____ single-parent family
20. _____ subjective caregiver burden
21. _____ system

a. its unit includes the nuclear family as well as other relatives such as aunts, uncles, cousins, and grandparents who are committed to maintaining family ties

b. a set of integrated, interacting parts that function as a whole, with structure and patterns of function that accomplish the work of the whole

c. an emotion that occurs when a person has difficulty meeting the demands of a role

d. health care that focuses on the health of the family as a unit, as well as the maintenance and improvement in the health and growth of each person in that unit

e. a system that exchanges matter, energy, and information with other systems and with the environment

f. households in which the children live with one parent, usually because of divorce, out-of-wedlock births, or the death of a spouse

g. a depletion of physical and mental energy caused by providing care for a chronically ill person over a long period

h. more than one generation of a family living together in one residence or within a small geographical area

i. two or more people united by a common goal to create a physical, cultural, spiritual, and nurturing bond

j. refers to the visible, tangible costs to the caregiver as measured in required behaviors or disruptions

k. one who provides care to a dependent or partially dependent family member or friend

l. incompatible expectations for behavior within a role, between two or more roles, or when a role is incongruent with a person's beliefs and values

m. composed of a husband, a wife, and their child/children living in a common household with one or both spouses gainfully employed

n. refers to strain or load borne by a family member who cares for an elderly, chronically ill, or disabled family member

o. refers to the caregiver's personal appraisal of a caregiving situation and the extent to which the person perceives it to be a burden

p. a set of integrated interacting parts that function as a whole and do not interact with other systems or the environment

q. the specific protective behaviors used by an individual or a family to respond to stressful situations

r. the ever-changing pattern of interaction among family members; it is the forces at work within the family that create patterns of behavior

s. a behavior of having regard for, cherishing, protecting, being responsible for, or attending to the needs of others

t. refers to the caregiver's reaction to physical, emotional, sociocultural, financial, and environmental stressors brought on by the caregiving experience

u. a family that cannot meet the needs of the family or functions in way that is harmful to its members

TRUE OR FALSE

22. _____ The family is the basic social unit of society and has needs as a unit.
23. _____ The healthy family is an open system with complex interactions both within the family and in the external world.
24. _____ An unhealthy family will show genuine interest in learning to help the client.
25. _____ The family may or may not recognize that their coping is compromised.
26. _____ An appropriate nursing intervention to establish a nurse-family relationship is active listening.
27. _____ Interventions provided when a family is stressed or not focused are more easily remembered and accepted.
28. _____ *Caregiver role strain* may be minimized when the recipient and the caregiver predetermine how and by whom the care will be provided.
29. _____ Caregivers are more likely to experience *Caregiver role strain* when they have adequate support systems.
30. _____ An example of a cue that a family is at risk for *Caregiver role strain* is resurfacing of childhood issues with siblings.
31. _____ Financial costs associated with caregiving can cause many families to experience financial difficulties.

FILL IN THE BLANKS

32. The nurse must assess the needs of the _____ as well as the ill family member.

33. The primary functions of a family include the_____, _____ and social placement, reproductive, economic, and _____ care functions.

34. Family _____ is the family unit's method of managing the stressors of family life.

35. Your first visit to the family is definitive in establishing a _____ relationship.

36. In many cases, caregivers enter their roles with _____ feelings.

37. Caregiver _____ refers to the caregiver's reaction to physical, emotional, sociocultural, financial, and environmental stressors brought on by the caregiving experience.

38. The caregiver's _____ of the burden, rather than the perception of other family members or health care providers, determines the impact on his or her life.

39. Many caregivers do not have _____ into the role responsibilities involved in the day-to-day care of a dependent care receiver.

EXERCISING YOUR CLINICAL JUDGMENT

40. Mrs. Roddy's daughter, the client from the chapter's case study, quit work to care for her ill mother. As a result, she is experiencing financial hardship. Her stress originates from which one of the following sources?
    1. Interfamily
    2. Extrafamily
    3. Intrafamily
    4. Community

41. Mrs. Roddy is deteriorating physically and mentally. She is currently hospitalized, but her daughter insists that she be discharged to her home as opposed to a skilled nursing facility. The daughter is going to have to learn how to care for her mother's tracheostomy, gastrostomy tube feedings, indwelling catheter, heparin lock, and multiple medications. Which of the following nursing diagnosis is most appropriate for her daughter?
    1. *Risk for caregiver role strain.*
    2. *Caregiver role strain.*
    3. *Risk for injury.*
    4. *Ineffective management of therapeutic regimen.*

42. As a home health nurse, you develop a plan of care with Mrs. Roddy's daughter that includes having a home health aide bathe Mrs. Roddy three times a week. This is an example of which nursing intervention?
    1. Engaging the assistance of family and friends
    2. Encouraging social support
    3. Setting realistic goals
    4. Providing direct assistance

TEST YOURSELF

43. A husband and wife could not agree on whose responsibility it was to clean their house. The husband believed it was his wife's responsibility to do the house cleaning, and his wife believed that the household duties should be shared. They are experiencing which one of the following stressors?
    1. Developmental stress
    2. Economic stress
    3. Role stress
    4. Role conflict

44. Your client is interested in learning about a low-salt diet. Both he and his wife have hypertension and want to change their eating habits. The most appropriate nursing diagnosis would be which of the following?
    1. *Impaired parenting*
    2. *Readiness for enhanced family coping*
    3. *Compromised family coping*
    4. *Disabled family coping*

45. An 80-year-old client has been living with her middle-aged son and his wife, who have been providing financial and emotional support. The relationship has been mutually satisfying and beneficial. Unfortunately, the client fell and fractured her hip. The family does not know how to manage the client's care. Which nursing diagnosis would be most appropriate?
    1. *Impaired parenting*
    2. *Readiness for enhanced family coping*
    3. *Compromised family coping*
    4. *Disabled family coping*

46. Your client is experiencing caregiver burnout. What is the recommended nursing intervention?
    1. Have her and the ill family member placed in a skilled nursing facility.
    2. Help her recognize her unrealistic expectation of herself and get respite care.
    3. Have her and the ill family member placed in an assisted living facility for respite care.
    4. Help her recognize that she is experiencing burnout, and then proceed with nursing intervention.

47. You praise your client's family caregiver for doing a good job in taking care of the client. This is an example of what type of nursing intervention to reduce *Caregiver role strain*?
    1. Promoting a realistic appraisal
    2. Allowing the client to ventilate
    3. Providing direct care
    4. Providing empathy

SUPPORTING SPIRITUALITY

PURPOSE

This chapter discusses key concepts that relate to the nursing diagnoses *Spiritual distress, Risk for spiritual distress*, and *Readiness for enhanced spiritual well-being*. It discusses the concepts of spirituality, religion, and faith with the idea of providing spiritual care in nursing.

MATCHING

1. _____ agnostic
2. _____ atheist
3. _____ faith
4. _____ hope
5. _____ monotheism
6. _____ polytheism
7. _____ religion
8. _____ religiosity
9. _____ spiritual distress
10. _____ spiritual health
11. _____ spiritual well-being
12. _____ spirituality

a. the experiences and expressions of one's spirit in a unique and dynamic process reflecting faith in God or a supreme being; connectedness with oneself, others, nature, or God; and integration of the dimensions of mind, body, and spirit

b. a belief system, including dogma, rituals, and traditions

c. the belief in the existence of one god who created and rules the universe

d. the belief in more than one god

e. a person who believes there is no God or a supreme being

f. a person who is undecided about the existence of God or a supreme being

g. belief in or commitment to something or someone greater than the self that helps a person realize purpose

h. the process of being and becoming by reflecting one's spirituality; it represents the totality of a person's inner resources, the wholeness of spirit and unifying dimension, a process of transcendence, and the perception of life as having meaning

i. an interpersonal process created through trust and nurtured by a trusting relationship with others, including God

j. a disruption that pervades the entire being and that integrates and transcends biological and social nature resulting in anguish of the human spirit

k. a person's dependence on and involvement in religious practices and behaviors

l. a state of wholeness of the spiritual dimension

TRUE OR FALSE

13. _____ Religion can mean a social institution in which people participate together, rather than an individual searching alone for meaning in life.

14. _____ Spiritual and religious expressions are synonymous.

15. _____ By definition, faith is belief with proof. Each person chooses what to believe.

16. _____ Several research studies confirm that nurses commonly address spirituality.

17. _____ The fundamental teachings of Judaism are grouped around the concept of monotheism.

18. _____ Children do not have spiritual crises in the same sense as adults.

19. _____ Clients who despair or feel hopeless are more likely to die, or die sooner, even when there is little physiological disease to justify the death.

FILL IN THE BLANKS

20. Religion can be viewed as a service to _____, organized within a specified set of beliefs and practices.

21. _____ is belief, expectancy, or trust that things will be better.

22. _____ believe in three gods, including the originator Lao Tzu.

23. Protestant churches have many _____ with a variety of differing beliefs.

24. Clients who are experiencing a crisis are susceptible to _____ distress.

25. Many clients use _____ as an effective coping strategy for dealing with health crises.

EXERCISING YOUR CLINICAL JUDGMENT

26. Mr. Guevara, the Mexican-American client from the chapter's case study, states that he is going to ask his pastor why God causes diseases like cancer. You ask him if his wife is going to be present when he discusses his feelings with the pastor. You tell him that you think he might be able to express himself more openly if his wife was not present during his conversation with the pastor. What were you taking into consideration during your discussion with Mr. Guevara?
    1. His religion
    2. His culture
    3. His family
    4. His psychological well-being

27. You ask Mr. Guevara what has bothered him most about being sick. This is an example of which element of a spiritual assessment?
    1. To determine a client's beliefs, values, and concept of God or divine being
    2. To determine a client's sources of hope and strength
    3. To determine a client's religious practices
    4. To determine a client's perceived relationship between spiritual beliefs and health

28. If the expected outcome for Mr. Guevara is to establish a meaningful relationship with himself, God, and others, the most likely nursing diagnosis is which of the following?
    1. *Ineffective individual coping*
    2. *Readiness for enhanced spiritual well-being*
    3. *Risk for spiritual distress*
    4. *Spiritual distress*

TEST YOURSELF

29. Activities such as prayer and going to church are examples of which characteristic of spirituality?
    1. General
    2. Being
    3. Knowing
    4. Doing

30. A person who is undecided about the existence of God or a supreme being is which of the following?
    1. An atheist
    2. A polytheist
    3. A monotheist
    4. An agnostic

31. Which nursing theorist stated that one assumption about the healing process is the premise that human nature is rooted in relatedness to the absolute truth of the creator?
    1. Watson
    2. Roy
    3. Travelbee
    4. Newman

32. If you help a client examine his or her life experiences to discover new meanings or reconnect to forgotten moments that represent significant meaning, which nursing intervention are you using?
    1. Life review
    2. Reminiscence
    3. Counseling
    4. Visualization

33. Your client who recently lost her infant expresses disbelief in God. Which nursing diagnosis would be most appropriate?
    1. *Ineffective individual coping*
    2. *Readiness for enhanced spiritual well-being*
    3. *Risk for spiritual distress*
    4. *Spiritual distress*

THE SURGICAL CLIENT

PURPOSE

This chapter describes the perioperative phases and factors that affect the surgical experience for a client. It discusses how you can use the nursing process to care for a client before, during, and after surgery.

MATCHING

1. _____ ambulatory surgery
2. _____ anesthesia
3. _____ anesthesiologist
4. _____ certified registered nurse anesthetist (CRNA)
5. _____ circulating nurse
6. _____ general anesthesia
7. _____ intraoperative phase
8. _____ local anesthesia
9. _____ malignant hyperthermia (MH)
10. _____ perioperative
11. _____ perioperative nursing
12. _____ postanesthesia care unit (PACU)
13. _____ postoperative phase
14. _____ preoperative phase
15. _____ regional anesthesia
16. _____ registered nurse first assistant (RNFA)
17. _____ scrub nurse

a. can be divided into two segments of care: the immediate and the ongoing periods

b. any agent that induces a temporary loss of feeling due to the inhibition of nerve endings in a specific part of the body

c. an area where clients remain until they regain consciousness from the effects of anesthesia; formerly called recovery room

d. a specialized area of practice that describes the provision of care for the surgical client throughout the continuum of care

e. a registered nurse with special qualifications that include knowledge of aseptic technique, instruments and equipment, anatomy and physiology, surgical procedures, and most importantly, promotion of client safety

f. a type of anesthesia in which medication is instilled into or around the nerves to block the transmission of nerve impulses in a particular area or region

g. a medical physician who specializes in anesthesiology

h. same-day or outpatient surgery that can be performed with general or local anesthesia; usually takes less than 2 hours, and requires less than a 3-hour stay in a recovery area

i. a rare autosomal dominant inherited syndrome that causes rigidity of the skeletal muscles and is life-threatening

j. begins when the decision for surgical intervention is made and ends when the client is safely transported into the operating room (OR) for the surgical procedure

k. an expanded nursing role requiring additional education, in which the perioperative nurse works as a first assistant during the surgical procedure

l. an advanced practice registered nurse who has been specifically educated in the administration of anesthetic agents

m. begins with the client's entry into the OR and ends when the client is transferred to the recovery room (postanesthesia care unit) or other areas such as the intensive care unit, where immediate postsurgical attention is given

n. the partial or complete loss of sensation with or without a loss of consciousness that results from administration of an anesthetic agent

o. produced by inhalation or by injection of anesthetic drugs into the bloodstream, or a combination of both, and causes the client to lose all sensation and consciousness

p. a registered nurse who assists the client to meet individual needs during all three phases of the surgical experience

q. the term used to describe the preoperative, intraoperative, and postoperative phases of the surgical experience

TRUE OR FALSE

18. _____ Collaborative and independent nursing care prevents complications and promotes optimal outcomes for the surgical client.

19. _____ The scrub nurse coordinates client care, is the client advocate, and manages all activities outside the sterile field.

20. _____ Prior to surgery, the surgeon is required to ask for informed consent to have the operative procedure performed.

21. _____ Normal tissue repair and resistance to infection after surgery depend on good nutrition.

22. _____ Clients are less anxious and participate more readily if they know the reasons for perioperative activities.

23. _____ Pain is an unexpected and abnormal response to the surgical procedure.

24. _____ Turning in bed postoperatively improves venous return and respiratory function.

25. _____ In addition to the skin incision, there are many other risk factors that can influence a surgical client's risk for infection.

26. _____ Acetaminophen (Tylenol) is the drug of choice to treat malignant hyperthermia.

27. _____ Urinary retention and urinary tract infections are two common postoperative complications of the urinary system.

FILL IN THE BLANKS

28. A surgery that is performed according to the client's preference with no ill effects occurring due to postponement would be classified as _____ surgery.

29. The _____ phase of anesthesia is begun as soon as the client is brought into the operating room.

30. One advantage of _____ anesthesia is that it can be used for clients of any age and for any surgical procedure.

31. It is the legal responsibility of the _____ to obtain the client's consent before a surgical procedure.

32. Latex allergies have become much more common since the late 1980s with the advent of _____ precautions.

33. Positioning the client for surgery is usually done _____ induction of anesthesia.

34. _____ is a respiratory emergency caused by reflex contractions of pharyngeal muscles, causing spasm of the vocal cords.

35. To encourage maximal lung expansion following surgery, a client should use an _____ _____.

36. A nurse should assess for bladder distention in a postoperative client if the client has not voided for _____ to _____ hours.

37. _____ and _____ instructions are given to a postoperative client before discharge.

EXERCISING YOUR CLINICAL JUDGMENT

Mr. Warren, a 61-year-old Afro-Caribbean client, has come to the United States for a second medical opinion after he was diagnosed with prostate cancer. His daughter, who is a nurse, lives in Atlanta.

38. Which of the following nursing diagnoses would you be sure to consider, knowing that Mr. Warren is undergoing surgery for cancer, a potentially incurable problem?
    1. *Anxiety*
    2. *Knowledge deficit*
    3. *Hopelessness*
    4. *Powerlessness*

39. You are providing instructions to Mr. Warren about leg exercises that he can do after surgery to reduce the risk of thrombus formation in his legs. How often should you tell him to perform them?
    1. 1 to 2 times every hour
    2. 5 to 6 times every 1 to 2 hours
    3. 10 to 12 times every 1 to 2 hours
    4. 20 to 25 times every 8 hours

40. Encouraging Mr. Warren to turn, cough, and breathe deeply (TCDB) helps him prevent:
    1. Being thirsty.
    2. Having alveolar collapse and moving secretions to large airway passages for easier expectoration.
    3. Having a low heart rate.
    4. Having no crackles in his lung fields.

41. You are assisting Mr. Warren to get out of bed for the first time since surgery. Knowing that he has an abdominal incision, you would be sure to use which of the following when helping him get up?
    1. A cane to steady himself against
    2. A walker to lean on in case of dizziness
    3. A pillow to use as a splint during movement
    4. A mechanical lift, because he should not stand at all

TEST YOURSELF

42. As part of client preparation just before surgery, you must check the consent form to verify that the client has signed it, have the client void, give preoperative medication, and assist the client onto the stretcher to go to the operating room. Which of the following would be best to do first?
    1. Have the client void.
    2. Put the client on the stretcher for needed rest.
    3. Administer the ordered medication.
    4. Verify that the client has signed the consent form.

43. The preoperative nurse would alert the anesthesiologist or surgeon regarding which of the following health problems that could cause cancellation of a client's elective surgery?
    1. Headache
    2. Sore throat
    3. Heart attack 1 year ago
    4. Chronic lung disease

44. The circulating nurse in the operating room notes that two sponges are missing near the end of a client's surgery. Which of the following actions should the nurse take first?
    1. Call for an x-ray.
    2. Ignore it because the sponges dissolve.
    3. Perform a second count.
    4. Search the floor around the operating table.

45. The nurse would teach the client about which of the following ordered pain medication administration methods that provides for the most continuous relief of pain?
    1. Patient-controlled analgesia
    2. Intermittent nurse-administered IV push medication
    3. Subcutaneous injections
    4. Intramuscular injections

46. A postoperative client with nausea has begun vomiting. The nurse would avoid giving antiemetic medication by which of the following routes?
    1. Intravenous
    2. Intramuscular
    3. Subcutaneous
    4. Oral

ANSWER KEY

CHAPTER 1

1. b
2. d
3. n
4. c
5. j
6. i
7. a
8. g
9. f
10. e
11. T
12. F. Nursing practice is governed by law, and standards are set forth by the profession.
13. T
14. T
15. T
16. F. A doctoral program is considered advanced practice education.
17. F. The nurse's role would be critical thinker.
18. T
19. T
20. F. The knowledge explosion in nursing is so great that today's nurse must use critical thinking and problem-solving skills to practice effectively.
21. Assessment, nursing diagnosis, planning, implementation, evaluation
22. Florence Nightingale
23. Nurse Informatics
24. Mary Adelaide Nutting
25. public health
26. African American, Hispanic
27. master's degree
28. professional licensure
29. state
30. 1. The Nurse Practice Act forms the legal basis for nursing practice in a specific state. The NLN focuses on the improvement of nursing services and education. The ARN is a specialty nursing organization, and the ANA is the professional organization for nurses.
31. 3. The client advocate role is one in which the nurse protects the rights of clients. In this instance, Kate is protecting the rights of the client whose privacy is being invaded.
32. 2. Many states require that nurses obtain CEUs in order to maintain their professional licensure in that state.
33. 2. A bachelor's degree is the minimum educational degree that must be held in order to become certified by the ANCC in nursing administration.
34. 1
35. 3
36. 2
37. 4
38. 4

CHAPTER 2

1. g
2. mm
3. l
4. q
5. ff
6. w
7. ii
8. aa
9. ee
10. a
11. f
12. m
13. r
14. x
15. bb
16. b
17. t
18. hh
19. u
20. nn
21. dd
22. c
23. h
24. oo
25. n
26. z
27. cc
28. jj
29. d
30. s
31. i
32. kk
33. o
34. y
35. e
36. qq
37. p
38. k
39. pp
40. v
41. gg
42. ll
43. j
44. T
45. F. It does include refusing to let clients leave the hospital against their wishes.
46. T
47. F. The nurse would be tried under criminal law.
48. T
49. F. An individual state has the power to change the Nurse Practice Act.
50. T
51. T
52. T
53. T

156 ANSWER KEY

54. F. A terminally ill client should be told of his or her prognosis.
55. F. An ethical dilemma exists when choices are unfavorable.
56. T
57. T
58. battery
59. procedural
60. certification
61. collective bargaining
62. informed consent
63. confidentiality, or privacy
64. incident report
65. ethics
66. culture, life experiences
67. privacy
68. Nonmaleficence
69. medical
70. 4. This is the only option that removes the client from the area and protects the confidentiality of the information being given in the report.
71. 1. The CDC is the federal agency responsible for issuing guidelines for infection control.
72. 2. The other options constitute documentation errors.
73. 3
74. 4
75. 2
76. 2
77. 3
78. 4
79. 2
80. 3
81. 3
82. 1
83. 2

CHAPTER 3

1. e
2. i
3. j
4. a
5. f
6. h
7. k
8. c
9. d
10. b
11. g
12. T

13. F. This is an example of stereotyping.
14. T
15. T
16. F. This refers to a person who is past-oriented.
17. T
18. T
19. T
20. T
21. F. Native Americans believe that illness is a price paid for a past or future event.
22. preservation, maintenance
23. accommodation, negotiation
24. Awareness
25. Environmental control
26. European
27. African
28. Mexican
29. Chinese
30. Navajo Indians
31. harmony
32. 3. An adult may choose to continue to closely identify with the group to which his or her parents belonged, or may adopt the ways of the larger culture around him or her.
33. 1. Religion is taken very seriously, and many African Americans actively participate in church-related activities and believe strongly in the power of prayer.
34. 4
35. 2
36. 3
37. 1
38. 4

CHAPTER 4

1. b
2. g
3. d
4. e
5. f
6. c
7. a
8. i
9. j
10. p
11. k
12. l
13. m
14. h

15. n
16. o
17. q
18. T
19. F. Advanced nurse practitioners include clinical nurse specialists and nurse practitioners. Physician assistants are health care professionals licensed to practice medicine with physician supervision.
20. F. The use of alternative health therapy is growing in typical health care settings.
21. F. Although there may be room for debate, many factors influence access and quality of hospital services. Among these factors, consider rural versus urban, system of financing, and types of services offered.
22. T
23. T
24. T. Respite care is designed to relieve the stress and burden of informal caregivers by providing temporary relief of caring for their ill family members.
25. F. The U.S. government's share of the national health care bill was 46%.
26. F. An HMO establishes standards for the quality of care provided.
27. F. Managed care organizations make decisions about what services will be reimbursed, thus rationing health care.
28. T. This is also the age-group with the greatest per capita expenditures for health care.
29. T. Hispanics, Asians, and Muslims are among the minority groups whose presence is visibly increasing in the United States.
30. T. As a nurse, you need to understand the economic forces putting pressure on the structure and function of the health care delivery system.

31. F. Cost of care and quality of care are highly interrelated.
32. Nurses
33. Pharmacists
34. inpatient
35. rural community hospital
36. Rehabilitation
37. Hospice
38. physician's office
39. Adult day care
40. United States
41. preferred provider organization
42. people over 65, disabled people, people with end-stage renal disease
43. Canada
44. 26
45. 2. Although none of these sources may provide this service, the goal of a health maintenance organization is most in keeping with this service.
46. 2. Although the managed care organization will make a decision about paying for the medication, a physician must prescribe this medication and will consider his medical history in making the decision.
47. 1. Option 1 is a definition of *rehabilitation*.
48. 3
49. 4
50. 3
51. 4

CHAPTER 5

1. k
2. m
3. j
4. f
5. g
6. d
7. e
8. a
9. i
10. b
11. c
12. h
13. l
14. T
15. F. It is acceptable when consensus of the nursing

profession is that the theory provides an adequate description of reality.
16. F. This is attributed to Leininger.
17. F. The T.H.I.N.K. model incorporates five modes of thinking used in combination or simultaneously.
18. T
19. F. A list of assessment questions is a tool to be used as a reminder and is never intended to be complete.
20. person, nursing
21. theory
22. nurse
23. overuse of the habit mode, anxiety, time, bias, lack of confidence
24. goals, nursing
25. physician's
26. North American Nursing Diagnosis Association
27. 4
28. 3
29. 4
30. 1
31. 1
32. 2
33. 4
34. 1
35. 4
36. 1

CHAPTER 6

1. w
2. z
3. x
4. q
5. u
6. e
7. r
8. v
9. y
10. s
11. t
12. h
13. o
14. f
15. j
16. p
17. n
18. m
19. g

20. i
21. k
22. l
23. d
24. b
25. aa
26. c
27. a
28. T
29. T
30. F. If the client wishes to maintain privacy or the family is not a reliable source, you would not collect data from the family.
31. T
32. T
33. F. The purpose is never only to collect a standard set of data.
34. F. You prepare for termination when you tell the client how much time the interview will take.
35. F. Biographical data may be helpful in accurately anticipating a medical diagnosis.
36. F. The medical history helps the nurse anticipate nursing needs.
37. T
38. T
39. F. Exercise tolerance is related to the respiratory and cardiovascular systems as well.
40. F. However, subjective data are documented in an objective manner, without including your opinions.
41. T
42. potential for, potential rate of, evidence of
43. location, quality, chronology, setting, severity, aggravating or alleviating factors, associated factors
44. chronology
45. nutritional-metabolic
46. activity-exercise
47. self-perception/self-concept
48. 4
49. 2
50. 2
51. 3

52. 1
53. 2
54. 2
55. 2
56. 3
57. 3

CHAPTER 7

1. d
2. h
3. e
4. i
5. j
6. k
7. g
8. n
9. t
10. q
11. s
12. a
13. r
14. f
15. o
16. l
17. p
18. c
19. b
20. m
21. F. Vital signs must be evaluated and compared with the client's baseline.
22. T
23. T
24. T
25. F. The oral thermometer must be placed in the pocket created by the frenulum under the tongue.
26. F. Clean from clean to dirty; that is, from the end to the bulb.
27. F. A heart rate of 100 with exercise or anxiety that returns to normal with rest is normal.
28. T
29. T
30. F. Head injuries can cause bradycardia.
31. F. The blood volume is also a factor.
32. F. The carotid is not routinely used to count the pulse. Massage of the carotid can cause a reflex slowing of the heart rate.

33. T
34. T
35. T
36. Vital signs
37. thermoregulation
38. glass
39. tympanic
40. higher
41. increase
42. pulsus paradoxus
43. resistance
44. contraction
45. relaxation
46. two thirds
47. 2
48. 1
49. 2
50. 1
51. 3
52. 3
53. 3
54. 1
55. 2
56. 3
57. 2
58. 1
59. 1
60. 4
61. 2
62. 1
63. 3
64. 3

CHAPTER 8

1. o
2. e
3. f
4. d
5. n
6. g
7. h
8. i
9. j
10. c
11. b
12. k
13. a
14. q
15. p
16. l
17. m
18. F. You can begin the physical exam in any position.
19. T
20. F. The heart is on the left side.

21. T
22. F. This information is a form of orientation to time, but can only be evaluated in the context of the information.
23. T
24. T
25. F. PERRLA tells you more about motor function than the ability to see clearly.
26. T
27. F. Angle the ophthalmoscope slightly toward the nose.
28. F. The thyroid should be rubbery.
29. T
30. T
31. T
32. T
33. F. An apical radial pulse deficit usually occurs with irregular cardiac rhythms.
34. T
35. F. A grade 6 is the loudest murmur.
36. F. A bruit is never normal.
37. T
38. F. Identifying hypoactive bowel sounds is a subjective judgment dependent on your ability to recognize normal sounds.
39. T
40. T
41. light palpation
42. percussion
43. auscultation
44. cognitive function
45. natural
46. Crepitus
47. 2, 30, 60
48. Rinne
49. gingivitis
50. Kussmaul
51. discontinuous
52. Deep tendon
53. Papanicolaou smear
54. varicocele
55. 1, 6, 10, and 11 are essential.
    1. Essential. Assessing for adventitious sounds will help you know the seriousness of her condition, anticipate complications, and monitor progress.

2. Nonessential. However, you will probably want to gather some information about her mental status such as orientation to person, place, and time. Gather enough information that you can recognize if her condition changes.

3. Nonessential. Assess the radial and pedal pulses. Assess the radial pulse to evaluate the rate and rhythm of the heart. If the rhythm is irregular, assess the apical pulse. Assess the pedal pulses to evaluate the circulation in the feet. It would not be surprising for a 90-year-old to have diminished circulation in the feet.

4. Nonessential. However, you do want to listen for bowel sounds and assess for abdominal distention. The stress of illness can slow the bowels and cause distention.

5. Nonessential. The rectal examination is never routine for a general duty nurse.

6. Essential. Skin assessment in the elderly is important especially when the person will be confined to bed.

7. Nonessential. However, you will want to note some information about range of motion and the ability to move about safely in the environment.

8. Nonessential. However, most nurses will usually note the condition of the toenails in the elderly. Health teaching needs can be met and sometimes a podiatrist referral can be made.

9. Nonessential. However, you do want to gather some information about the client's functional

level of vision and hearing and the use of glasses or hearing aids.

10. Essential. Cardiac and respiratory problems are closely interrelated and should always be assessed together.

11. Essential. Anytime you listen to the heart one of the things you are listening for is murmurs. The presence of most murmurs will not appreciably change your nursing care.

56. 4
57. 2
58. 3
59. 1
60. 3
61. 1
62. 3
63. 2
64. 2
65. 4
66. 4
67. 2
68. 3
69. 3
70. 3
71. 2
72. 3
73. 2
74. 2
75. 1
76. 2
77. 3
78. 2
79. 2

CHAPTER 9

1. g
2. j
3. h
4. i
5. n
6. b
7. d
8. m
9. l
10. e
11. c
12. f
13. a
14. k

15. T
16. T
17. F. NANDA
18. T
19. F. A shared diagnostic language fostered critical thinking by placing the emphasis on nursing care to solve the client's problem
20. T
21. T
22. T
23. T
24. F. Nursing diagnoses should be discussed with the client.
25. second
26. Omaha
27. diagnostic label
28. wellness
29. clusters
30. differentiating
31. defining characteristic
32. value judgment
33. overdiagnosing
34. 1. This is an actual nursing diagnosis, not "risk for," and lists specific related factors.
35. 2. The client cannot retain urine with a catheter in place.
36. 2. This would be a "risk for" diagnosis. The "related to" factors must relate to the client's situation.
37. 4. The diagnosis would be written as *Risk for infection.*
38. 4
39. 1
40. 2
41. 1
42. 3

CHAPTER 10

1. t
2. b
3. m
4. s
5. v
6. r
7. l
8. e
9. k
10. a

11. f

12. p

13. h

14. n

15. j

16. c

17. o

18. d

19. i

20. g

21. u

22. q

23. F. Planning is ongoing throughout the client's health care experience.

24. F. Each care plan is individualized.

25. F. Whereas other disciplines may in some cases assume primary responsibility for some aspects of the client's care, the nurse has a role in the provision of that care.

26. T

27. F. Physical needs may be secondary to other needs at different stages of the client's experience.

28. T

29. T

30. T

31. T

32. F. Outcomes or nursing diagnoses may also be revised.

33. F. The client and family must be asked.

34. T

35. T

36. T

37. changes

38. physiological integrity

39. nursing, multidisciplinary

40. accountable

41. sensitive

42. expected outcomes

43. communication

44. partially

45. resolved

46. barrier

47. 2

48. 4

49. 2

50. 4

51. 4

52. 3

53. 4

54. 1

55. 2

56. 3

57. 2

58. 2

CHAPTER 11

1. d

2. f

3. k

4. g

5. p

6. a

7. i

8. e

9. o

10. q

11. j

12. b

13. l

14. c

15. h

16. n

17. m

18. T

19. F. Errors are documented in the client's chart.

20. F. Abbreviations vary from geographical area or specialty.

21. F. Charting should be brief and concise.

22. T

23. T

24. T

25. communication

26. standards

27. Black

28. client's

29. client

30. orientation

31. observations

32. 1. Narrative charting is a method of charting that provides information in the form of statements that describe events surrounding client care.

33. 2. Recording of information should be sequential.

34. 3. A discharge note is done when the client is released from the hospital.

35. 3

36. 4

37. 4

38. 2

39. 1

CHAPTER 12

1. c

2. s

3. p

4. m

5. t

6. h

7. g

8. r

9. d

10. i

11. k

12. e

13. l

14. n

15. o

16. f

17. b

18. a

19. q

20. j

21. T

22. F. This is Travelbee's theory.

23. T

24. F. A person's personal space is culturally determined.

25. T

26. T

27. F. You should ask the client to consider what might be the best thing to do.

28. T

29. ethical, professional

30. Positive

31. body language

32. presenting reality

33. talking

34. silence

35. Active

36. 1. The nurse asks "why" of the client, thereby asking for a reason for feelings and behaviors when the client may not know the reason.

37. 3. The nurse lets the client know that what was said was unclear.

38. 1. The nurse invites the client to select a topic.

39. 1

40. 1

41. 4
42. 1
43. 4

CHAPTER 13

1. e
2. c
3. f
4. b
5. g
6. a
7. d
8. h
9. T
10. T
11. F. Clients may only be able to comprehend the steps of a carefully prescribed routine.
12. F. Literacy is an important consideration when using written instructions.
13. T
14. T
15. F. Written supplemental materials reinforce learning.
16. F. Some clients prefer not to know.
17. F. Other nursing diagnoses can also apply.
18. T
19. T
20. individual
21. group
22. printed
23. reinforce learning
24. active participant
25. short-term
26. long-term
27. 3. Adult learning is purposeful.
28. 3. For adults, learning must have a purpose.
29. 1. Motivation is greatest in clients who recognize their learning needs and perceive the available teaching as meaningful.
30. 2
31. 1
32. 1
33. 1
34. 2
35. 2
36. 1
37. 1
38. 3

CHAPTER 14

1. a
2. e
3. l
4. w
5. y
6. f
7. m
8. g
9. h
10. o
11. n
12. c
13. aa
14. z
15. q
16. k
17. p
18. r
19. i
20. b
21. x
22. d
23. s
24. u
25. j
26. bb
27. t
28. v
29. T
30. T
31. F. A mission statement is written.
32. T
33. T
34. T
35. T
36. F. policy manual
37. concurrent
38. improved
39. leaders
40. quality
41. outcomes
42. Policies, procedures
43. cost
44. 1. The nurse-manager can delegate this task to the charge nurse, who is responsible for the daily operation of the unit. Although the nurse-manager role involves managing personnel, this usually involves evaluation of performance and possibly hiring and firing personnel. The other options

do not address the immediate problem in an effective manner.
45. 2. Because the change enhanced the level of service rendered to the client, this is an example of an improvement in quality.
46. 2
47. 3
48. 4
49. 3
50. 1
51. 4
52. 3

CHAPTER 15

1. a
2. h
3. b
4. g
5. c
6. d
7. e
8. m
9. l
10. f
11. i
12. o
13. j
14. n
15. k
16. p
17. r
18. q
19. s
20. T
21. T
22. T
23. F. Ethical guidelines should still be followed.
24. T
25. F. There is a relationship, but not necessarily causation.
26. F. The abstract is a short summary only.
27. T
28. T
29. T
30. F. It can.
31. T
32. F. Valuable information can still be obtained.
33. T
34. T
35. T
36. Nursing research

37. human subjects
38. case study
39. variables
40. random
41. reduction
42. extraneous
43. maturation
44. 1
45. 4
46. 2
47. 1
48. 4
49. 1
50. 1
51. 2

CHAPTER 16

1. j
2. h
3. d
4. k
5. g
6. c
7. b
8. a
9. e
10. i
11. l
12. f
13. T
14. T
15. F. Tasks can derive from cultural patterns as well.
16. T
17. T
18. T
19. F. The preschool child gains weight more slowly.
20. T
21. F. Children of this age-group have many fears.
22. T
23. head, heel
24. 4
25. separation anxiety
26. 12
27. ectomorphic, endomorphic
28. preschool-aged
29. head
30. 5 years
31. 4. The other toys are best used with children younger than 12 months of age.
32. 2. The other strategies should be avoided.

33. 3. A nap should be planned around lunchtime.
34. 3
35. 3
36. 1
37. 2
38. 3
39. 4
40. 3
41. 3
42. 2

CHAPTER 17

1. j
2. d
3. e
4. a
5. i
6. h
7. g
8. c
9. T
10. F. Boys are affected more than girls.
11. F. Most cases of short stature result from heredity.
12. T
13. T
14. T
15. F. Each adult's development is unique and complex and is influenced by many factors including genetics, socioeconomic status, ethnic group, religious faith, and societal expectation.
16. T
17. F. Of this age-group, more than 30% do not have health insurance.
18. identity, identity diffusion
19. health care
20. morals, values
21. homicide, suicide, and intentional injuries
22. half
23. nonjudgmental
24. comply
25. intimacy, isolation
26. individualized
27. small changes, large
28. activity
29. health, illness
30. 1. Adolescents try to figure out who they are but are confused

as to which of the many roles to adopt.
31. 3. It is important for the client to recognize the connection between her diet and physical activity changes and her blood sugar levels.
32. 2. The adolescent who is unable to cope with a lifestyle change may experience stress and demonstrate substance abuse behaviors or depression.
33. 1
34. 3
35. 2
36. 4
37. 3
38. 1
39. 1

CHAPTER 18

1. a
2. i
3. h
4. f
5. d
6. e
7. c
8. g
9. b
10. T
11. T
12. F. This is the middle adult stage.
13. T
14. F. It is usually difficult to detect.
15. F. One in every five deaths is related to cigarette smoking.
16. T
17. T. This is especially true for clients in high-risk groups.
18. T
19. generativity, stagnation
20. seasons
21. infectious diseases
22. Ageism
23. depressed
24. Poverty
25. heart disease, cerebrovascular diseases, chronic respiratory diseases, Alzheimer's disease, pneumonia
26. health care
27. incontinence

28. 3. The individual must balance the feeling that life is personally satisfying and socially meaningful with the feeling that life is without meaning.
29. 3. Disengagement pertains to adults past the age of 65 and the theory that they gradually disengage from societal roles as a natural response to lessened capabilities and interest.
30. 3. To persuade clients to change their behaviors, it is first necessary to identify their beliefs relevant to the high-risk behavior and to provide information based on this foundation.
31. 4
32. 3
33. 2
34. 1
35. 1

CHAPTER 19

1. g
2. j
3. i
4. k
5. a
6. d
7. c
8. b
9. f
10. o
11. m
12. h
13. l
14. p
15. e
16. p
17. T
18. T
19. F. Health is a fundamental right of all people.
20. F. Not all diseases can be cured.
21. T
22. F. Population health addresses the five determinants of health: biology, behaviors, physical environment, social environment, and public policies and interventions.

23. T
24. T
25. World Health Organization
26. quality, years
27. choice, passively
28. diagnosis
29. health-illness continuum
30. population
31. perception
32. health
33. 1
34. 1
35. 2
36. 4
37. 2
38. 1

CHAPTER 20

1. d
2. f
3. o
4. i
5. m
6. k
7. h
8. c
9. p
10. e
11. a
12. b
13. q
14. l
15. g
16. j
17. n
18. T
19. T
20. F. They do interfere.
21. T
22. F. They may conflict with interventions.
23. T
24. T
25. T
26. F. Client and family should also be involved.
27. T
28. reasoned action
29. risk factors
30. lifestyle, family
31. medical
32. knowledge
33. Values clarification
34. reinforcing, motivating
35. denial
36. Discharge

37. social
38. 1. In this stage, the person does not intend to change a high-risk behavior in the foreseeable future.
39. 2. He disliked having to go to the bathroom so frequently because of medication effects.
40. 3. An educational plan must be focused on increasing awareness of the relationships between the client's specific unhealthy lifestyles and the development of health problems.
41. 4. The single most influential factor in increasing participation in effective management of a therapeutic regimen is the relationship with the health care provider.
42. 1
43. 3
44. 2
45. 4
46. 3

CHAPTER 21

1. d
2. z
3. p
4. a
5. y
6. w
7. o
8. l
9. b
10. k
11. u
12. m
13. e
14. q
15. t
16. x
17. g
18. v
19. n
20. c
21. i
22. j
23. f
24. r
25. s
26. h
27. T

28. T
29. F. The drugs reach the liver first, called the first-pass effect.
30. T
31. F. It varies according to facility policy.
32. T
33. T
34. F. Sufficient body fluid is needed to transport drugs and their metabolites.
35. T
36. Drug Enforcement
37. Drug tolerance
38. Enteric-coated
39. X
40. body weight
41. *Constipation, Diarrhea*
42. superinfection
43. 30
44. 3. The client should develop and use a reminder system, if needed, because omitted doses can jeopardize health. The statements in the other options are false.
45. 2. Standing or sitting up slowly allows the blood vessels time to adjust in caliber to the position change and may help decrease adverse symptoms. Options 1 and 3 will make dizziness worse. The client should take the medication at bedtime if dizziness is a chronic problem.
46. 4. The term *sublingual* means "under the tongue," making it the only correct response.
47. 1. Adverse medication effects are more likely to occur with increasing age because the body may not metabolize and excrete them as easily.
48. 1
49. 3
50. 2
51. 4
52. 2
53. 3, 2, 1, 4
54. 1, 3, 2, 4
55. 4, 2, 3, 1

CHAPTER 22

1. w
2. i
3. h
4. e
5. a
6. k
7. n
8. u
9. p
10. t
11. q
12. b
13. v
14. m
15. o
16. d
17. j
18. l
19. x
20. g
21. c
22. s
23. r
24. f
25. T
26. T
27. F. Chickenpox is an airborne infection.
28. T
29. T
30. F. It is a left shift.
31. T
32. F. Anxiety can reduce protection.
33. T
34. T
35. convalescence
36. reservoir
37. Opportunistic
38. environmental
39. localized
40. dirty
41. hand hygiene
42. steam
43. Droplet
44. 1. The others are localized signs of infection.
45. 3. The environment has other children, and hand-washing is a fundamental procedure to reduce transmission of organisms.
46. 2. Viruses, such as influenza, require droplet precautions.
47. 4. The stool should be recultured, or new sites of infection should be looked for.
48. 1
49. 1
50. 4
51. 2
52. 3
53. 1, 3, 2, 4
54. 3, 4, 1, 2
55. 4, 2, 3, 1
56. 2, 1, 4, 3

CHAPTER 23

1. b
2. f
3. e
4. a
5. h
6. i
7. g
8. d
9. c
10. T
11. T
12. F. Cigarette smoking is the leading cause of fatal residential fires.
13. T
14. F. Most back injuries develop slowly over time.
15. T
16. T
17. T
18. F. The child's age is also a consideration when buying a car seat.
19. T
20. falls
21. choking, aspiration
22. Poisons
23. accidental
24. occupational
25. financial resources
26. infants, toddlers
27. prevention
28. grounded
29. rescue, alarm, confine, extinguish
30. 2. Measures to promote home safety may include using nonskid rugs or tacking down throw rugs to prevent slips and falls.
31. 2. Safety practices to prevent burns, such as positioning pans with handles toward the back of the stove while cooking, should be in place.
32. 4. A person's cognitive and perceptual abilities are crucial to promoting safety.

33. 3. Multipurpose extinguishers are for type A, B, and C fires.
34. 3
35. 4
36. 2
37. 2, 1, 4, 3
38. 4, 1, 2, 3
39. 3, 1, 4, 2

CHAPTER 24

1. i
2. a
3. d
4. b
5. s
6. q
7. c
8. m
9. n
10. g
11. e
12. r
13. f
14. o
15. h
16. j
17. p
18. l
19. k
20. T
21. F. Most digestion and absorption occur in the small intestine.
22. T
23. F. A high-fiber diet contains cereals and raw fruits and vegetables.
24. F. Positive nitrogen balance and anabolism occur when the body is storing protein.
25. T
26. T
27. F. The RDA is meant to meet the needs of healthy individuals.
28. T
29. T
30. T
31. Digestion
32. fiber
33. 4
34. Vitamins
35. minerals
36. diet history
37. MyPyramid

38. protein
39. Nutrition Facts food label
40. grains, vegetables, fruits, milk, meat/beans
41. Polyphenols
42. 2. During a 24-hour recall, the client is asked to recall everything eaten the previous day or within the last 24 hours.
43. 2 and 4. Joan's diet is lacking in fruits, vegetables, and diary with the exception of the cheese she snacks on during the day.
44. 2. Fat intake should be less than 30% of the total caloric intake with saturated fats less 10% of calories. Overall clients should modify fat intake to keep the cholesterol level below 200 mg/dL.
45. 4. The MyPyramid uses a graphic design that is useful in teaching clients about the types and amounts of foods to include in the daily diet. It is easy to understand and follow.
46. 1
47. 2
48. 4
49. 3
50. 2
51. 1
52. 3, 1, 2, 4
53. 1, 2, 4, 3
54. 4, 3, 2, 1

CHAPTER 25

1. d
2. e
3. a
4. f
5. g
6. b
7. c
8. T
9. F. Ketones are positive, and nitrogen balance is negative.
10. T
11. F. It occurs over months or years.
12. T
13. T
14. T
15. F. At least 2 pounds per month is considered successful.
16. T
17. F. They should be avoided.

18. medulla
19. B$_{12}$
20. iron
21. 32 to 34
22. 10
23. pharyngeal
24. 170
25. clear
26. 2
27. limited or restricted
28. 3. Zinc is the element that has an effect of increasing the ability to taste. The other minerals listed do not have this property.
29. 1. Clients with cancer and AIDS tend to eat better in the morning.
30. 2. These foods can cause further irritation.
31. 4. Both hemoglobin and hematocrit will reflect increased iron intake.
32. 1
33. 3
34. 2
35. 4
36. 2
37. 2, 1, 4, 3
38. 1, 2, 3, 4
39. 3, 2, 4, 1

CHAPTER 26

1. a
2. u
3. f
4. c
5. e
6. b
7. h
8. g
9. j
10. q
11. t
12. s
13. o
14. n
15. r
16. p
17. k
18. m
19. i
20. d
21. w
22. v
23. l
24. T

25. T
26. T
27. F. Hypokalemia is a result of high-volume urine output.
28. T
29. T
30. F. It cannot be measured.
31. T
32. T
33. F. It's given primarily for fluid replacement.
34. F. Sodium is present in this solution (0.45%).
35. T
36. T
37. T
38. retention
39. water-soluble
40. decompression, obstruction
41. third spacing
42. high Fowler's
43. Normal saline
44. distal
45. 18
46. at the site, away from
47. blood return
48. 3. Others represent deficient fluid volume.
49. 1. Sodium would be low; others show normal or high values.
50. 1. Crackles are consistent with overload.
51. 2. 20 times 60 divided by 60 = 20.
52. 3. Weight is a reliable indicator of fluid status.
53. 4
54. 3
55. 3
56. 1
57. 1
58. 2
59. 2
60. 2
61. 3
62. 2
63. 4, 3, 2, 1
64. 2, 4, 3, 1
65. 2, 3, 1, 4

CHAPTER 27

1. f
2. k
3. i
4. l
5. b

6. j
7. c
8. h
9. r
10. d
11. g
12. m
13. q
14. n
15. e
16. o
17. p
18. a
19. F. They may or may not be related.
20. F. Yellow indicates that a wound is not ready to heal.
21. T
22. T
23. F. Wounds cannot heal when infected.
24. F. Yellow drainage does not always mean the wound is infected.
25. T
26. Protection
27. red, yellow, black
28. pressure ulcer
29. nutrition
30. clock
31. sutures, staples
32. enterostomal
33. 2. A Stage II ulcer may look like a blister or shallow crater.
34. 2. The erythrocyte sedimentation rate can help assess the client's inflammation, infectious, or necrotic processes.
35. 4. *Impaired skin integrity:* It is a state in which an individual has altered body tissue.
36. 3
37. 1
38. 4
39. 2
40. 1
41. 3, 4, 1, 2
42. 2, 1, 4, 3
43. 2, 3, 4, 1

CHAPTER 28

1. f
2. h
3. c

4. a
5. g
6. d
7. e
8. b
9. F. Fever may also be caused by inflammation without infection.
10. T
11. T
12. T
13. F. Hypothermic clients exhibit a high alcohol or other drug intake.
14. T
15. T
16. T
17. F. Besides identifying bacteria in the blood (bacteremia), blood cultures can identify viruses in the blood (viremia).
18. F. Blood cultures are drawn through a central line IV site only if the central line is suspected to be the source of the infection.
19. T
20. F. Convulsions in infants are associated with a temperature of 102° to 104° F or higher.
21. T
22. T
23. F. Hypothermia is the result.
24. T
25. T
26. effervescence, plateau, defervescence
27. 10%
28. increased
29. dry skin, hypotension, tachycardia, vomiting, diarrhea
30. warmth, shivering, vasodilation
31. Chronic fever
32. tinnitus, bruising
33. liver
34. conduction
35. convection
36. hyperthermia
37. Defervescence
38. hypothalamus
39. antipyretics, physical cooling
40. abdominal distention, bowel sounds, nausea
41. 1. If the client has an elevated temperature, monitoring every 4 hours is usually sufficient.

42. 1. Fever is a host defense response that frequently occurs in hospitalized clients either from the primary diagnosis or from complications.
43. 2
44. 2
45. 3
46. 1
47. 4, 1, 2, 3
48. 1, 2, 4, 3
49. 4, 1, 2, 3

CHAPTER 29

1. f
2. h
3. g
4. i
5. r
6. o
7. b
8. c
9. e
10. n
11. q
12. p
13. d
14. l
15. m
16. a
17. j
18. k
19. T
20. T
21. F. It can be done with a consistent bowel training program.
22. T
23. F. Exercise can prevent constipation.
24. T
25. F. Motor sensory disturbances can lead to constipation and fecal incontinence.
26. T
27. T
28. F. Mental depression can contribute by slowing bodily processes.
29. fiber
30. loosen
31. Diverticulosis
32. mastication
33. fat, fiber
34. liquid
35. 40

36. flatulence
37. person or individual
38. dependence
39. 3
40. 4
41. 2
42. 1
43. 1
44. 3
45. 2
46. 4
47. 4, 2, 1, 3
48. 2, 4, 3, 1
49. 1, 2, 3, 4

CHAPTER 30

1. m
2. u
3. k
4. l
5. a
6. y
7. h
8. t
9. v
10. b
11. r
12. s
13. e
14. n
15. g
16. d
17. i
18. p
19. q
20. w
21. c
22. f
23. o
24. j
25. x
26. F. The bladder is under voluntary control of the sympathetic nervous system.
27. T
28. T
29. F. Urinary incontinence is not normal.
30. T
31. F. It is under control of the sympathetic nervous system.
32. T
33. T
34. T
35. F. Small amounts of blood are not visible.

36. F. A minimum of 10 cc is needed.
37. F. Antibiotics are not always indicated.
38. vesicoureteral
39. detrusor
40. urea, creatinine, uric acid, bilirubin, metabolites of hormones
41. sodium, potassium
42. peristalsis
43. inflammation, infection, obstruction
44. frequency
45. 150, 500
46. Voiding urogram
47. Creatinine
48. Stress
49. total
50. prompted voiding
51. habit training
52. Kegel exercises
53. 1. Indwelling urinary catheters are a major cause of urinary tract infection in hospitalized clients. For this reason, it is important to remove the catheter as soon as possible after surgery.
54. 2. Taking a deep breath relaxes the abdominal muscles, which may make catheter removal easier. Each of the other options represents an activity in which the client could bear down, which could increase discomfort.
55. 3. Clients are expected to void no later than 8 hours after catheter removal. It is very important to calculate the appropriate time for each client.
56. 4. Increasing fluid intake will increase the volume of blood filtered in the kidneys, resulting in increased urine output. The larger volume of urine often makes it easier to void following catheter removal.
57. 2
58. 1
59. 4
60. 1
61. 4

62. 4
63. 2
64. 3
65. 2
66. 1
67. 3, 2, 4, 1
68. 4, 1, 2, 3
69. 3, 2, 1, 4

CHAPTER 31

1. f
2. b
3. a
4. e
5. c
6. g
7. h
8. d
9. F. The melanocyte, which is located at the base of the epidermis, produces melanin, one of the pigments responsible for skin color.
10. T
11. F. Thick, yellow nails could indicate a fungal infection.
12. F. It would reinforce a client's dependence.
13. T
14. T
15. T
16. T
17. Self-care
18. vitamin D
19. systemic
20. caries
21. blood
22. carcinomas
23. bed bath
24. wide-toothed, pick
25. 2. *Bathing/hygiene self-care deficit:* Impaired ability to perform or complete bathing/hygiene activities for oneself
26. 2. A hot-water bath helps relieve muscle spasm and muscle tension.
27. 4. *Disturbed thought processes* related to loss of memory.
28. 2
29. 1
30. 2
31. 1
32. 4
33. 3, 2, 1, 4

34. 1, 3, 4, 2
35. 4, 3, 2, 1

CHAPTER 32

1. j
2. h
3. g
4. l
5. m
6. i
7. o
8. f
9. c
10. b
11. e
12. d
13. n
14. k
15. a
16. T
17. F. Vertebral bone decreases in postmenopausal women.
18. T
19. T
20. F. A slight limitation of ROM is acceptable.
21. T
22. T
23. osteoclastic
24. atrophy
25. metatarsus varus
26. muscle weakness
27. Crepitus
28. Physical
29. Rehabilitation
30. 1. *Impaired physical mobility* related to healing hip fracture.
31. 2. The physical therapist focuses on increasing mobility skills.
32. 1. ROM exercises are isotonic exercises.
33. 1
34. 3
35. 1
36. 3
37. 3
38. 1, 2, 4, 3
39. 4, 3, 2, 1
40. 3, 2, 4, 1

CHAPTER 33

1. c
2. b
3. d

4. o
5. r
6. k
7. e
8. j
9. v
10. p
11. a
12. x
13. h
14. l
15. u
16. m
17. f
18. g
19. n
20. q
21. i
22. w
23. t
24. s
25. T
26. T
27. F. The longer the person is immobile, the higher the risk of complications of disuse.
28. F. Local circulation is impaired.
29. F. Orthostatic intolerance is a drop in systolic blood pressure.
30. T
31. T
32. Disuse
33. longer
34. energy
35. ulcers
36. orthostatic hypotension
37. calculi
38. 1, 2, hours
39. 1. In a friction injury, the epidermal layer of the skin is rubbed off.
40. 2. For moderate *Risk for disuse syndrome*, assess and intervene every 2 to 4 hours.
41. 3. *Risk for disuse syndrome:* A state in which an individual is at risk for deterioration of body systems as the result of prescribed or unavoidable musculoskeletal inactivity.
42. 4
43. 2
44. 1
45. 2

46. l
47. 3, 2, 1, 5, 4, 6
48. 1, 4, 3, 2
49. 3, 4, 1, 2

CHAPTER 34

1. b
2. c
3. i
4. d
5. a
6. h
7. j
8. f
9. e
10. g
11. k
12. r
13. o
14. v
15. q
16. m
17. l
18. n
19. u
20. p
21. s
22. t
23. T
24. T
25. F. Tidal volume is the amount of air moved with normal flow of air in and out of the lungs.
26. T
27. F. Sitting or standing straight without support is the optimum position.
28. T
29. F. Nicotine patches, along with counseling and support, have a 30% success rate.
30. F. The pain of fractured ribs restricts the chest wall movement.
31. T
32. T
33. F. In a stable client in a home environment, clean technique is appropriate.
34. F. Always ask if the client has COPD when starting oxygen at greater than 2 L/min.
35. diaphragm
36. Elastic recoil
37. Surfactant
38. Sighing

39. Dead space
40. glottis
41. complete blood count
42. forced vital capacity
43. 90
44. Obtundation
45. Thick, tenacious
46. Altered breathing pattern
47. deoxygenated hemoglobin
48. Naloxone (Narcan)
49. 2. Because this is a low-flow oxygen system, the client needs to breathe additional air in order to inhale sufficient air to meet the needs of the lungs. The other responses are incorrect rationales for this question.
50. 1. With hypoventilation, the lungs do not expand as fully as necessary, and because of this, the respiratory rate increases in an attempt to compensate.
51. 3. The inhaler should be activated at the same time as the client takes a deep breath so that the medication is dispersed well into the respiratory tree and does not accumulate in the mouth and upper airway.
52. 2
53. 3
54. 1
55. 1
56. 4
57. 4
58. 1
59. 1
60. 4
61. 1
62. 2
63. 2
64. 4, 3, 2, 1
65. 3, 4, 2, 1
66. 3, 2, 6, 5, 1, 4
67. 2, 1, 4, 3, 5, 6

CHAPTER 35

1. f
2. g
3. p
4. a
5. r
6. i
7. b
8. j

9. l
10. m
11. o
12. d
13. n
14. h
15. q
16. e
17. c
18. k
19. T
20. F. Greater stroke volume is produced.
21. T
22. F. Decreased blood flow to tissues and decreased oxygen-carrying capacity of hemoglobin results.
23. T
24. T
25. F. They cause inflammation and scarring of cardiac tissue.
26. T
27. T
28. T
29. 5, 6
30. Cocaine, amphetamines
31. atherosclerosis
32. 140/90
33. cerebrovascular accident
34. left
35. Iron
36. heparin
37. vasoconstriction
38. diet, exercise, smoking
39. 1. Rest periods should be interspersed with activities.
40. 3. Sauces often contain salt.
41. 4. This will help to prevent orthostatic hypotension, a risk of this type of medication.
42. 2. Any activity that tenses abdominal or chest muscles can cause the Valsalva maneuver.
43. 1
44. 4
45. 3
46. 4
47. 1
48. 4, 1, 2, 6, 3, 5
49. 1, 5, 2, 3, 4
50. 3, 2, 1, 4
51. 3, 1, 6, 5, 2, 4

CHAPTER 36

1. k
2. a
3. m
4. s
5. c
6. h
7. q
8. t
9. n
10. p
11. e
12. r
13. f
14. w
15. i
16. v
17. g
18. b
19. d
20. l
21. o
22. x
23. t
24. F. A depressed client may stay in bed an adequate number of hours but may feel mentally drained.
25. T
26. F. It is one of the most Common.
27. T
28. zeitgeber
29. Melatonin
30. caffeine
31. REM
32. 2
33. back
34. 1. Because it has such a long half-life, caffeine taken late in the day may increase insomnia and nighttime arousals.
35. 4. Because the half-life of nicotine is 1 to 2 hours, the person who smokes more than one cigarette within an hour of bedtime may delay sleep onset.
36. 2. The client should go to bed only when sleepy, refrain from daytime naps, and set the alarm for the same time each day.
37. 4. They are practiced for 20 minutes, can be used during the night as well, and may be enhanced with deep breathing exercises.

38. 2
39. 1
40. 4
41. 3
42. 2
43. 1, 3, 2, 5, 4
44. 3, 5, 4, 2, 1
45. 4, 2, 1, 3

CHAPTER 37

1. s
2. dd
3. l
4. hh
5. m
6. u
7. y
8. t
9. ff
10. w
11. aa
12. bb
13. ii
14. v
15. n
16. h
17. d
18. b
19. c
20. ee
21. k
22. j
23. cc
24. i
25. a
26. r
27. x
28. p
29. jj
30. q
31. g
32. z
33. e
34. gg
35. o
36. f
37. T
38. F. This refers to somatic pain.
39. T
40. T
41. T
42. F. Pain is the same in the elderly as for any other population and is not a normal part of the aging process.
43. T

44. diagnostic, response
45. Referred
46. learned
47. Chronic
48. pain rating scale
49. neuropathic
50. neuropathic
51. 3. Cultural expectations can mold the meaning of pain and the subsequent behaviors; your lack of understanding of those expectations can interfere with an accurate pain assessment.
52. 4. The correct nursing diagnosis is *Chronic pain* related to malignant disease progression.
53. 4. Rescue dosing involves giving as-needed doses of an immediate-release analgesic in response to the breakthrough pain in addition to the scheduled analgesic dosage.
54. 2
55. 2
56. 4
57. 3
58. 2
59. 3, 2, 1, 4
60. 4, 2, 3, 1
61. 1, 2, 3, 4

CHAPTER 38

1. i
2. j
3. m
4. l
5. c
6. b
7. g
8. f
9. e
10. a
11. n
12. d
13. k
14. h
15. F. Sensory deficits occur most commonly in older adults.
16. T
17. T
18. T
19. F. They are tests to determine conduction or sensorineural hearing loss.
20. T

21. F. A hearing aid may be damaged from radiation.
22. 85
23. Strabismus
24. conductive
25. age
26. Snellen
27. staining
28. overload
29. 1. Night blindness is one of the most distressing symptoms of cataracts because it interferes with night driving and seeing in darkened rooms.
30. 3. *Disturbed sensory perception: visual* cataracts causing visual problems for her
31. 2. *Risk for injury:* teaching client how to care for eye to prevent it from becoming injured.
32. 3
33. 1
34. 2
35. 2
36. 1
37. 1, 3, 4, 2, 5
38. 5, 1, 3, 2, 4
39. 3, 6, 1, 5, 2, 4

CHAPTER 39

1. i
2. d
3. k
4. g
5. l
6. a
7. h
8. j
9. b
10. e
11. f
12. m
13. c
14. T
15. F. Nonverbal communication, such as eye contact, facial expression, and head movements, may have different meanings in different cultures.
16. T
17. T
18. T
19. T
20. T
21. F. Psychiatric illness can affect communication with others.

22. T
23. F. A risk is that both think they understand each other when in fact they do not.
24. neurological
25. Telegraphic
26. global
27. dysphonia
28. tracheostomy
29. Broca's
30. esophageal
31. receptive
32. Powerlessness
33. physical
34. 1. If there is incongruity between behavior and the spoken word, it requires further assessment.
35. 3. When using an interpreter, always direct your questions and attention to the client, not the interpreter.
36. 4. The client may not understand explanations of procedures and treatment, and it raises an ethical concern if the client cannot fully understand a consent form or completely understand the teaching related to an informed consent solicited before a test, procedure, or surgery.
37. 2. Expected outcome appropriate for diagnosis of *Impaired communication* in this situation is that he expresses satisfaction with the communication process.
38. 1
39. 1
40. 3
41. 4
42. 1
43. 2, 1, 3, 4
44. 2, 3, 1, 4
45. 1, 3, 2, 4

CHAPTER 40

1. e
2. g
3. n
4. f
5. l
6. j
7. i
8. a

9. o
10. c
11. k
12. r
13. m
14. p
15. b
16. s
17. d
18. h
19. q
20. F. Confusion can occur in younger people, although incidence increases with age.
21. T
22. T
23. F. The client may not be able to judge safety issues with any degree of insight.
24. T
25. T
26. T
27. F. Attention span is included in the assessment.
28. T
29. F. Bright colors or symbols should be used to identify room and/or bathroom for a client with chronic confusion.
30. frontal, temporal
31. acute
32. night
33. circadian
34. Alzheimer's
35. agnosia
36. fever
37. remote
38. injury
39. 2. The other options could increase the risk of injury.
40. 3. The other options could increase anxiety, which could worsen confusion.
41. 1. The other options could impair the client's ability to get restful sleep.
42. 4. Appropriate lighting and visible reminders are most helpful.
43. 4
44. 2
45. 3
46. 1
47. 2
48. 1, 3, 2, 4

49. 1, 4, 3, 2
50. 3, 4, 2, 1

CHAPTER 41

1. e
2. c
3. f
4. b
5. a
6. d
7. T
8. T
9. T
10. T
11. F. This demonstrates a positive correlation.
12. T
13. F. Socioeconomic status has a direct relationship to self-concept.
14. T
15. T
16. F. This is done only when indicated, such as with health problems that typically affect self-concept.
17. body image
18. self-actualization
19. identity
20. power, control
21. emotional, cognitive, perceptual
22. parenting
23. self-esteem
24. Chronic
25. Disturbed body image
26. 2. This often results from long-standing negative evaluations or feelings about the self.
27. 2. It is helpful to include people who have meaning to the client.
28. 1. Shock and disbelief is the first stage of the grieving process.
29. 3. It may help to talk to someone who has lived through and coped with the experience.
30. 4. Encouraging choices in care promotes a sense of power and control.
31. 1
32. 2
33. 3
34. 4
35. 3
36. 1

CHAPTER 42

1. e
2. d
3. a
4. b
5. h
6. c
7. f
8. g
9. T
10. T
11. T
12. F. Anxiety disorders are common.
13. T
14. T
15. F. It is a learned behavior that is a conditioned response to a specific stimulus.
16. T
17. T
18. F. A panic attack is sudden.
19. biological, ego
20. vulnerability
21. severe
22. pathological
23. obsession
24. environmental
25. obsessive, compulsive
26. economic
27. 2. *Powerlessness* is associated with a perceived lack of control over situations or life events.
28. 1. This is an early goal. The others would be achieved later.
29. 3. Active listening involves listening to feelings as well as words.
30. 4
31. 3
32. 4

CHAPTER 43

1. s
2. t
3. b
4. i
5. l
6. m
7. f
8. o
9. p
10. q
11. h
12. g
13. r
14. c
15. a
16. e
17. n
18. d
19. j
20. k
21. T
22. F. Low, not high, socioeconomic status is a factor.
23. T
24. T
25. F. Hope can be present.
26. T
27. T
28. risk, health
29. housing
30. Social status
31. Social
32. energy
33. control
34. self-determination
35. 4. Social needs are also concerned with the social or environmental structures, such as the assessment of the risk of neighborhood violence and neighborhood resources, affecting the client's life.
36. 2. Helping a person to have a sense of relatedness to others, such as helping her contact her parents, can instill hope.
37. 2. To evaluate interventions for *Hopelessness*, assess for a change in the way the client thinks about the self in relation to others, the environment, and the self.
38. 1
39. 4
40. 3
41. 1
42. 1

CHAPTER 44

1. c
2. g
3. h
4. i
5. b
6. d

7. e
8. f
9. a
10. j
11. T
12. T
13. T
14. F. This refers to an orthotist.
15. F. These are long-term care facilities.
16. T
17. T
18. F. This client would have unilateral neglect.
19. injury, mental conditions
20. physical, bowel, skin
21. coping
22. Assisted
23. Americans, Disabilities
24. Functional Independence Measure
25. maximizing, complications
26. 2. The physical therapist assesses a client's range of motion, mobility, strength, balance, and gait.
27. 4. Respite care is a temporary service enabling informal caregivers to take a break.
28. 1. *Self-care deficit* is applicable to people experiencing impaired ability to perform any one of the basic self-care activities.
29. 2
30. 3
31. 3
32. 3
33. 4

CHAPTER 45

1. d
2. n
3. a
4. f
5. q
6. k
7. j
8. s
9. e
10. h
11. m
12. o
13. l
14. i
15. r

16. p
17. c
18. g
19. b
20. T
21. F. This is a result of dysfunctional grieving.
22. T
23. T
24. T
25. F. Many people experience these feelings of relief or emancipation.
26. F. This refers to the person who is uncomfortable facing the reality of his or her own death.
27. religious, condolences, burial
28. self
29. recognition
30. reflection
31. family
32. presence
33. Condemnation
34. 2. Recognition: shock and denial: somatic responses: These may include gastrointestinal symptoms and cardiopulmonary reactions.
35. 1. This is the act of choosing when and to whom a person will give attention to a loss and allow thoughts and feelings to enter the conscious mind.
36. 3. This is an unexpected, involuntary resurgence of acute grief-related emotions and behaviors triggered by routine events.
37. 2
38. 3
39. 4
40. 4

CHAPTER 46

1. f
2. m
3. j
4. b
5. c
6. e
7. h
8. q
9. i
10. o

11. n
12. l
13. p
14. d
15. g
16. k
17. r
18. a
19. T
20. F. Gender identity is an internal sense.
21. F. Sexual patterns may not precisely fit with prevailing expectations.
22. T
23. F. At least one third of nurses never assess their client's sexual health.
24. T
25. T
26. biological, cultural
27. adolescence
28. Orgasm
29. emotional, love
30. embarrassment
31. sexual
32. touch
33. 1. The correct diagnosis is *Ineffective sexuality patterns:* the state in which an individual expresses concern regarding his or her sexuality.
34. 2. Because of the additional information about not having sexual relations with her husband for the last 3 months, the nurse should also consider the diagnosis of *Sexual dysfunction.*
35. 1. The first step in the PLISSIT model is *permission* to discuss sexual issues.
36. 1
37. 2
38. 2
39. 4
40. 1

CHAPTER 47

1. l
2. n
3. k
4. g
5. i
6. c
7. j

8. b
9. m
10. a
11. d
12. f
13. e
14. h
15. T
16. F. It is the exhaustion stage.
17. T
18. F. This refers to rationalization.
19. T
20. T
21. F. Stress is highly individualized.
22. F. This defines transference.
23. T
24. alarm reaction
25. crisis
26. developmental, situational
27. projection
28. genetics, developmental stage
29. sympathetic
30. coping
31. adulthood
32. denial
33. 2. He is drinking and does not acknowledge that his wound is infected.
34. 3. A therapeutic relationship is necessary to build trust and is a precursor to other interventions.
35. 4. Knowledge and control are best achieved by helping him learn how to manage his health status.
36. 1. Relaxation and music can be used together. The other methods are cognitive coping methods.
37. 2
38. 3
39. 1
40. 1

CHAPTER 48

1. k
2. n
3. g
4. t
5. s
6. p
7. q
8. u
9. a

10. i
11. d
12. r
13. h
14. m
15. j
16. e
17. l
18. c
19. f
20. o
21. b
22. T
23. T
24. F. This occurs in a healthy family.
25. T
26. T
27. F. Interventions may not be remembered or may be rejected.
28. T
29. F. They are more likely to when they have inadequate support systems.
30. T
31. T
32. caregiver
33. affective, socialization, health
34. coping
35. trusting
36. ambivalent
37. stress
38. perception
39. insight
40. 2. An example of an extrafamily stressor is when a caregiver quits work to care for a family member and then experiences a financial hardship.
41. 1. She is vulnerable for felt difficulty in performing the family caregiver role.
42. 4. Providing direct assistance helps the caregiver identify professional resources.
43. 4
44. 2
45. 3
46. 2
47. 4

CHAPTER 49

1. f
2. e
3. g
4. i

5. c
6. d
7. b
8. k
9. j
10. l
11. h
12. a
13. T
14. F. They are not necessarily synonymous.
15. F. Faith is belief without proof.
16. F. Nurses commonly avoid addressing spirituality.
17. T
18. T
19. T
20. God
21. Hope
22. Taoists
23. denominations
24. spiritual
25. prayer
26. 2. Mexican Americans have a tendency toward traditional values of family roles, including men heading the family.
27. 4. Asking a client "What has bothered you most about being sick?" helps you assess the client's perceived relation between spiritual beliefs and health.
28. 4. The diagnosis is *Spiritual distress:* disruption in the life principle that pervades a person's entire being and that integrates and transcends one's biological and psychological nature.
29. 4
30. 4
31. 2
32. 2
33. 4

CHAPTER 50

1. h
2. n
3. g
4. l
5. p
6. o
7. m
8. b
9. i

10. q

11. d

12. c

13. a

14. j

15. f

16. k

17. e

18. T

19. F. These are duties of the circulating nurse.

20. T

21. T

22. T

23. F. Pain is expected and normal.

24. T

25. T

26. F. The drug of choice is dantrolene sodium.

27. T

28. elective

29. preinduction

30. general

31. surgeon

32. standard

33. after

34. Laryngospasm

35. incentive spirometer

36. 6, 8

37. Verbal, written

38. 1. *Anxiety* is expected due to the uncertain outcome of the surgery.

39. 3. They should be done 10 to 12 times every 1 to 2 hours for best effect.

40. 2. It will help him prevent alveolar collapse and move secretions to large airway passages for easier expectoration.

41. 3. Splinting the incision makes movement more comfortable.

42. 4

43. 2

44. 3

45. 1

46. 4

PERFORMANCE CHECKLISTS

Name _____ Specific Skill Performed _____

Date _____ Attempt Number _____

Instructor _____ PASS _____ FAIL _____

Performance Checklist 7-1: Assessing Temperature

	S	U	Comments
1. Performed preliminary actions.	_____	_____	_____
2. Selected an appropriate route and obtained corresponding thermometer.	_____	_____	_____
3. Prepared the thermometer.	_____	_____	_____

GLASS THERMOMETER

a. Ensured that glass thermometer was clean and free of defects. Followed agency policy for storage and cleaning. Cleansed thermometer with an alcohol wipe between uses, wiping from the stem to the bulb using a rotating motion. Thoroughly rinsed away any disinfectant in cool water before use. _____ _____ _____

b. Ensured that liquid was confined to the bulb. Held thermometer firmly by the tip and using a flicking wrist motion; shook the thermometer to force the liquid into the bulb. Checked the reading on the thermometer to ensure that it was below body temperature. _____ _____ _____

ELECTRONIC OR TYMPANIC THERMOMETER

a. If using an electronic thermometer, turned on the device by removing the probe. If using a tympanic thermometer, turned on the unit. _____ _____ _____

b. Place a disposable sheath or cover over the probe. _____ _____ _____

4. Measured the temperature. _____ _____ _____

ORAL ROUTE

a. Placed the thermometer or electronic probe under the client's tongue, in the sublingual pocket next to the frenlum linguae, for 2 to 4 minutes or according to facility policy (glass thermometer) or until unit beeped (electronic thermometer). _____ _____ _____

b. Had client close mouth and hold thermometer in place with lips, making sure the bulb remained in direct contact with the sublingual tissue. Warned client not to bite on the thermometer. _____ _____ _____

RECTAL ROUTE

a. Positioned client in the side-lying (left Sims') position and draped for privacy. _____ _____ _____

b. Put on clean gloves. _____ _____ _____

c. Lubricated the bulb of the thermometer with water-soluble jelly. _____ _____ _____

d. Gently inserted the thermometer about 1.5 inches into the rectum, angling the thermometer toward the client's umbilicus during insertion. _____ _____ _____

e. Held the thermometer in place for 2 to 4 minutes or according to facility policy. _____ _____ _____

AXILLARY ROUTE

a. Placed the thermometer in the center of the client's axilla and left it in place for 8 to 10 minutes or according to facility policy. Made sure the thermometer was secure and the bulb remained in contact with the axillary skin. Had client cross his or her arm across the chest. _____ _____ _____

TYMPANIC ROUTE

a. Pulled client's auricle back and gently obtained the temperature measurement. _____ _____ _____

b. Placed athe probe into the ear canal, pointing the tip of the probe toward the client's nose and directing the probe toward the tympanic membrane. _____ _____ _____

c. Held the probe steady and quickly pressed the activation button. _____ _____ _____

d. Listened for the buzzer to sound when the temperature had been measured. _____ _____ _____

5. Read the temperature measurement. _____ _____ _____

a. After an appropriate time or after the electronic thermometer beeped, removed the thermometer from the client's mouth, axilla, ear canal, or anus. _____ _____ _____

b. After removing a glass rectal thermometer, wiped it with a tissue using a rotating motion from stem to bulb. Discarded the tissue or moved the disposable sheath. _____ _____ _____

6. Documented the client's temperature in the medical record as soon at the reading was obtained. Noted whether the reading was oral, rectal, or axillary by writing oral, R, or Ax next to the measurement. Reported an abnormal temperature to a charge nurse or physician. _____ _____ _____

• Performed completion actions. _____ _____ _____

Additional Comments:

Name _____   Specific Skill Performed _____

Date _____   Attempt Number _____

Instructor _____   PASS _____   FAIL _____

Performance Checklist 7-2: Assessing Radial and Apical Pulse

	S	U	Comments

ASSESSING RADIAL PULSE

1. Performed preliminary actions. ___ ___ _____

2. Prepared the client for pulse measure. ___ ___ _____

   a. Placed the client in a comfortable position and had the client relax. ___ ___ _____

3. Measured the pulse. ___ ___ _____

RADIAL PULSE MEASUREMENT

   a. Placed the client's arm across his or her abdomen or in another relaxed, comfortable position. Located the client's radial pulse. ___ ___ _____

   b. Placed the pad of the middle fingers on the inside of the client's wrist. ___ ___ _____

   c. Compressed the radial artery firmly against the underlying bone. ___ ___ _____

   d. Occluded the pulse and then gradually released pressure until the pulse became palpable. ___ ___ _____

   e. Assessed the quality and rhythm of the client's radial pulse while counting the pulse. If the radial pulse was irregular or weak, assessed the client's apical pulse. If the pulse was regular and of normal strength, counted the number of beats for 30 seconds and multiplied by 2. If the pulse was irregular, counted for a full minute. ___ ___ _____

APICAL PULSE MEASUREMENT

   a. Placed the client in the supine position and located the apical pulse at the fifth intercostal space to the left of the midclavicular line of the anterior thorax. ___ ___ _____

   b. Kept the client covered and appropriately exposed the chest only as needed. ___ ___ _____

   c. If necessary, lifted a female's breast to find her apical pulse. ___ ___ _____

   d. Placed the ear pieces of the stethoscope in the ears and the diaphragm firmly against the client's chest. Avoided rubbing it against clothing or linens. ___ ___ _____

   e. Assessed the rate and rhythm of the client's apical pulse. Counted the apical pulse for 1 full minute. ___ ___ _____

4. Documented the rate and any abnormality of rhythm or strength as soon as the reading was obtained. Reported an abnormal pulse to a charge nurse or physician. _____ _____ _____

- Performed completion actions. _____ _____ _____

Additional Comments:

Name _____   Specific Skill Performed _____

Date _____   Attempt Number _____

Instructor _____   PASS _____ FAIL _____

Performance Checklist 7-3: Assessing Respiration

	S	U	Comments
1. Performed preliminary actions.	____	____	_____
2. Made sure client was relaxed and quiet, either sitting or lying down. Made sure the client's anterior thorax was easily visible and that the lungs could complete the full excursion of respiratory movement without hindrance.	____	____	_____
3. Made sure the client did not know the respirations were being counted.	____	____	_____
4. Watched the rise and fall of the client's chest, counting each cycle of inhalation and exhalation as one breath If necessary, placed one hand on the client's lower thorax or abdomen to palpate the movement.	____	____	_____
5. Counted the client's respirations. For a client with a regular rhythm, counted for 30 seconds and multiplied the result by 2. For an infant, child, or adult with an irregular rhythm, counted for one full minute.	____	____	_____
6. Documented the respirations as soon as the reading was obtained.	____	____	_____
7. Reported abnormal respirations to a charge nurse or physician.	____	____	_____
• Performed completion actions.	____	____	_____

Additional Comments:

Name _____   Specific Skill Performed _____

Date _____   Attempt Number _____

Instructor _____   PASS _____   FAIL _____

Performance Checklist 7-4: Assessing Oxygen Saturation

	S	U	Comments
1. Performed preliminary actions.	_____	_____	_____
2. Chose site with adequate capillary refill.	_____	_____	_____
3. Chose proper sensor according to location and client's size and weight.	_____	_____	_____
4. Cleansed site with alcohol, and removed nail polish if dark or contained blue pigments.	_____	_____	_____
5. Attached sensor probe to site and to pulse oximeter if not already connected.	_____	_____	_____
6. Turned on power to activate unit; observed pulse waveform on screen, and listened to audible beep.	_____	_____	_____
7. Waited for machine to display consistent reading, and recorded value.	_____	_____	_____
8. Shut off machine and removed probe if single reading was obtained. Left probe in place if continuous monitoring was required.	_____	_____	_____
9. Reported abnormal reading to a charge nurse or physician.	_____	_____	_____
• Performed completion actions.	_____	_____	_____

Additional Comments:

Name _____ Specific Skill Performed _____

Date _____ Attempt Number _____

Instructor _____ PASS _____ FAIL _____

Performance Checklist 7-5: Assessing Blood Pressure

	S	U	Comments
1. Performed preliminary actions.	_____	_____	_____
2. Selected a cuff of correct size for the client and the limb being used.	_____	_____	_____
a. Selected a bladder that fit almost completely around the client's arm.	_____	_____	_____
b. Selected a cuff width about two-thirds the length of the client's upper arm.	_____	_____	_____
3. Chose the arm on which to take the BP reading; avoided an arm being used for hemodialysis or that had a shunt, burn, cast, IV lines, or traumatic injury or was contiguous with the site of breast or axillary surgery. If unable to use on of the client's arms, used on a leg and measured the BP at the popliteal artery.	_____	_____	_____
4. Positioned the client's arm level with the heart, palm up and in a relaxed and comfortable fashion.	_____	_____	_____
5. If the client was changing from a lying to a sitting position, waited at least 2 minutes before taking the BP measurement.	_____	_____	_____
6. Affixed the cuff onto the client's arm.	_____	_____	_____
a. Did not place the cuff over clothing and did not push clothing up so it constricted the brachial artery.	_____	_____	_____
b. Placed the bottom edge of the cuff 1 inch above the client's antecubital fossa.	_____	_____	_____
c. Placed the center of the cuff directly over the brachial artery.	_____	_____	_____
d. Wrapped the cuff snugly around the client's arm while allowing space to place the stethoscope over the brachial artery.	_____	_____	_____
7. Positioned the sphygmomanometer at eye level, with the liquid in the manometer or the needle of an aneroid gauge at zero.	_____	_____	_____
8. Obtained a palpated systolic blood pressure if client's BP was being read for the first time.	_____	_____	_____
a. Palpated the brachial or radial pulse.	_____	_____	_____
b. Inflated the cuff until the pulse disappeared.	_____	_____	_____
c. Released the pressure slowly until the pulse returned and noted this reading.	_____	_____	_____
d. Quickly released the cuff.	_____	_____	_____
9. Obtained the BP reading without talking during the measurement.	_____	_____	_____
a. Waited 30 to 60 seconds after obtaining the palpated BP.	_____	_____	_____
b. Placed the bell of the stethoscope lightly over the brachial artery.	_____	_____	_____

    c. Tightened the screw clamp and quickly inflated the cuff
to 30 mm Hg above the palpated systolic reading.   _____ _____ _____

    d. Deflated the cuff slowly and steadily at 2 to 3 mm Hg
per second until a soft tapping sound was heard.   _____ _____ _____

    e. Continued deflating the cuff, slowly, listening for a murmur,
swishing sounds, clear tapping, and a muffling of sound.   _____ _____ _____

    f. Continued deflating the cuff, slowly listening for sounds to stop. _____ _____ _____

10. Deflated the cuff at a moderate rate and completely. If necessary
to take another BP reading, waited 1 to 2 minutes before doing so.   _____ _____ _____

11. Documented the client's BP in the medical record as soon as
the reading was obtained. If an aucultory gap was identified,
documented the reading in mm Hg that corresponded to
the length of the silence.   _____ _____ _____

12. Reported an abnormal blood pressure to a charge nurse or physician. _____ _____ _____

• Performed completion actions.   _____ _____ _____

Additional Comments:

Name _____   Specific Skill Performed _____

Date _____   Attempt Number _____

Instructor _____   PASS _____   FAIL _____

Performance Checklist 21-1: Administering Oral Medications

	S	U	Comments
1. Performed preliminary actions.	_____	_____	_____
2. Assessed client to verify that oral route was appropriate. Notified physician if oral medications were contraindicated.	_____	_____	_____
3. Confirmed medication order sheet against original physician orders.	_____	_____	_____
a. Clarified inconsistencies if found.	_____	_____	_____
b. Checked client's record for allergies.	_____	_____	_____
c. Determined and performed assessments needed prior to dose being given (e.g., blood pressure or pulse).	_____	_____	_____
4. Dispensed medications one at a time, for one client at a time.	_____	_____	_____
a. Unlocked drawer of medication cart or storage area.	_____	_____	_____
b. Selected correct medication, and compared its label with order sheet.	_____	_____	_____
c. Correctly calculated dose needed.	_____	_____	_____
d. Rechecked dose to ensure that it was correct.	_____	_____	_____
e. Placed solid medication in disposable soufflé cup.	_____	_____	_____
f. For partial dose, used gloved hand or cutting device to spit a scored medication in half, and discarded unused half of divided tablet.	_____	_____	_____
g. When removing dose from bottle, poured correct number of tablets into bottle cap and transferred them into a clean medicine cup without touching tablets. Returned untouched extra tablets in cap to bottle. Used a new cup for each medication.	_____	_____	_____
h. Left unit dose medications in their original packaging and placed them together in one cup. Kept medication requiring special assessments in a separate cup.	_____	_____	_____
i. Poured liquid medication into a calibrated, disposable medication cup.	_____	_____	_____
(1) Mixed liquid medication thoroughly. Discarded medication if it had changed color or become cloudy.	_____	_____	_____
(2) Removed lid from bottle or container, and placed it upside down to prevent contamination.	_____	_____	_____
(3) Held bottle with label facing up under palm of hand.	_____	_____	_____
(4) Held medication cup at eye level, and used thumbnail to mark level of correct dose. Poured medication into cup until bottom of meniscus reached level of thumbnail. Discarded excess medication.	_____	_____	_____

(5) Wiped lip of container with clean paper towel before recapping.   _____ _____ _____

(6) Took unit dose of liquid to bedside without opening unless client required partial dose.   _____ _____ _____

5. For medications of all types, rechecked medication and dose after it was poured but before it was given to client.   _____ _____ _____

6. Locked medication cart or storage area, and took medications to client.   _____ _____ _____

7. Identified client.   _____ _____ _____

   a. Read client's name on identification bracelet.   _____ _____ _____

   b. Asked an alert, cooperative client to state his or her name.   _____ _____ _____

   c. Verified client's identity with another staff member familiar with the client if the client did not have an identification bracelet or was confused or unable to communicate.   _____ _____ _____

8. Performed final assessments, and explained purpose of medications to client.   _____ _____ _____

9. Gave medications to client.   _____ _____ _____

   a. Allowed client to choose taking one medication at a time or in a certain order.   _____ _____ _____

   b. Rechecked the accuracy of any medications that the client questioned.   _____ _____ _____

   c. Removed unit dose medications from wrappers. Gave medications to client in a cup or client's hand, depending on client's preference.   _____ _____ _____

   d. Offered a full glass of liquid. Had client moisten mouth with fluid and bow head slightly to aid swallowing. Followed medications with an additional 60 to 100 mL of fluid if client not on fluid restriction.   _____ _____ _____

   e. Gave liquids, chewable medications, lozenges, sublingual medications, and/or buccal medications separately from oral tablets, pills, or capsules.   _____ _____ _____

   f. Ensured that client had swallowed all medications by questioning client or checking client's mouth. Stayed with client until all medications had been taken.   _____ _____ _____

10. Documented medication administration promptly on client's medication administration record or computerized medication record.   _____ _____ _____

11. Rechecked client after medication had time to take effect, and assessed client's response to medication.   _____ _____ _____

• Performed completion actions.   _____ _____ _____

Additional Comments:

Name _____   Specific Skill Performed _____

Date _____   Attempt Number _____

Instructor _____   PASS _____   FAIL _____

Performance Checklist 21-2: Withdrawing Medication From an Ampule

	S	U	Comments
1. Performed preliminary actions.	_____	_____	_____
2. Opened ampule.	_____	_____	_____
a. Tapped upper chamber of ampule until fluid dropped into lower chamber.	_____	_____	_____
b. Wrapped alcohol swab or gauze pad around ampule neck.	_____	_____	_____
c. Snapped neck so it opened away from the body.	_____	_____	_____
3. Placed ampule upright on flat surface and withdraw medication into syringe.	_____	_____	_____
a. Attached filter needle (if used) to syringe. Held ampule while inserting filter needle into center of the opening on the ampule. Did not allow tip or shaft to touch the rim of the ampule.	_____	_____	_____
b. Gently pulled back on plunger to aspirate medication into the syringe.	_____	_____	_____
c. Tilted ampule as needed to keep the needle tip below the level of medication.	_____	_____	_____
d. If air entered syringe, did not inject into ampule. Removed needle from ampule. Held syringe with needle pointing upward and ejected air (not fluid). Reinserted needle into center of ampule and withdrew fluid again.	_____	_____	_____
4. Ejected excess air or fluid as needed.	_____	_____	_____
5. Replaced needle or filter needle with a new needle, and secured tightly. Discarded used filter needle properly.	_____	_____	_____
6. Compared volume of fluid in syringe with dose ordered.	_____	_____	_____
• Performed completion procedures.	_____	_____	_____

Additional Comments:

Name _____   Specific Skill Performed _____

Date _____   Attempt Number _____

Instructor _____   PASS _____   FAIL _____

Performance Checklist 21-3: Withdrawing Medication From a Vial

	S	U	Comments
1. Performed preliminary actions.	_____	_____	_____
2. Prepared vial.	_____	_____	_____
a. Removed plastic or metal top of new vial to expose rubber seal.	_____	_____	_____
b. Cleansed rubber seal with alcohol swab.	_____	_____	_____
c. Checked expiration date of a previously opened vial; did not use medication opened longer than stated in manufacturer's directions. Checked for appropriate color and clarity.	_____	_____	_____
3. Prepared syringe.	_____	_____	_____
a. Checked for a tight connection between needle hub and syringe barrel.	_____	_____	_____
b. Removed needle cover.	_____	_____	_____
c. Drew back on plunger to fill syringe with a volume of air equal to the dose of medication to be given.	_____	_____	_____
4. Withdrew medication.	_____	_____	_____
a. Inserted needle into center of vial's rubber seal.	_____	_____	_____
b. Injected air from syringe into vial.	_____	_____	_____
c. Inverted vial holding it with first two fingers of nondominant hand.	_____	_____	_____
d. Withdrew medication slowly while holding vial at eye level. Kept tip of needle in solution at all times.	_____	_____	_____
e. Removed excess air by tapping side of syringe with finger, and pushed air back into vial. Removed additional fluid if needed to ensure full dose.	_____	_____	_____
f. Returned vial to upright position, and removed needle by pulling back on syringe barrel, not plunger. Removed excess air if present.	_____	_____	_____
5. Replaced needle with a new one, and secured tightly discarded used needle properly.	_____	_____	_____
6. Compared volume of fluid in syringe with ordered dose.	_____	_____	_____
• Performed completion actions.	_____	_____	_____

Additional Comments:

Name _____   Specific Skill Performed _____

Date _____   Attempt Number _____

Instructor _____   PASS _____   FAIL _____

Performance Checklist 21-4: Mixing Insulins in a Single Syringe

	S	U	Comments
1. Performed preliminary actions.	____	____	_____
2. If insulin in suspension, rotated vial between palms of hands.	____	____	_____
3. Prepared vials.	____	____	_____
a. Removed metal covers if using new vials.	____	____	_____
b. Wiped rubber seals with alcohol swabs.	____	____	_____
c. Checked expiration dates.	____	____	_____
4. Added air to both vials.	____	____	_____
a. Removed needle cover.	____	____	_____
b. Drew up volume of air equal to dose of modified (NPH) insulin and injected into NPH vial without letting needle touch solution. Removed needle from vial.	____	____	_____
c. Drew up volume of air equal to dose of unmodified (Regular) insulin and injected into Regular insulin vial. Left needle in vial.	____	____	_____
5. Removed insulin from two vials.	____	____	_____
a. Inverted vial of Regular insulin and withdrew correct dose without air bubbles present. Turned vial upright, and removed needle from vial.	____	____	_____
b. Cleansed rubber seal of NPH insulin vial and inserted needle. Inverted vial and withdrew correct dose. Turned vial upright again and removed needle.	____	____	_____
c. Recapped needle using scoop technique, did not contaminate needle.	____	____	_____
6. Double-checked dose. Asked another licensed nurse to check dose. Returned vials to storage area. Administered within 5 minutes of preparation.	____	____	_____
• Performed completion actions.	____	____	_____

Additional Comments:

Name _____   Specific Skill Performed _____

Date _____   Attempt Number _____

Instructor _____   PASS _____ FAIL _____

Performance Checklist 21-5: Administering an Intradermal Injection

	S	U	Comments
1. Performed preliminary actions.	____	____	_____
2. Checked medication order, and noted client allergies.	____	____	_____
3. Withdrew medication from vial as described in Procedure 21-3. Took syringe and supplies to client's room, and placed medication on a clean, flat surface.	____	____	_____
4. Prepared client for intradermal injection.	____	____	_____
a. Checked client identity using identification bracelet or other accepted means.	____	____	_____
b. Explained procedure to client.	____	____	_____
c. Put on disposable gloves and opened swab(s) and gauze package using aseptic technique.	____	____	_____
d. Provided privacy, and positioned client comfortably. Selected and exposed injection site.	____	____	_____
5. Prepared injection site and syringe.	____	____	_____
a. Chose an area free from bruises, redness, or lesions.	____	____	_____
b. Cleansed skin with alcohol swab skin, wiping from top to bottom. Allowed alcohol to air-dry.	____	____	_____
c. Removed needle guard or cap.	____	____	_____
d. Checked that volume of medication was correct and that syringe was free of air bubbles.	____	____	_____
6. Injected medication.	____	____	_____
a. Held syringe in dominant hand, and spread skin taut with nondominant hand.	____	____	_____
b. Inserted needle bevel up at a 10- to 15-degree angle into skin for ⅛-inch or until bevel disappeared from view. Ensured needle was visible below skin surface, and resistance was felt.	____	____	_____
c. Injected medication slowly while watching for wheal formation. If none appeared, withdrew needle slightly and continued injecting.	____	____	_____
d. Withdrew needle at same angle as used for insertion.	____	____	_____
e. Used gauze pad to pat dry without massaging.	____	____	_____
7. Disposed of equipment properly, and cleaned area.	____	____	_____
a. Discarded needle and syringe in rigid container without recapping. Disposed of other used materials in trash receptacle.	____	____	_____
b. Positioned client comfortably.	____	____	_____

   c.   Removed gloves and discarded in proper receptacle. Performed hand hygiene. _____ _____ _____

8.   Documented the procedure. _____ _____ _____

   a.   Observed site for an immediate allergic reaction. _____ _____ _____

   b.   Circled area of wheal with skin pencil or ballpoint pen. _____ _____ _____

   c.   Documented date, time, substance, and site of injection in client medication administration order. Documented the date and time of follow-up observations. _____ _____ _____

•   Performed completion actions. _____ _____ _____

Additional Comments:

Name _____   Specific Skill Performed _____

Date _____   Attempt Number _____

Instructor _____   PASS _____   FAIL _____

Performance Checklist 21-6: Administering a Subcutaneous Injection

	S	U	Comments
1. Performed preliminary actions.	___	___	___
2. Checked medication order, and noted any client allergies.	___	___	___
3. Checked medication for appropriate color and clarity, and withdrew medication from ampule or vial as described in previous procedures.	___	___	___
4. Took syringe and other supplies to client's room, and placed them on a clean, flat surface.	___	___	___
5. Prepared client for injection.	___	___	___
a. Checked client identity using an identification bracelet or other agency accepted means.	___	___	___
b. Explained procedure to client in a calm and confident manner.	___	___	___
c. Put on disposable gloves, and opened alcohol swab wrapper using aseptic technique.	___	___	___
d. Provided privacy, and positioned client comfortably. Selected and exposed injection site.	___	___	___
6. Prepared injection site and syringe.	___	___	___
a. Chose an area free from bruises, redness, or lesions.	___	___	___
b. Identified exact site of injection. Cleaned skin with alcohol swab using circular motion outward from injection site. Allowed alcohol to air-dry. Left swab in clean area for use when withdrawing needle.	___	___	___
c. Removed needle guard or cap with nondominant hand by pulling it straight off.	___	___	___
d. Checked syringe to ensure that volume of medication was correct and contained no air bubbles.	___	___	___
7. Injected medication.	___	___	___
a. Held syringe in dominant hand between thumb and forefinger.	___	___	___
b. Pinched or bunched up subcutaneous tissue between thumb and forefinger of nondominant hand. If client had ample subcutaneous tissue or if injecting an anticoagulant drug, spread skin taut.	___	___	___
c. Quickly inserted needle up to hub at a 45- or 90-degree angle, depending on needle length.	___	___	___
d. Released tissue and grasped distal end of syringe with nondominant hand.	___	___	___

e. Unless injecting insulin or heparin, aspirated for blood return by pulling back gently on tip of plunger with thumb and forefinger of dominant hand. _____ _____ _____

f. If blood return was noted, pulled needle from injection site, discarded syringe and needle, and began procedure again. _____ _____ _____

g. If no blood return was noted, injected medication slowly and steadily. _____ _____ _____

h. Withdrew needle quickly at same angle used for insertion, and massaged area with alcohol swab unless insulin or heparin was given. _____ _____ _____

8. Disposed of equipment properly. _____ _____ _____

a. Discarded needle and syringe in rigid container without recapping needle. Disposed of alcohol swab, wrapper, and other used materials in trash receptacle. _____ _____ _____

b. Positioned client comfortably. _____ _____ _____

c. Removed gloves, and discarded them in proper receptacle; performed hand hygiene. _____ _____ _____

9. Documented procedure carefully. _____ _____ _____

a. Recorded date, time, substance, and site of injection on client's medication administration record. _____ _____ _____

b. Checked client within 30 minutes to assess effects of medication. _____ _____ _____

• Performed completion actions. _____ _____ _____

Additional Comments:

Name _____   Specific Skill Performed _____

Date _____   Attempt Number _____

Instructor _____   PASS _____ FAIL _____

Performance Checklist 21-7: Administering an Intramuscular Injection

	S	U	Comments
1. Performed preliminary actions.	_____	_____	_____
2. Checked medication order, and noted any client allergies.	_____	_____	_____
3. Checked medication for color and clarity, and withdrew medication from ampule or vial as described in previous procedures. Took syringe and other supplies to client's room and placed them on a clean, flat surface.	_____	_____	_____
4. Prepared client for injection.	_____	_____	_____
a. Identified client using an identification bracelet or other accepted means.	_____	_____	_____
b. Explained procedure to client in a calm and confident manner.	_____	_____	_____
c. Put on disposable gloves, and opened an alcohol swab wrapper using aseptic technique.	_____	_____	_____
d. Provided privacy, and positioned client comfortably. Selected and exposed injection site.	_____	_____	_____
5. Prepared injection site and syringe.	_____	_____	_____
a. Chose an area free from bruises, redness, or lesions.	_____	_____	_____
b. Identified exact site of injection. Cleaned site with alcohol swab using circular motion outward from injection site. Allowed alcohol to air-dry. Left swab in clean area for use when withdrawing needle.	_____	_____	_____
c. Removed needle guard or cap with nondominant hand by pulling it straight off.	_____	_____	_____
d. Checked syringe to ensure that volume of medication was correct.	_____	_____	_____
6. Injected medication.	_____	_____	_____
a. Held syringe in dominant hand between thumb and forefinger.	_____	_____	_____
b. Spread skin taut between thumb and forefinger of nondominant hand, or displaced tissue using Z-track technique.	_____	_____	_____
c. Inserted needle quickly at a 90-degree angle up to hub.	_____	_____	_____
d. Released skin, and grasped distal end of syringe with nondominant hand.	_____	_____	_____
e. Aspirated for blood return by pulling back gently on plunger with thumb and forefinger of dominant hand.	_____	_____	_____
f. If blood return noted, removed needle, discarded syringe, and began procedure again.	_____	_____	_____

g.   If no blood return noted, injected medication slowly and
     steadily, taking about 10 seconds to inject each 1 mL.   _____ _____ _____

h.   Waited a few seconds, and then withdrew needle quickly
     at same angle used for injection. Applied gentle pressure
     to site with alcohol swab or with 2-by-2–inch gauze.   _____ _____ _____

7.   Disposed of equipment.   _____ _____ _____

a.   Discarded needle and syringe in a rigid container without
     recapping needle. Disposed of alcohol swab, wrapper,
     and other used materials in trash receptacle.   _____ _____ _____

b.   Positioned client comfortably. If medication was injected
     into a leg muscle, encouraged client to flex and extend
     leg muscles.   _____ _____ _____

c.   Removed gloves, and discarded them in proper receptacle.
     Performed hand hygiene.   _____ _____ _____

8.   Documented procedure carefully.   _____ _____ _____

a.   Recorded date, time, substance, and site of injection on
     client's medication administration record.   _____ _____ _____

b.   Checked on client at an appropriate time after giving
     injection to assess client's response to the medication.

•   Performed completion actions.   _____ _____ _____

Additional Comments:

Name _____   Specific Skill Performed _____

Date _____   Attempt Number _____

Instructor _____   PASS _____   FAIL _____

Performance Checklist 21-8: Adding Medication to an IV Bag

	S	U	Comments
1. Performed preliminary actions.	_____	_____	_____
2. Checked medication order.	_____	_____	_____
3. Drew up medication from vial or ampule as described in procedures 21–2 and 21-3.	_____	_____	_____
4. Injected medication into bag of IV solution.	_____	_____	_____
a. Closed roller clamp on tubing attached to IV solution.	_____	_____	_____
b. Wiped medication port of bag containing IV solution.	_____	_____	_____
c. Inserted needle into center of medication port and injected medication from syringe into solution bag.	_____	_____	_____
d. Withdrew needle, and discarded needle and syringe without recapping needle into approved receptacle.	_____	_____	_____
e. Rotated solution bag gently but thoroughly.	_____	_____	_____
f. Wrote the name and dose of medication, date, time, and nurse's initials on a medication label. Affixed label to IV bag without obstructing name of the solution or IV time tape.	_____	_____	_____
g. Disposed of medication container, alcohol swab, wrapper, and any other used materials in appropriate receptacle.	_____	_____	_____
5. Primed tubing, took container to client's room, and hung solution according to standard procedure. Set drip rate carefully, and followed all procedures needed to monitor IV therapy properly.	_____	_____	_____
6. Documented date, time, IV solution used, and additive used on client's medication administration record or other IV charting form.	_____	_____	_____
• Performed completion actions.	_____	_____	_____

Additional Comments:

Name _____   Specific Skill Performed _____

Date _____   Attempt Number _____

Instructor _____   PASS _____ FAIL _____

Performance Checklist 21-9: Administering an IV Medication by Intermittent Infusion

	S	U	Comments
1. Performed preliminary actions.			
2. Checked medication order, and assessed client's allergies.			
3. Prepared medication at the medication cart or another designated area. Labeled IV medication bag/bottle if the pharmacy had not done so.			
4. Administered medication.			

ADMINISTRATION THROUGH AN EXISTING IV LINE (IVPB OR TANDEM SETUP)

	S	U	Comments
a. Attached secondary tubing to IV bag or bottle that contains the medication according to standard IV therapy protocol.			
b. Used nonvented tubing for an IV bag and vented tubing for an IV bottle. Closed roller clamp on tubing before attaching tubing.			
c. Primed and labeled secondary bag and tubing with date, time, and nurse's initials.			
d. Took medication administration record, IV bag with medication, needle or needleless device, alcohol swab, metal hook, gloves, and tape to client's room.			
e. Identified client using an identification bracelet or other agency accepted means.			
f. Assessed IV site, and donned gloves if required by facility.			
g. Removed cap from distal end of IV tubing, and attached needle or needleless device.			
h. Wiped IV additive port on primary IV line with alcohol swab, and attached needle or needleless device. Attached medication above flow regulator clamp on primary line. Taped connection if needed for stability.			
i. Lowered primary IV solution below level of IV medication bag using hook provided with secondary tubing set.			
j. Regulated IV medication drip rate, or set infusion pump rate and volume as ordered. Checked to make sure that solution was running, and monitored client.			
k. Returned when medication had infused, and reset drip rate on primary line.			
l. Reassessed IV site and client's tolerance of medication.			

ADMINISTRATION THROUGH AN INTERMITTENT INFUSION DEVICE (SALINE LOCK)

a. Closed roller clamp and attached tubing of adequate length to IV medication bag or bottle according to standard IV therapy protocol. Used nonvented tubing for an IV bag; used vented tubing for an IV bottle. Primed tubing. _____ _____ _____

b. Using standard procedure, withdrew 3 mL sterile normal saline solution into a 3-mL syringe (or another solution or amount according to facility policy). _____ _____ _____

c. Took medication administration record, IV medication bag, needle or needleless device, syringe with flush, alcohol swab, gloves, and tape to client's room. _____ _____ _____

d. Identified client using an identification bracelet or other agency accepted means. _____ _____ _____

e. Assessed IV site, and put on gloves if required by facility. _____ _____ _____

f. Removed cap from distal end of IV tubing. Attached needle or needleless device, and primed tubing. _____ _____ _____

g. Wiped port of intermittent infusion device with alcohol swab. _____ _____ _____

h. Assessed site, and flushed infusion device port with sterile saline or other ordered solution. _____ _____ _____

i. Attached IV medication bag to the infusion device port using needle or needleless device. Taped connection if needed. _____ _____ _____

j. Regulated drip rate of IV medication as ordered. Monitored client to ensure that client was tolerating medication. _____ _____ _____

k. After medication had infused, closed roller clamp and removed tubing from port. Recapped or attached a clean needle or needleless device to tubing according to facility policy. _____ _____ _____

l. Reassessed IV site, and flushed infusion port with a second syringe filled with ordered flush solution. Evaluated client response to medication. _____ _____ _____

5. Documented date, time and IV medication on client's medication administration record or computerized medication record. _____ _____ _____

• Performed preliminary actions. _____ _____ _____

Additional Comments:

Name _____   Specific Skill Performed _____

Date _____   Attempt Number _____

Instructor _____   PASS _____   FAIL _____

Performance Checklist 21-10: Administering an IV Push Medication

	S	U	Comments
1. Performed preliminary actions.	_____	_____	_____
2. Checked medication order and assessed client allergies. Checked compatibility of medication with current IV fluid if IV infusing.	_____	_____	_____
3. Prepared medication at the medication cart or other designated area.	_____	_____	_____
4. Administered medication.	_____	_____	_____

ADMINISTRATION THROUGH AN EXISTING IV LINE

	S	U	Comments
a. Drew up medication from an ampule or vial as described in previous procedures. Checked that medication was labeled for IV use. Recapped needle using one-handed technique. Labeled syringe with medication and dose.	_____	_____	_____
b. Removed capped needle, and attached needleless device if needleless system in use.	_____	_____	_____
c. Took medication administration record, IV medication, alcohol swab, and gloves to client's room.	_____	_____	_____
d. Checked client identity, using an identification bracelet or other agency accepted means.	_____	_____	_____
e. Assessed IV site, and donned gloves if required by facility.	_____	_____	_____
f. Wiped IV additive port of primary line with alcohol swab using port nearest to client.	_____	_____	_____
g. Inserted needle into port, and pinched off tubing above injection port. Drew a small amount of IV fluid into syringe to check for precipitation if incompatible.	_____	_____	_____
h. Injected medication slowly and steadily at manufacturer's recommended rate, using watch with second hand to ensure accurate timing. Assessed IV site during injection.	_____	_____	_____
i. Released tubing, removed syringe, and assessed client's tolerance of medication.	_____	_____	_____

ADMINISTRATION THROUGH AN INTERMITTENT INFUSION DEVICE (HEPARIN LOCK)

	S	U	Comments
a. Drew up sterile normal saline (or another ordered flush solution) into two syringes of 3 mL each (or another ordered volume) according to facility policy, using Procedure 21-3. Labeled syringes.	_____	_____	_____

b. Drew up ordered medication into syringe from an ampule
or vial. Recapped needle using one-handed technique.
Labeled syringe.   _____ _____ _____

c. Took IV medication, needle or needleless devices, syringes
with flush solution, alcohol swabs, and gloves to client's
room.   _____ _____ _____

d. Identified client using identification bracelet or other
agency-accepted means.   _____ _____ _____

e. Assessed IV site and put on gloves if required by facility.   _____ _____ _____

f. Wiped port of intermittent infusion device with alcohol swab.   _____ _____ _____

g. Inserted one syringe filled with flush solution, and injected
slowly into client. Removed syringe.   _____ _____ _____

h. Wiped port again with alcohol swab.   _____ _____ _____

i. Inserted syringe with medication and injected it slowly and
steadily at manufacturer's recommended rate, using watch
with second hand to ensure accurate timing. Assessed IV
site during injection.   _____ _____ _____

j. Wiped port again with another alcohol swab.   _____ _____ _____

k. Inserted second syringe containing flush solution, and
injected slowly into client. Removed syringe, and continued
to assess client's tolerance of medication.   _____ _____ _____

l. Disposed of supplies properly, and discarded syringe in
rigid needle-disposal container.   _____ _____ _____

5. Documented date, time, and IV medication given on medication
administration record or computerized medication record.   _____ _____ _____

• Performed completion actions.   _____ _____ _____

Additional Comments:

Name _____   Specific Skill Performed _____

Date _____   Attempt Number _____

Instructor _____   PASS _____ FAIL _____

Performance Checklist 21-11: Administering an Eye Medication

	S	U	Comments
1. Performed preliminary actions.	_____	_____	_____
2. Checked medication order. Noted eye to be treated. Noted client allergies.	_____	_____	_____
3. Prepared client for medication instillation.	_____	_____	_____
a. Checked client's identity using an identification bracelet or other accepted means.	_____	_____	_____
b. Explained procedure to client in a calm and confident manner. Assisted client to sit or lie down with head slightly hyperextended. Put on gloves.	_____	_____	_____
c. Assessed condition of eye and washed away exudate, wiping from inner to outer canthus.	_____	_____	_____
4. Administered medication.	_____	_____	_____

EYEDROPS

	S	U	Comments
a. Removed cap from bottle and placed it on its side. Filled medicine dropper (if used) to prescribed amount.	_____	_____	_____
b. Placed nondominant hand on client's cheekbone under eyelid, and pulled downward against bony orbit to expose lower conjunctival sac. Held tissue or cotton ball under eyelid, and applied slight pressure to inner canthus.	_____	_____	_____
c. Rested dominant hand against client's forehead, and held medication bottle or dropper ½ to ¾ of an inch above conjunctival sac.	_____	_____	_____
d. Asked client to look up at ceiling, and instilled prescribed number of drops into lower conjunctival sac.	_____	_____	_____
e. Asked client to gently close eye and move it around. Applied gentle pressure over lacrimal duct for 1 minute or asked client to do so.	_____	_____	_____

EYE OINTMENT

	S	U	Comments
a. Removed cap from tube and placed on its side. Squeezed and discarded small bead of medication.	_____	_____	_____
b. Separated client's eyelids with thumb and forefinger of nondominant hand, pulling lower eyelid over bony prominence of cheek (or drew upper lid up and away from eyeball if instilling in upper lid).	_____	_____	_____

   c. Asked client to look up for instillation in lower
lid or down for instillation in upper lid.   _____ _____ _____

   d. Applied thin layer of ointment along inside edge of
lower or upper lid, moving from inner to outer canthus.   _____ _____ _____

   e. Asked client to gently close eye and move it around.   _____ _____ _____

MEDICATED EYE DISK

   a. Opened package and pressed tip of index finger of
dominant hand against convex part of disk.   _____ _____ _____

   b. Pulled client's lower eyelid away from eye with nondominant
hand, and asked client to look up.   _____ _____ _____

   c. Placed disk horizontally in conjunctival sac between
iris and lower lid.   _____ _____ _____

   d. Pulled lower lid out, up, and over disk. Asked client
to blink a few times. Repeated if disk still visible. Had client
place fingers against closed lids and press without rubbing
eyes or moving disk.   _____ _____ _____

   e. If disk fell out, rinsed with cool water and reinserted it.   _____ _____ _____

   f. Removed disk by inverting lower eyelid to see disk.
Used thumb and index finger of dominant hand to pinch
disk and lift it from conjunctival sac. Stroked closed eyelid
with fingertip in gentle, long, circular motions to lower a
disk in the upper eye. Asked client to open eye and
checked corner of eye for disk. Slid disk to lower lid
and removed.   _____ _____ _____

5. Removed gloves and performed hand hygiene   _____ _____ _____

6. Documented medication administration on the
medication administration record or computerized medication
record.   _____ _____ _____

• Performed completion actions.   _____ _____ _____

Additional Comments:

Name _____   Specific Skill Performed _____

Date _____   Attempt Number _____

Instructor _____   PASS _____   FAIL _____

Performance Checklist 21-12: Irrigating an Eye

	S	U	Comments
1. Performed preliminary actions.	____	____	_____
2. Prepared client for irrigation.	____	____	_____
a. Identified client using an identification bracelet or other accepted means.	____	____	_____
b. Explained procedure to client in a calm and confident manner.	____	____	_____
c. Helped client sit or lie with head tilted toward eye to be irrigated. Placed waterproof pad under affected side, and donned gloves.	____	____	_____
d. Poured irrigant into container and drew up into syringe using aseptic technique.	____	____	_____
e. Cleaned eyelids and eyelashes with cotton ball moistened with irrigant or normal saline. Wiped from inner to outer canthus using a new cotton ball with each pass.	____	____	_____
f. Positioned curved basin under affected cheek, and asked client to hold if possible.	____	____	_____
3. Irrigated the eye.	____	____	_____
a. Used nondominant hand to hold client's upper lid open and expose lower conjunctival sac.	____	____	_____
b. Held irrigation syringe 1 inch above eye without touching eye and pushed fluid gently into conjunctival sac, directing flow from inner canthus to outer canthus.	____	____	_____
c. Repeated irrigation until secretions were gone or irrigant was used up. Allowed client to close eyes intermittently during procedure as needed.	____	____	_____
d. Dried area with cotton balls, and offered client a towel to dry face and neck.	____	____	_____
4. Removed gloves, and performed hand hygiene.	____	____	_____
5. Documented the irrigation promptly in client's medical record including the appearance of the eye, characteristics of the drainage, and client's response to treatment.	____	____	_____
• Performed completion actions.	____	____	_____

Additional Comments:

Name _____   Specific Skill Performed _____

Date _____   Attempt Number _____

Instructor _____   PASS _____   FAIL _____

Performance Checklist 21-13: Administering an Ear Medication

	S	U	Comments
1. Performed preliminary actions.	_____	_____	_____
2. Checked medication order and noted client allergies.	_____	_____	_____
3. Prepared client for medication instillation.	_____	_____	_____
a. Checked client's identity using an identification bracelet or other agency-accepted means.	_____	_____	_____
b. Explained procedure and helped client to lie with affected ear upward. Put on gloves.	_____	_____	_____
c. Assessed condition of ear and washed away cerumen or exudates with cotton-tipped applicators.	_____	_____	_____
4. Administered medication.	_____	_____	_____
a. Removed cap from bottle and placed cap on its side. Filled medication dropper (if applicable) to prescribed amount.	_____	_____	_____
b. Pulled the pinna up and back for an adult or down and back for a child.	_____	_____	_____
c. Held dropper ½ inch above ear canal, and instilled ordered number of drops.	_____	_____	_____
d. Asked client to maintain side-lying position for 2 to 3 minutes. Used finger to apply gentle pressure to tragus of ear, or asked client to do so.	_____	_____	_____
e. Placed a cotton ball into outermost portion of ear canal.	_____	_____	_____
5. Removed gloves, and performed hand hygiene.	_____	_____	_____
6. Documented the medication administration promptly in the medication administration record or computerized medication record.	_____	_____	_____
7. Checked on client in 15 minutes to remove cotton ball from ear, assess condition, and reposition.	_____	_____	_____
• Performed completion actions.	_____	_____	_____

Additional Comments:

Name _____ Specific Skill Performed _____

Date _____ Attempt Number _____

Instructor _____ PASS _____ FAIL _____

Performance Checklist 21-14: Administering an Intranasal Medication

	S	U	Comments
1. Performed preliminary actions.	___	___	___
2. Checked the medication order, and noted any client allergies.	___	___	___
3. Prepared client for instillation of medication.			
a. Identified client using an identification bracelet or other accepted means.	___	___	___
b. Explained procedure to client, mentioning that the solution could cause choking, stinging, or burning as it drips into the throat. Put on gloves.	___	___	___
c. Asked client to blow nose unless contraindicated. Assessed resulting discharge.	___	___	___
4. Administered the medication.	___	___	___

ADMINISTRATION OF NASAL SPRAY

	S	U	Comments
a. Removed cap from bottle and placed cap on its side.	___	___	___
b. Asked an adult client to tilt head backward, and supported head with nondominant hand. Kept a child's head in upright position.	___	___	___
c. Held medication container just inside tip of nostril without touching nasal tissue. Asked client to occlude other nostril and inhale while spray was administered.	___	___	___
d. Assisted client to a comfortable position.	___	___	___

ADMINISTRATION OF NASAL DROPS

	S	U	Comments
a. Removed cap from bottle, and placed cap on its side.	___	___	___
b. Positioned client to accommodate intended site of action. Supported head with nondominant hand.	___	___	___
c. Held tip of dropper just above intended nostril, and pointed toward midline of ethmoid bone. Instilled ordered number of drops with client breathing through mouth, and without touching nasal tissue with dropper.	___	___	___
d. Asked client to maintain head position for 5 minutes and then assisted to a comfortable position.	___	___	___
5. Removed gloves, and performed hand hygiene.	___	___	___
6. Documented the medication administration promptly on the medication administration record or computerized medication record.	___	___	___

7. Washed nasal spray devices daily in luke warm water.
    If used for infection, discarded when no longer needed.   _____ _____ _____

•   Performed completion actions.   _____ _____ _____

Additional Comments:

Name _____   Specific Skill Performed _____

Date _____   Attempt Number _____

Instructor _____   PASS _____   FAIL _____

Performance Checklist 21-15: Administering a Vaginal Medication

	S	U	Comments
1. Performed preliminary actions.	_____	_____	_____
2. Checked the medication order.	_____	_____	_____
3. Prepared client for medication instillation.	_____	_____	_____
a. Identified client using an identification bracelet or other accepted means.	_____	_____	_____
b. Explained procedure to client and offered client opportunity to void. Closed curtain or door, and assisted client to supine position with abdomen and legs draped.	_____	_____	_____
c. Put on gloves.	_____	_____	_____
d. Inspected client's external genitalia, and provided perineal hygiene as needed.	_____	_____	_____
4. Administered medication using clean technique.	_____	_____	_____

ADMINISTRATION OF A SUPPOSITORY

	S	U	Comments
a. Removed suppository from wrapper and inserted into applicator, if used.	_____	_____	_____
b. Lubricated rounded end of suppository with water-soluble lubricant. Lubricated index finger of gloved dominant hand if not using applicator.	_____	_____	_____
c. Separated client's labia with nondominant hand, and inserted rounded end of suppository along posterior vaginal wall for entire finger length.	_____	_____	_____
d. Withdrew finger or applicator and wiped away excess lubricant from client's genitals.	_____	_____	_____

ADMINISTRATION OF A FOAM, JELLY, OR CREAM

	S	U	Comments
a. Filled applicator with medication per package directions.	_____	_____	_____
b. Separated client's labia with nondominant hand, pointed applicator toward client's sacrum, and used dominant hand to insert applicator 2 to 3 inches into vagina.	_____	_____	_____
c. Depressed plunger on applicator to push medication out of applicator.	_____	_____	_____
d. Withdrew applicator and placed it on tissue or paper towel. Wiped away excess medication from genitals.	_____	_____	_____

5. Assisted client to comfortable position and asked her to remain supine for 5 to 10 minutes or time frame recommended in medication directions. Offered perineal pad if needed. _____ _____ _____

6. Washed applicator with soap and water and stored for future use. _____ _____ _____

7. Removed gloves, and performed hand hygiene. _____ _____ _____

8. Documented the medication administration promptly on the medication administration record or computerized medication record. _____ _____ _____

•   Performed completion actions. _____ _____ _____

Additional Comments:

Name _____   Specific Skill Performed _____

Date _____   Attempt Number _____

Instructor _____   PASS _____   FAIL _____

Performance Checklist 21-16: Administering a Rectal Medication

	S	U	Comments
1. Performed preliminary actions.	____	____	_____
2. Checked medication order.	____	____	_____
3. Prepared client for medication instillation.	____	____	_____
a. Identified client using an identification bracelet or other accepted means.	____	____	_____
b. Explained procedure, and offered opportunity to void; closed curtain or door.	____	____	_____
c. Put on gloves. Assisted client to left lateral Sims' position with upper leg flexed, and draped client to expose on the anal area.	____	____	_____
d. Put on gloves, inspected area, and provided perineal hygiene as needed.	____	____	_____
4. Administered medication using clean aseptic technique.	____	____	_____
a. Removed suppository from packaging. Lubricated rounded end of suppository and index finger of gloved, dominant hand.	____	____	_____
b. Instructed client to breathe slowly and deeply through mouth.	____	____	_____
c. Separated buttocks with gloved, nondominant hand. Used dominant hand to insert rounded end of suppository 4 inches into rectal canal along rectal wall. Inserted suppository 2 inches for child.	____	____	_____
d. Withdrew finger and wiped away fecal material or excess lubricant from client's anus.	____	____	_____
e. Asked client to remain on side for 5 to 30 minutes depending on medication. Provided immobile client with the call bell and asked client to call when needing to have a bowel movement.	____	____	_____
5. Removed gloves, and performed hand hygiene.	____	____	_____
6. Returned after 5 minutes to see if suppository was expelled reinserted if it was expelled.	____	____	_____
7. Documented medication administration on the medication administration record or computerized medication record.	____	____	_____
8. Returned after 30 minutes to assess effectiveness and assisted client as needed.	____	____	_____
• Performed completion actions.	____	____	_____

Additional Comments:

Name _____   Specific Skill Performed _____

Date _____   Attempt Number _____

Instructor _____   PASS _____   FAIL _____

Performance Checklist 22-1: Hand Washing

	S	U	Comments
1. Performed preliminary actions.	___	___	___
2. Turned on faucet so warm water was running.	___	___	___
3. Wet hands and lower arms under running water while holding hands lower than elbows.	___	___	___
4. Rubbed all surfaces of hands and wrists with soap, working soap into a foamy lather while rubbing hands together in a circular motion.	___	___	___
5. Paid special attention to areas between fingers, at creases and breaks in skin, at nail beds, and under fingernails. Spent 15 to 30 seconds performing hand hygiene.	___	___	___
6. Rinsed hands with warm running water under faucet; allowed water to wash down hands and over fingertips.	___	___	___
7. Dried hands thoroughly with a paper towel.	___	___	___
8. If sink was not foot operated, turned off faucet with used paper towel and discard towel in appropriate receptacle.	___	___	___
• Performed completion actions.	___	___	___

Additional Comments:

Name _____   Specific Skill Performed _____

Date _____   Attempt Number _____

Instructor _____   PASS _____ FAIL _____

Performance Checklist 22-2: Caring for a Client on Isolation Precautions

	S	U	Comments

APPLICATION OF BARRIERS

1. Performed preliminary actions.

2. Put on gown.

    a. Picked up gown by collar and allowed it to unfold without touching floor.

    b. Put arms through sleeves, and pulled gown up over shoulders.

    c. Fastened neckties.

    d. Fastened Waist ties, making sure gown lapped over itself at back.

3. Put on mask by positioning over nose and mouth.

    a. Positioned mask or face shield without touching the outside.

    b. Bent nose bar over bridge of nose.

    c. Fastened it in place with elastic or strings.

4. Put on protective eyewear, if indicated, after mask was in place.

5. Put on disposable gloves.

    a. Pulled cuff of each glove over edge of gown sleeve.

    b. Interlaced fingers as needed to adjust fit of gloves.

6. Administered care to client. After disposing of soiled items used in client care, tied bag securely.

REMOVAL OF BARRIERS

1. At door to client's room and next to trash container untied gown at waist only.

2. Removed gloves.

    a. Grasped outside cuff of one glove and pulled glove inside out over hand.

    b. Tucked ungloved finger inside the cuff of remaining glove.

    c. Discarded both gloves, and pulled second glove off inside out over first glove.

3. Removed gown.

    a. Untied gown at neck and allowed it to fall forward from shoulders.

   b.   Slid hands through sleeves, and removed them without
        touching outside of gown.   _____ _____ _____

   c.   Held gown at inside shoulder seams away from body,
        turned it inside out, and folded it with contaminated
        side to the inside.   _____ _____ _____

   d.   Discarded gown in proper receptacle.   _____ _____ _____

4. Discarded both gloves, and pulled second glove off inside out
    over first glove.   _____ _____ _____

5. Removed mask or respirator.   _____ _____ _____

   a.   Pulled elastic or untying strings without
        touching outside surface.   _____ _____ _____

   b.   Placed mask or respirator in appropriate receptacle.   _____ _____ _____

6. Performed hand hygiene.   _____ _____ _____

•   Performed completion actions.   _____ _____ _____

Additional Comments:

Name _____   Specific Skill Performed _____

Date _____   Attempt Number _____

Instructor _____   PASS _____   FAIL _____

Performance Checklist 22-3: Donning and Removing Sterile Gloves

	S	U	Comments
1. Performed preliminary actions.	_____	_____	_____

DONNING STERILE GLOVES

	S	U	Comments
1. Removed rings with stones or irregular surfaces.	_____	_____	_____
2. Grasped package at tabs above sealed edge, peeled down, and discarded outer wrapper.	_____	_____	_____
3. Placed inner package on flat surface, opened inner package at first fold, touched outside of folded edge, and pulled outward.	_____	_____	_____
• Opened next fold, pulling edge outward without touching inside of package.	_____	_____	_____
4. Donned first glove.	_____	_____	_____
a. Grasped folded edge of cuff of one glove.	_____	_____	_____
b. Lifted glove above wrapper and away from body.	_____	_____	_____
c. Did not adjust cuff or fingers at this time or let ungloved hand touch outside of glove.	_____	_____	_____
d. Placed thumb inside top cuffed edge and stretched glove over fingertips.	_____	_____	_____
5. Donned second glove.	_____	_____	_____
a. Picked up second glove by sliding sterile gloved fingers under cuff edge. Kept gloved thumb off cuff of second glove.	_____	_____	_____
b. Slid fingers of opposite hand into glove and keeping fingers straight. Let go of edge when hand in glove.	_____	_____	_____
c. Adjusted for comfort and fit. Kept sterile surface to sterile surface.	_____	_____	_____

REMOVING STERILE GLOVES

	S	U	Comments
1. Grasped outside of first glove just below the wrist.	_____	_____	_____
2. Folded glove over and peeled it back, turning it inside out. Once glove was almost off, held it in palm of gloved hand.	_____	_____	_____
3. Slid ungloved thumb or fingers inside second glove and removed it pulling it inside out also.	_____	_____	_____
4. Discarded into appropriate receptacle.	_____	_____	_____
5. Performed hand hygiene.	_____	_____	_____
• Performed completion actions.	_____	_____	_____

Additional Comments:

Name _____   Specific Skill Performed _____

Date _____   Attempt Number _____

Instructor _____   PASS _____ FAIL _____

Performance Checklist 22-4: Preparing a Sterile Field by Opening a Tray Wrapped in a Sterile Drape

	S	U	Comments
1. Performed preliminary actions.	_____	_____	_____
2. Checked integrity of package; noted if nondisposable items were sterilized and removed kit from outer wrapper.	_____	_____	_____
3. Positioned inner package in center of work surface with outer flap facing away from nurse.	_____	_____	_____
4. Reached around (not over) package to open flap away from nurse, touching outside of flap only.	_____	_____	_____
5. Opened side flaps one at a time, uppermost side first, and in same manner as first. Did not let hands cross over sterile field.	_____	_____	_____
6. Opened innermost flap last and stood back far enough throughout procedure to avoid flap touching nurse while opening.	_____	_____	_____
• Performed completion actions.	_____	_____	_____

Additional Comments:

Name _____   Specific Skill Performed _____

Date _____   Attempt Number _____

Instructor _____   PASS _____   FAIL _____

Performance Checklist 22-5: Preparing a Sterile Field

	S	U	Comments
1. Performed preliminary actions.	____	____	_____
2. Established clean, dry, flat, uncluttered work area at waist level and close to client.	____	____	_____
3. Checked expiration date on supplies, and checked for integrity of all packages.	____	____	_____
4. Set up a drape as a sterile field on a surface at least 2 inches larger on all sides than area needed to work with supplies.	____	____	_____
a. Prepared a sterile field or			
(1) Opened outer wrapping of sterile cloth drape, and kept drape sterile.	____	____	_____
(2) Picked up drape by loose corner edge, and lifted drape up and away from body.	____	____	_____
(3) With other hand, grasped another corner edge and spread drape in air.	____	____	_____
(4) Decided which surface should remain sterile, and spread drape on table with sterile side facing up.	____	____	_____
5. Added sterile supplies.	____	____	_____
a. Peel-apart packages	____	____	_____
(1) Opened peel-apart package by grasping edges designed to peel open with both hands.	____	____	_____
(2) Opened package over sterile field so material fell freely from package onto field without touching the hands.	____	____	_____
b. Sterile liquids	____	____	_____
(1) Removed or loosened cap without touching inside of cap or rim of bottle. Placed cap face-up on flat, nonsterile surface.	____	____	_____
(2) Labeled bottle with date and time.	____	____	_____
(3) If container that held liquid needed to be adjusted, put on sterile glove.	____	____	_____
(4) Picked up liquid with ungloved hand so label was in palm of hand.	____	____	_____
(5) Held bottle of solution 10 cm (4 inches) above container. Poured without spills or splashes. Avoided touching field with bottle lid.	____	____	_____
(6) Replaced lid on both tightly.	____	____	_____
(7) Donned second sterile glove or both sterile gloves.	____	____	_____

c. Wrapped Packages

(1) Held object in one hand or by underside of wrapping. _____ _____ _____

(2) Unwrapped first corner away from body, then each side, then opened last corner toward body. _____ _____ _____

(3) Stabilized corners against wrist. _____ _____ _____

(4) Turned object onto sterile field, and dropped it onto field without touching sterile field. _____ _____ _____

- Performed completion actions. _____ _____ _____

Additional Comments:

Name _____   Specific Skill Performed _____

Date _____   Attempt Number _____

Instructor _____   PASS _____   FAIL _____

Performance Checklist 22-6: Performing a Surgical Hand Scrub

	S	U	Comments
1. Performed preliminary actions.	___	___	_____
2. Applied surgical attire (shoe covers, cap or hood, face mask, protective eyewear).	___	___	_____
3. Turned on water using control lever, and adjusted to comfortably warm temperature.	___	___	_____
4. Wet hands and arms, keeping elbows flexed with hands higher than elbows, and allowing water to flow off arms at elbows.	___	___	_____
5. Cleaned under fingernails on both hands.	___	___	_____
6. Applied antimicrobial liquid or alcohol-based foam or gel.	___	___	_____
7. Washed hands and forearms for amount of time recommended by manufacturer (usually 2 to 6 minutes) if antibacterial soap used.	___	___	_____
8. If an alcohol-based product was used, prewashed hands with soap and water and dried hands completely. Used product according to manufacturer's instructions.	___	___	_____
9. If an antimicrobial soap was used, walked backward into operating room with hands elevated in front of and away from body.	___	___	_____
10. Picked up sterile towel without dripping water onto sterile field. Used one end of the towel to dry one hand completely, using a rotating motion and moving from fingers to elbow.	___	___	_____
11. Used other end of the towel to repeat with other hand. Discarded towel into designated area or assistant's hand.	___	___	_____
• Performed completion actions.	___	___	_____

Additional Comments:

Name _____   Specific Skill Performed _____

Date _____   Attempt Number _____

Instructor _____   PASS _____   FAIL _____

Performance Checklist 22-7: Donning a Sterile Gown and Closed Gloving

	S	U	Comments
1. Performed preliminary actions.	____	____	_____
2. Donned surgical attire and scrubbed hands and arms.	____	____	_____
3. Had circulating nurse or other designated person opened sterile gown and gloves.	____	____	_____
4. Donned gown.	____	____	_____
a. Held arms out straight and let scrub nurse slip gown over hands and arms. If no scrub nurse available:	____	____	_____
(1) Identified inner surface of gown and picked it up beneath neckband without touching sterile field or outer surface of gown.	____	____	_____
(2) Ensured control of all folded layers to avoid contact with nonsterile surfaces.	____	____	_____
(3) Moved away from table, held gown away from body at arm's length, and allowed it to unfold from the top down without touching floor.	____	____	_____
(4) Held gown below neckband near shoulders, and slid both hands into sleeves until fingers were at end of cuffs but not through them.	____	____	_____
(5) Had someone tie gown.	____	____	_____
5. Put on gloves.			
a. Applied first sterile glove.	____	____	_____
(1) With hands covered by sterile gown cuffs, opened inner sterile glove package and picked up first glove by cuff.	____	____	_____
(2) Positioned glove on forearm of dominant hand so cuff faced hand and fingers faced elbow.	____	____	_____
(3) Began to put opposite hand into glove. Held cuff edge of glove with sleeve cover of hand to be gloved. Grasped back of glove cuff with sleeve-covered second hand and turned cuff over sleeve.	____	____	_____
(4) Pushed fingers into glove.	____	____	_____
b. Donned second sterile glove.	____	____	_____
(1) Used sterile hand to pick up second glove.	____	____	_____
(2) Positioned and donned it in same manner as first.	____	____	_____
c. Adjusted both gloves for comfort and fit.	____	____	_____
• Performed completion actions.	____	____	_____

Additional Comments:

Name _____ Specific Skill Performed _____

Date _____ Attempt Number _____

Instructor _____ PASS _____ FAIL _____

Performance Checklist 23-1: Using Protective Restraints

	S	U	Comments
1. Performed preliminary actions.	___	___	_____
2. Assessed need for restraint.	___	___	_____
3. Considered alternatives.	___	___	_____
4. Chose least restrictive restraint.	___	___	_____
5. Applied restraint correctly.	___	___	_____
a. Approached client in calm reasoning manner.	___	___	_____
b. Explained need to client if able to understand.	___	___	_____
c. If client did not understand need for restraint, proceeded by applying in gentle but firm manner.	___	___	_____
d. Padded skin under restraint, especially over bony prominences.	___	___	_____
e. Allowed room for two fingers to be inserted between restraint and limb to prevent circulatory constriction.	___	___	_____
f. Avoided obstructing client's breathing.	___	___	_____
g. Allowed freedom to turn in bed, if possible.	___	___	_____
h. Used slipknot to tie restraint to bed frame rather than side rail.	___	___	_____
i. Placed it where client could not reach it, but where attendant could quickly release in an emergency.	___	___	_____
j. Used a slip knot for quick release. Did not tape a restraint knot.	___	___	_____
6. Monitored client and took action to prevent complications.	___	___	_____
a. Observed client every 30 minutes.	___	___	_____
b. Checked client's circulatory status every 30 minutes.	___	___	_____
c. Provided a regular schedule of toileting.	___	___	_____
d. Repositioned client, every 2 hours.	___	___	_____
e. Reoriented client with each contact.	___	___	_____
f. Assessed client's respiration, cough, and deep breathing every 2 hours.	___	___	_____
g. Reassessed need for restraint every 2 hours.	___	___	_____
h. Provided for food and fluid intake as needed.	___	___	_____
7. Documented	___	___	_____
a. The rationale or behavior that lead to restraint.	___	___	_____
b. Type and time of application.	___	___	_____

    c.   Ongoing assessments and interventions.   _____ _____ _____

    d.   Time of removal and client response.   _____ _____ _____

- Performed completion actions.   _____ _____ _____

Additional Comments:

Name _____   Specific Skill Performed _____

Date _____   Attempt Number _____

Instructor _____   PASS _____   FAIL _____

Performance Checklist 25-1: Administering an Enteral Feeding

	S	U	Comments
1. Performed preliminary actions.			
2. Ensured that client was comfortable and had privacy. Raised head of bed 30 to 45 degrees.			
3. Assessed client.			
a. Listened to bowel sounds.			
b. Observed for abdominal distention or distress.			
c. Inquired about diarrhea, and checked with other assigned caregiver if client was nonverbal.			
4. Prepared for feeding.			
a. Made sure formula was at room temperature and within its expiration date.			
b. Confirmed tube placement and checked for residual volume. With tube clamped, inserted syringe into end of tube. Unclamped tube, and aspirated residual fluid from client's stomach. Returned gastric aspirate to the stomach.			
c. Tested pH of gastric fluid.			
5. Flushed tube with water using syringe with plunger removed. For small-bore tubes, injected water slowly using syringe.			
6. Gave bolus feeding.			
a. Using barrel of syringe as a funnel, filled barrel with feeding solution and let it instill by gravity.			
b. Refilled syringe when it was almost empty, and repeated until total amount had been instilled. Did not force feedings using the plunger.			
c. Instilled 50 mL water (or other amount as ordered by physician) after the feeding was complete.			
d. Clamped tube.			
e. Removed syringe, washed with tap water, and stored for future use.			
f. Covered end of tube with clean gauze.			
7. Gave an intermittent feeding with a bag and tubing.			
a. After instilling water into the tube in step 5, clamped tube and attached feeding bag tubing.			
b. Filled feeding bag with prescribed amount of formula, and primed tubing.			
c. Hung feeding bag on an IV stand.			

    d.   Unclamped feeding tube. _____ _____ _____

    e.   Regulated the flow so that the formula instilled over 20 minutes. _____ _____ _____

    f.   When formula had finished, clamped tube, removed feeding bag, and instilled 50 mL of water into the feeding tube. _____ _____ _____

    g.   Washed feeding bag with tap water, and stored for future use. _____ _____ _____

    h.   When hanging a new feeding bag, labeled it with time, date, and nurse's initials. _____ _____ _____

8. Gave continuous feeding as outlined in steps 1 to 7 above, but used an infusion pump to regulate the flow of formula. _____ _____ _____

    a.   Threaded tubing from feeding bag through infusion pump (according to manufacturer's directions). _____ _____ _____

    b.   Set infusion pump at prescribed rate. _____ _____ _____

9. Before administering medications given through a nasogastric tube, ensured that it was in liquid form or could be finely crushed. _____ _____ _____

10. If necessary, cleaned and dressed entrance site of gastrostomy or jejunostomy tube. _____ _____ _____

    a.   Used clean technique to clean entrance site unless client was in immediate postoperative period. Used soap and water to remove all leakage of gastric contents and crusty drainage. Dried the area well. _____ _____ _____

    b.   Observed for and reported any unusual drainage, redness, puffiness, or pain at the site. _____ _____ _____

    c.   Dressed the site using a precut 4-by-4–inch gauze pad, or cut middle of a pad and placed pad around tube so tube protruded from middle of pad. Used nonallergenic tape to affix pad in place. _____ _____ _____

11. Monitored the client. _____ _____ _____

    a.   Ensured that tube was taped securely to client's nose and pinned safely to the gown when finished with feeding. _____ _____ _____

    b.   Assessed client for gastric distress, distention, cramping, and diarrhea. _____ _____ _____

12. Tidied client's environment and discarded any unused materials. Discarded gloves, and performed hand hygiene. _____ _____ _____

13. Documented on an intake and output sheet the amount and type of feeding delivered, time of feeding, assessment findings, residual gastric contents, pH, and client's daily weight. _____ _____ _____

•   Performed completion actions. _____ _____ _____

Additional Comments:

Name _____   Specific Skill Performed _____

Date _____   Attempt Number _____

Instructor _____   PASS _____   FAIL _____

Performance Checklist 25-2: Administering Parenteral Nutrition Through a Central Line

	S	U	Comments
1. Performed preliminary actions.	___	___	___
2. Confirmed physician order, and checked order against listed ingredients on bag of solution and appearance.	___	___	___
3. Checked solution.			
a. Removed solution from refrigerator at least 1 hour before use.	___	___	___
b. Observed solution for cloudiness, turbidity, particles, or cracks in container.	___	___	___
c. Returned solution to pharmacy if lipid emulsion has separated from solution, giving an appearance of a brown layer.	___	___	___
4. Assessed client.	___	___	___
a. Noted client's potassium, phosphorus, and glucose values.	___	___	___
b. Observed for signs of inflammation or swelling at infusion site.	___	___	___
c. Assessed client's frame of mind, and reassured client that procedure was not painful.	___	___	___
5. Prepared tubing in infusion pump.	___	___	___
a. Connected tubing, filter, and extension tubing.	___	___	___
b. If tubing did not have Luer-Lok connections, taped all connections.	___	___	___
c. Primed and clamped tubing.	___	___	___
d. Threaded tubing through infusion pump.	___	___	___
e. Timed and dated new tubing.	___	___	___
6. Prepared central line catheter.	___	___	___
a. Flushed catheter according to facility policy with saline.	___	___	___
b. Put on sterile gloves.	___	___	___
c. Cleaned catheter cap with alcohol.	___	___	___
d. Used aseptic technique to insert needle into injection cap.	___	___	___
e. Unclamped tubing.	___	___	___
7. Set infusion pump at prescribed rate. Started flow slowly, and monitored rate carefully.	___	___	___

8. Did not use single-lumen line to infuse blood or draw blood. Avoided giving IV medication during parenteral nutrition. Before adding a piggyback medication to parenteral nutrition, check with pharmacist to make sure it was compatible. Did not add medication to a parenteral nutrition solution. _____ _____ _____

9. Monitored and documented VS, lab values, glucose levels, daily weight, urine output, and catheter site. Used sterile technique for dressing changes. _____ _____ _____

10. Documented on intake and output sheet the type of solution used, time and date bag was hung, client's response, and amount of solution added. _____ _____ _____

• Performed completion actions. _____ _____ _____

Additional Comments:

Name _____   Specific Skill Performed _____

Date _____   Attempt Number _____

Instructor _____   PASS _____   FAIL _____

Performance Checklist 26-1: Inserting and Maintaining a Nasogastric Tube

	S	U	Comments
1. Performed preliminary actions.	____	____	_____
2. Prepared equipment	____	____	_____
a. Arranged all equipment on a small table or bedside stand.	____	____	_____
b. Prepared the dressing needed to secure tube to client's nose.	____	____	_____
c. Checked suction apparatus, and attached collection device and tubing; Confirmed a pressure of 80 to 100 mm Hg.	____	____	_____
3. Prepared the client.	____	____	_____
a. Positioned client to enable swallowing, usually a high Fowler's position.	____	____	_____
b. Assessed nostrils to determine which was best to use by inspecting for septal deviation, asking about history of broken nose, and occluding one nostril at a time and having client breathe through other nostril.	____	____	_____
4. Passed the tube.	____	____	_____
a. Measured length correctly (from client's nose to earlobe and then to xiphoid process).	____	____	_____
b. Marked length of tube to be passed with small piece of tape partially around tube, and lubricated final 3 inches of tube.	____	____	_____
c. With head in neutral position, inserted tube through client's patent nostril and passed it to the nasopharynx. Asked client to bend head forward while holding the water glass in one hand. Grasped lubricated tube with dominant hand 6 inches from the end with the forefinger on top and thumb on the bottom. Bent the tube with the thumb and forefinger after reaching the posterior part of the nostril to advance the tube past the sharp curvature of the nasopharynx.	____	____	_____
d. After cleaning the epiglottis, asked client to bend the head forward, touching the chin to the chest. Advanced tube until it reached tape marker. Instructed client to sip water through straw while advancing tube with each swallow.	____	____	_____
5. Connected tube to suction, and ensured client safety.	____	____	_____
a. Secured tube properly to nose.	____	____	_____
b. Verified tube placement in client's stomach by aspirating for gastric secretions. Advanced tube and additional 2 inches if no gastric secretions appeared on initial aspiration. Repeated attempt to aspirate gastric secretions.	____	____	_____

    c. Checked for gastric pH using a pH test strip to assess aspirated stomach contents.

    d. Used a five-in-one connector to attach distal end of tube to tubing marked "to patient" on lid of suction collection device.

    e. Finished taping tube to client's nose using method preferred by facility.

    f. Attached tube to gown with rubber band and safety pin, leaving slack to prevent accidental pulling on tube with head movement.

    g. Set suction to prescribed level.

6. Finished procedure

    a. Documented reason for NG tube, collaboration with physician, procedure, and client's response.

    b. Provided comfort care to client's nose and mouth at least every 8 hours and as needed. Assessed amount and characteristics of nasogastric drainage.

7. Monitored the client.

    a. Inspected client's abdomen and auscultated bowel sounds at least every 8 hours with suction tubing pinched during auscultation.

    b. Monitored and documented amount and characteristics of client's NG output and manifestations of deficient fluid volume (e.g., low electrolyte levels or plasma levels).

    c. Notified physician if NG output exceeded 100 mL/hr, if total output exceeded total intake, or there were new or worsening signs of deficient fluid volume.

    d. If NG tube stopped draining well, assessed equipment for function errors and if necessary contacted physician for an irrigation order. Irrigated tube as ordered.

    e. Removed gloves, and performed hand hygiene.

4. Documented procedure, findings, and client's tolerance.

• Performed completion actions.

Additional Comments:

Name _____   Specific Skill Performed _____

Date _____   Attempt Number _____

Instructor _____   PASS _____   FAIL _____

Performance Checklist 26-2: Removing a Nasogastric Tube

	S	**U**	**Comments**
1. Performed preliminary actions.	_____	_____	_____
2. Prepared client.	_____	_____	_____
a. Assessed client, and determined presence of bowel sounds before removing tube.	_____	_____	_____
b. Placed emesis basin and opened plastic bag on table. Put on gloves, and placed towel across client's chest.	_____	_____	_____
c. Turned off suction machine, and disconnected nasogastric tube from suction tubing.	_____	_____	_____
d. Unpinned tube from client's gown or untaped it from cheek.	_____	_____	_____
e. Instilled 20 mL of air into tube to displace secretions back into client's stomach or pinched tube.	_____	_____	_____
f. Loosened tape on client's nose while holding distal end of tube.	_____	_____	_____
3. Removed tube. Instructed client to hold breath, and withdrew tube in one steady motion. Noted intactness of tip of tube.	_____	_____	_____
4. Finish	_____	_____	_____
a. Assisted with or provided skin and mouth care.	_____	_____	_____
b. Documented present bowel sounds, tube removal procedure, and client's response.	_____	_____	_____
c. Continued to monitor bowel state.	_____	_____	_____
• Performed completion actions.	_____	_____	_____

Additional Comments:

Name _____   Specific Skill Performed _____

Date _____   Attempt Number _____

Instructor _____   PASS _____   FAIL _____

Performance Checklist 26-3: Initiating Peripheral Intravenous Therapy

	S	U	Comments
1. Performed preliminary actions.	_____	_____	_____
2. Prepared for IV therapy.	_____	_____	_____
a. Verified the six rights, investigated client allergies, and checked for incompatibility between solutions or IV medications. Read facility procedure manual for specific instructions.	_____	_____	_____
b. Obtained and marked an IV time-tape strip, and placed it on IV bag.	_____	_____	_____
c. Selected IV tubing and closed roller clamp. Removed protective covers on IV bag injection port and IV spike, keeping both sites sterile. Spiked IV port, and primed IV tubing and chamber.	_____	_____	_____
d. Primed chamber ⅓ to ½ full by pressing it between thumb and index finger. Primed tubing on a gravity system by opening roller clamp and allowing IV fluid to completely displace air in tubing, and then closing the roller clamp. Primed IV tubing for use on a pump according to manufacturer's directions.	_____	_____	_____
3. Started IV line.	_____	_____	_____
a. Determined appropriate gauge catheter for client's condition.	_____	_____	_____
b. Put on gloves, and assessed client for appropriate site to start new IV line, using the most distal vein possible and avoiding an arm with previous lymphatic problems, surgery, or a fistula.	_____	_____	_____
c. Lowered client's arm to below heart level, and applied tourniquet at least 6 inches above projected site. Selected a vein that was straight without sclerotic or tortuous feel/appearance. Avoided sites near a point of flexion. Used nondominant hand or arm if possible.	_____	_____	_____
d. Implemented strategies to dilate the vein and ease insertion (such as a warm moist pack) as needed.	_____	_____	_____
e. Prepped skin using alcohol, povidone-iodine (Betadine), or chlorhexidine (Hibiclens) according to facility policy, starting at insertion point and wiping in an enlarging spiral (3-inch circle). Alternatively, used two pledgets, using friction and multidirectional cleansing with the first pledget, and using the second as described above.	_____	_____	_____
f. Removed needle or catheter from protective cover and held it bevel-up with dominant hand at a 30-degree angle to skin, directly over or parallel to vein.	_____	_____	_____

g. Pierced through skin with one quick motion, decreasing angle of needle or catheter to 15 degrees. Continued advancing until blood return obtained, then advanced another ¼ inch to ensure that it was well into vein. (If needle used, advanced until entire needle within vein.) If inserting a catheter, used one hand to advance the catheter and the other to stabilize the guidewire. Removed needle guidewire while applied pressure over catheter tip.   _____ _____ _____

h. Released tourniquet.   _____ _____ _____

i. Attached primed IV tubing.   _____ _____ _____

   (1) Attached primed saline lock device if ordered.   _____ _____ _____

4. Dressed site following facility's procedural guidelines.   _____ _____ _____

5. Stabilized tubing with additional piece of tape.   _____ _____ _____

6. Labeled IV site with catheter size, date, and nurse's signature if required by facility policy.   _____ _____ _____

7. Labeled IV tubing and bag, if these were attached, with the date and the nurse's initials.   _____ _____ _____

8. Regulated flow of IV as ordered.   _____ _____ _____

9. Monitored and maintained ongoing drip rate.   _____ _____ _____

• Performed completion actions.   _____ _____ _____

Additional Comments:

Name _____   Specific Skill Performed _____

Date _____   Attempt Number _____

Instructor _____   PASS _____   FAIL _____

Performance Checklist 26-4: Discontinuing Peripheral Intravenous Therapy

	S	U	Comments
1. Performed preliminary actions.	_____	_____	_____
2. Prepared to discontinue IV therapy and donned clean gloves.	_____	_____	_____
3. Removed tape and dressing covering insertion site.	_____	_____	_____
4. Removed catheter.	_____	_____	_____
a. Stabilized catheter.	_____	_____	_____
b. Held alcohol swab or cotton ball over IV insertion site without applying pressure.	_____	_____	_____
c. Slid catheter out of vein, and promptly applied pressure to site. Held pressure for 1 to 2 minutes until vein no longer leaked blood.	_____	_____	_____
d. Applied bandage (such as Band-Aid) to site.	_____	_____	_____
• Performed completion actions.	_____	_____	_____

Additional Comments:

Name _____ Specific Skill Performed _____

Date _____ Attempt Number _____

Instructor _____ PASS _____ FAIL _____

Performance Checklist 26-5: Changing the Dressing on a Central Line

	S	U	Comments
1. Performed preliminary actions.	___	___	_____
2. Removed soiled dressing.	___	___	_____
a. Put on face mask, washed hands and put on and clean gloves.	___	___	_____
b. Removed old dressing with dominant hand while stabilizing central line device with nondominant hand. Removed dressing in direction toward catheter insertion site.	___	___	_____
c. Held old dressing in dominant hand, and used nondominant hand to pull glove of dominant hand over old dressing. Removed other glove and discarded both in plastic bag.	___	___	_____
d. Performed hand hygiene.	___	___	_____
3. Cleaned the site.	___	___	_____
a. Set up sterile field. If kit available, opened kit to create a sterile field. Put on sterile gloves, and tore open Betadine and alcohol swabs. Alternatively, if not using kit, opened sterile gloves, used inside of package as sterile field. Opened Betadine and alcohol swabs and placed on corner of sterile field. Plastic bag to side of sterile field and put on sterile gloves.	___	___	_____
b. With elbow of nondominant hand, held packaging of alcohol swab in place while grasping swab with dominant hand.	___	___	_____
c. Started at site of IV access, and used alcohol wipe to clean skin in circular motion outward 3 inches from insertion site. Discarded swab in plastic bag. Repeated with two additional alcohol swabs.	___	___	_____
d. After alcohol evaporated (15 seconds), repeated cleansing with three Betadine swabs.	___	___	_____
4. Dressed site.	___	___	_____
a. Applied gauze (if used) and taped according to policy. Alternatively, applied transparent occlusive dressing so that IV access device was in center of dressing.	___	___	_____
b. Used fingers of one hand to smooth the dressing from the center outward to make a tight seal. Labeled dressing with initials, date, and time of dressing change.	___	___	_____
• Performed completion actions.	___	___	_____

Additional Comments:

Name _____ Specific Skill Performed _____

Date _____ Attempt Number _____

Instructor _____ PASS _____ FAIL _____

Performance Checklist 27-1: Irrigating a Wound

	S	U	Comments
1. Performed preliminary actions.	_____	_____	_____
2. Prepared client for procedure.	_____	_____	_____
a. Checked wound care order and specific order for irrigant.	_____	_____	_____
b. Premedicated client for pain if necessary.	_____	_____	_____
c. Performed hand hygiene, and applied protective eyewear and gown if splashing was anticipated.	_____	_____	_____
d. Placed underpad and/or clean basin to catch irrigating fluid.	_____	_____	_____
e. Determined whether or not procedure should be clean or sterile. Set up clean or sterile field by opening irrigation tray. Opened packages of sterile dressings.	_____	_____	_____
f. Poured irrigant into sterile basin.	_____	_____	_____
3. Removed old dressing using clean gloves.	_____	_____	_____
a. Removed outer layer, moistened dressing if stuck to granulation tissue.	_____	_____	_____
b. Removed any packing from wound. Disposed of old dressing according to agency policy.	_____	_____	_____
4. Irrigated wound.	_____	_____	_____
a. Applied sterile gloves.	_____	_____	_____
b. Filled syringe with solution. With tip of needle about 2 inches above wound bed, flushed with slow continuous pressure. Repeated as needed.	_____	_____	_____
5. Redressed the wound.	_____	_____	_____
a. Redressed wound with wet-to-moist packing, and dry outer dressing as needed.	_____	_____	_____
b. Disposed of used supplies according to standard precautions.	_____	_____	_____
6. Documented client's tolerance of wound irrigation and dressing change. Documented description of wound bed.	_____	_____	_____
• Performed completion actions.	_____	_____	_____

Additional Comments:

Name _____   Specific Skill Performed _____

Date _____   Attempt Number _____

Instructor _____   PASS _____ FAIL _____

Performance Checklist 27-2: Removing a Dressing

	S	U	Comments
1. Performed preliminary actions.	_____	_____	_____
2. Performed hand hygiene and applied gloves.	_____	_____	_____
3. Gently removed old dressing by pulling tape toward dressing and parallel to skin. Simultaneously applied pressure to client's skin at edge of tape to prevent skin from being pulled with tape.	_____	_____	_____
4. Observed removed dressing for drainage, especially noting amount, color, and odor (if any) of drainage.	_____	_____	_____
5. Disposed of dressing according to agency policy and government regulations.	_____	_____	_____
6. Documented odor, color, amount, and consistency of drainage. Described appearance of wound.	_____	_____	_____
• Performed completion actions.	_____	_____	_____

Additional Comments:

Name _____ Specific Skill Performed _____

Date _____ Attempt Number _____

Instructor _____ PASS _____ FAIL _____

Performance Checklist 27-3: Dressing a Simple Wound

	S	U	Comments
1. Performed preliminary actions.	_____	_____	_____
2. Answered client's questions about procedure.	_____	_____	_____
3. Confirmed dressing order.	_____	_____	_____
4. Assembled supplies needed for dressing change.	_____	_____	_____
5. Performed hand hygiene, and applied gloves.	_____	_____	_____
6. Removed dressing from its package and applied it to center of wound, covering the wound and 1 inch beyond with the dressing.	_____	_____	_____
7. Secured edges of dressing to client's skin with tape; used least amount of tape necessary.	_____	_____	_____
8. Stated that if dressing will be changed frequently or if client has sensitive or impaired skin, to consider using Montgomery straps rather than tape.	_____	_____	_____
9. Removed gloves and performed hand hygiene.	_____	_____	_____
• Performed completion actions.	_____	_____	_____

Additional Comments:

Name _____ Specific Skill Performed _____

Date _____ Attempt Number _____

Instructor _____ PASS _____ FAIL _____

Performance Checklist 27-4: Culturing a Wound

	S	U	Comments
1. Performed preliminary actions.	_____	_____	_____
2. Rinsed or irrigated wound thoroughly with sterile normal saline before obtaining culture.	_____	_____	_____
3. Swabbed entire wound bed using a zigzag technique, starting at top of wound and proceeding to bottom of wound.	_____	_____	_____
4. Placed swab in culture tube. Sent specimen to laboratory.	_____	_____	_____
• Performed completion actions.	_____	_____	_____

Additional Comments:

Name _____ Specific Skill Performed _____

Date _____ Attempt Number _____

Instructor _____ PASS _____ FAIL _____

Performance Checklist 27-5: Applying a Wet-to-Moist Dressing

	S	U	Comments
1. Performed preliminary actions.	_____	_____	_____
2. Confirmed physician's order, and assembled needed supplies.	_____	_____	_____
3. Used sterile normal saline solution (or another ordered solution) to dampen dressing that will be placed into the wound.	_____	_____	_____
4. Put on sterile gloves. Twisted dressing so it remained wet, but not dripping. Opened dressing fully and fluffed it open.	_____	_____	_____
5. Gently placed dressing into wound. Did not pack wound tightly.	_____	_____	_____
6. Covered damp dressing with dry sterile dressing; secured it with tape or Montgomery straps, if needed.	_____	_____	_____
• Performed completion actions.	_____	_____	_____

Additional Comments:

Name _____   Specific Skill Performed _____

Date _____   Attempt Number _____

Instructor _____   PASS _____   FAIL _____

Performance Checklist 27-6: Applying a Hydrocolloid Dressing

	S	U	Comments
1. Performed preliminary actions.	_____	_____	_____
2. Confirmed physician order.	_____	_____	_____
3. Cleaned wound by irrigating it or lightly swabbing it with gauze soaked in sterile normal saline solution.	_____	_____	_____
4. Selected a hydrocolloid dressing of an appropriate size.	_____	_____	_____
5. Applied dressing from one side of wound to other side. Used hand pressure to hold dressing in place for 1 minute.	_____	_____	_____
6. Placed hypoallergenic tape around edges of dressing to secure it if needed.	_____	_____	_____
7. Stated to leave dressing in place for 3 to 5 days, but to remove and change it if it leaks or begins to peel off.	_____	_____	_____
• Performed completion actions.	_____	_____	_____

Additional Comments:

Name _____   Specific Skill Performed _____

Date _____   Attempt Number _____

Instructor _____   PASS _____   FAIL _____

Performance Checklist 29-1: Testing Feces for Occult Blood

	S	U	Comments
1. Performed preliminary actions.	_____	_____	_____
2. Instructed client about purpose of test and had client defecate, without voiding, into collection container.	_____	_____	_____
3. Put on clean gloves.	_____	_____	_____
4. Obtained small specimen using applicator, and smeared thin layer in first box of Hemoccult slide while noting stool characteristics.	_____	_____	_____
5. Repeated procedure using opposite end of applicator and another area of stool specimen.	_____	_____	_____
6. Closed slide cover, and turned it over to reverse side. Opened flap on card, and applied two drops of developing solution.	_____	_____	_____
7. Observed for bluish discoloration on guaiac paper 30 to 60 seconds after drop application.	_____	_____	_____
8. Disposed of slide in hazardous container, removed gloves, performed hand hygiene, and completed documentation.	_____	_____	_____
9. Documented characteristics of client's feces and results of guaiac test in the client's chart.	_____	_____	_____
• Performed completion actions.	_____	_____	_____

Additional Comments:

Name _____   Specific Skill Performed _____

Date _____   Attempt Number _____

Instructor _____   PASS _____   FAIL _____

Performance Checklist 29-2: Preparing and Administering a Large-Volume Enema

	S	U	Comments
1. Performed preliminary actions.	_____	_____	_____
2. Set up equipment. Closed door or drew curtain. Positioned client on left side or on bedpan if client was unable to retain enema. Draped client to expose only buttocks.	_____	_____	_____
3. Checked that temperature of enema solution was warm (40.5° C or 105° F), lubricated tip of enema tube with water-soluble lubricant, and inserted it 2 to 3 inches into rectum.	_____	_____	_____
4. Held bag 18 inches above rectum, and allowed 500 to 750 mL of solution to flow in slowly over 10 minutes.	_____	_____	_____
5. Encouraged client to retain enema for up to 15 minutes.	_____	_____	_____
6. Assisted client to bathroom or commode, or assisted onto bedpan for evacuation.	_____	_____	_____
7. Cleansed perineum, assisted client to position of comfort.	_____	_____	_____
8. If physician ordered enemas until clear, administered up to 3 large-volume enemas as described. Verbalized to consult physician if three enemas did not produce clear results, if enemas ordered until clear.	_____	_____	_____
• Performed completion actions.	_____	_____	_____

Additional Comments:

Name _____   Specific Skill Performed _____

Date _____   Attempt Number _____

Instructor _____   PASS _____   FAIL _____

Performance Checklist 30-1: Collecting Urine From an Indwelling (Foley) Catheter

	S	U	Comments
1. Performed preliminary actions.	___	___	_____
2. Observed for presence of urine at port site, and clamped catheter distal to port for 30 minutes or until urine visible at site if necessary.	___	___	_____
3. Cleaned collection port with an alcohol wipe.	___	___	_____
4. Used 10 mL syringe with needle attached, inserted into port, and withdrew 10 mL of urine.	___	___	_____
5. Injected urine into sterile container; discarded needle in sharps container.	___	___	_____
6. Labeled specimen with client's name, date, and time of collection. Sent immediately to laboratory; removed equipment and made client comfortable.	___	___	_____
7. Documented date, amount and characteristics of urine, and time sent to laboratory.	___	___	_____
• Performed completion actions.	___	___	_____

Additional Comments:

Name _____   Specific Skill Performed _____

Date _____   Attempt Number _____

Instructor _____   PASS _____ FAIL _____

Performance Checklist 30-2: Applying a Condom Catheter

	S	U	Comments
1. Performed preliminary actions.			
2. Positioned client on back, and draped client to expose only the penis.			
3. Cleaned genitals with soap and water and dried thoroughly.			
4. Applied skin-protecting cream packaged with catheter to penis and allowed it to dry.			
5. Wrapped adhesive spirally around shaft of penis, being careful not to apply too tightly.			
6. Placed rolled condom over glans penis and unrolled condom over adhesive liner and shaft of penis.			
7. Attached catheter to collection system and taped tubing to leg.			
8. Documented date, time of application, and assessment of shaft of penis, glans, and foreskin. Assessed penis after applying condom to detect potential urine leakage, edema, and changes in skin color.			
• Performed completion actions.			

Additional Comments:

Name _____   Specific Skill Performed _____

Date _____   Attempt Number _____

Instructor _____   PASS _____   FAIL _____

Performance Checklist 30-3: Inserting an Indwelling Catheter

	S	U	Comments
1. Performed preliminary actions.	___	___	___
2. Selected catheter of appropriate size and material.	___	___	___
3. Positioned client.	___	___	___
a. Positioned a female client in supine position with knees flexed and separated.	___	___	___
b. Positioned a male client in supine position.	___	___	___
4. Draped client for privacy.	___	___	___
a. Exposed only labia in females; used sheet as drape between legs.	___	___	___
b. Used gown or blanket to cover upper body to penis.	___	___	___
5. Established sterile field.	___	___	___
a. Opened prepackaged catheter tray, and placed it in convenient position.	___	___	___
b. Held drape by corner only, and allowed it to fall open; placed it under buttocks of female client still touching only corners.	___	___	___
c. Put on sterile gloves. Placed fenestrated upper drape in place.	___	___	___
d. Inflated catheter balloon to test it for leaks.	___	___	___
6. Cleaned area around urinary meatus.	___	___	___
a. Poured antiseptic on all three cotton balls.	___	___	___
b. For female client, spread labia with nondominant hand while holding cotton ball with forceps in dominant hand.	___	___	___
c. Used first cotton ball to clean from top to bottom on right side of urinary meatus and discarded; used second cotton ball to clean left side from top to bottom and discarded; used third cotton ball to clean down the center directly over meatus and discarded.	___	___	___
d. For male client, used at least two cotton balls, the first to clean around the glans penis and the second over the meatus. Retracted the foreskin in uncircumcised males.	___	___	___
7. Lubricated and inserted catheter.	___	___	___
a. Held catheter 1 to 2 inches from tip, lubricated tip, and inserted into urinary meatus. In male client, used nondominant hand to hold penis perpendicular to client's body and used fingers to gently encircle and stabilize penis.	___	___	___

b.   Inserted catheter until urine began to flow (2 to 3 inches in females and 6 to 8 inches in males).

_____ _____ _____

c.   After urine began to flow, inserted 1 inch more.

_____ _____ _____

8. Inflated balloon by injecting 8 to 10 mL of water via syringe or according to manufacturer's directions.

_____ _____ _____

9. Taped catheter to inner aspect of thigh.

_____ _____ _____

10. Established drainage system.

_____ _____ _____

a.   Leg bag: Attached catheter to inner thigh.

_____ _____ _____

b.   Gravity drainage: Attached bag to bed frame below level of bladder.

_____ _____ _____

11. Completed procedure.

_____ _____ _____

a.   Discarded all trash.

_____ _____ _____

b.   Made client comfortable. Blotted or rinsed excess solution from perineum.

_____ _____ _____

c.   Documented date and time of catheter insertion, amount and characteristics of urine, and size of catheter and balloon.

_____ _____ _____

•   Performed completion actions.

_____ _____ _____

Additional Comments:

Name _____   Specific Skill Performed _____

Date _____   Attempt Number _____

Instructor _____   PASS _____ FAIL _____

Performance Checklist 31-1: Giving the Client a Bath

	S	U	Comments
1. Performed preliminary actions.	_____	_____	_____
2. Checked physician's orders for activity and any special positioning needs or contraindications.	_____	_____	_____
• Assessed client's ability to participate in bath even if on a limited scale.	_____	_____	_____
• Evaluated client's need for teaching relative to skin care, and planned to incorporate teaching into procedure.	_____	_____	_____
• Assessed for presence of IV lines, catheters, tubes, casts, and dressing.	_____	_____	_____
• Assessed client's range of motion (ROM).	_____	_____	_____
3. Prepared the environment.	_____	_____	_____
a. Performed hand hygiene and applied gloves if needed.	_____	_____	_____
b. Gathered equipment and took to bedside.	_____	_____	_____
c. Raised bed to comfortable working height. Kept side rail on side of bed opposite from side on which individual was working. Ensured privacy by closing door or curtains, and regulated temperature of the room for comfort.	_____	_____	_____
d. Placed articles on over-bed table, within easy reach.	_____	_____	_____
4. Prepared client.	_____	_____	_____
a. Assisted client to use bedpan, commode, or urinal.	_____	_____	_____
b. Placed bath blanket over client covering top linen.	_____	_____	_____
c. Loosened top linen at foot of bed and removed from under bath blanket. Placed dirty linen in laundry hamper or bag.	_____	_____	_____
d. Placed bath towel under head, and removed pillow.	_____	_____	_____
e. Helped client move to side of bed nearest nurse or placed towel over pillow. Made sure that side rail on opposite side of bed was in raised position.	_____	_____	_____
f. Removed client's gown or pajamas.	_____	_____	_____
5. Washed client's face and neck.	_____	_____	_____
a. Filled washbasin ½ to ⅔ full of warm water. Tested temperature of water with bath thermometer or with wrist.	_____	_____	_____
b. Put on clean gloves if exposure to body fluids possible.	_____	_____	_____
c. Made a mitt with washcloth.	_____	_____	_____

d. Washed client's eyes with clear water from inner
    canthus outward using a different area of the
    washcloth for each eye dried thoroughly.

    _____ _____ _____

e. Washed client's face using clear water or mild soap as
    desired.

    _____ _____ _____

f. Washed forehead, cheeks, nurse, and perioral areas.

    _____ _____ _____

g. Washed, rinsed, and dried postauricular area. Cleaned
    anterior and posterior ear with tip of washcloth.

    _____ _____ _____

h. Washed front and back of client's neck.

    _____ _____ _____

i. Removed towel from beneath client's neck.

    _____ _____ _____

6. Washed client's arms.

    _____ _____ _____

a. Placed towel lengthwise under upper arm and axilla.
    Washed upper surface of arm from fingers to axilla.

    _____ _____ _____

b. Grasped client's wrist firmly and elevated arm to wash
    lower surface of arm.

    _____ _____ _____

c. Washed axilla.

    _____ _____ _____

d. Washed client's hands, immersed hands in warm water
    and allowed to soak. Dried client's hands, and performed
    ROM with client's fingers. Cleaned nails and applied lotion.

    _____ _____ _____

7. Washed client's chest.

    _____ _____ _____

a. Folded bath blanket down to umbilicus.

    _____ _____ _____

b. For female client, covered chest with a towel.

    _____ _____ _____

• Washed, rinsed, and dried chest and under breasts.

    _____ _____ _____

• Assessed breasts and taught breast self-examination if
    appropriate.

    _____ _____ _____

8. Washed client's abdomen.

    _____ _____ _____

a. Exposed only areas being washed, kept remaining areas
    covered with towel.

    _____ _____ _____

b. Used firm strokes to wash abdomen from
    side to side, including umbilicus.

    _____ _____ _____

c. Observed for signs of distention or visible peristalsis.

    _____ _____ _____

d. Re-covered client with bath blanket.

    _____ _____ _____

9. Washed client's legs.

    _____ _____ _____

a. Exposed one leg at a time.

    _____ _____ _____

b. Used firm distal-to-proximal strokes to wash, rinse,
    and dry leg.

    _____ _____ _____

c. Placed client's foot in basin for a few minutes to soak.
    Did ROM with toes. Inspected feet and nails.

    _____ _____ _____

d. Dried foot thoroughly, especially between toes.

    _____ _____ _____

e. Repeated process with other leg and foot.

    _____ _____ _____

10. Provided perineal care.

    _____ _____ _____

a. Placed client in a supine position. If client was able to wash genitalia without assistance, placed basin of water, washcloth, and towel within reach and provided privacy. If client was unable to wash perineal area, draped area with bath blanket so that only genitalia exposed.   _____ _____ _____

b. Washed perineal area as explained in Procedure 31-2.   _____ _____ _____

c. Changed bathwater and washcloth.   _____ _____ _____

11. Washed, rinsed and dried back, buttocks, and perianal area.   _____ _____ _____

a. Placed client in side-lying position.   _____ _____ _____

b. Placed towel lengthwise along client's back and buttocks, keeping client covered with bath blanket.   _____ _____ _____

c. Washed, rinsed, and dried client's back and buttocks, moving from shoulders to buttocks and upper thighs.   _____ _____ _____

d. Performed back massage with lotion (this may also be done at completion of bath).   _____ _____ _____

12. Helped client don a clean gown or pajamas.   _____ _____ _____

a. While client is still on one side, placed one arm in sleeve of gown.   _____ _____ _____

b. Turned client to back and placed other arm in sleeve.   _____ _____ _____

13. Assisted with hair care.   _____ _____ _____

14. Assisted with oral care, as explained in Procedure 31-6.   _____ _____ _____

15. Made bed with clean linens, as explained in Procedures 31-4 and 31-5.   _____ _____ _____

16. Left client's environment clean and uncluttered.   _____ _____ _____

17. Documented significant observations and assessment findings.   _____ _____ _____

•   Performed completion actions.   _____ _____ _____

Additional Comments:

Name _____   Specific Skill Performed _____

Date _____   Attempt Number _____

Instructor _____   PASS _____ FAIL _____

Performance Checklist 31-2: Providing Perineal Care

	S	U	Comments

FOR A FEMALE CLIENT

1. Performed preliminary actions.

2. Prepared for procedure.

   a. Organized necessary equipment and donned clean gloves.

   b. Placed protective pad or towel under client before placing client on bedpan if doing perineal care in bed.

   c. Placed client in comfortable position on bedpan, toilet, or commode chair, or on bedpan in semi-Fowler's position if necessary.

   d. If care was given in bed, asked client to bend knees and separate legs.

   e. Draped with bath blanket.

3. Cleaned perineum.

   a. Washed from front to back. Removed fecal debris with toilet paper and disposed of it in toilet. Cleansed buttocks and anus; rinsed and dried; changed water and gloves; washed hands.

   b. Poured water or prescribed solution over perineum.

   c. Washed labia majora; cleaned from perineum to rectum; rinsed and dried.

   d. Separated labia with one hand to expose urethral and vaginal openings. With free hand, wiped from front to back in a downward motion with either washcloth or cotton balls.

   e. Turned client to a side-lying position and washed anal area. Changed gowns.

   f. Patted dry with second towel.

4. Made client comfortable.

   a. Removed equipment and covered client.

   b. Positioned for comfort.

FOR A MALE CLIENT

1. Performed preliminary actions.

2. Prepared for procedure.

   a. Organized necessary equipment and donned clean gloves.

    b.   Covered client with bath blanket.   _____ _____ _____

3.   Cleaned perineum.   _____ _____ _____

    a.   If client was uncircumcised, retracted foreskin to remove smegma.   _____ _____ _____

    b.   Held shaft of penis firmly but gently with one hand. With other hand, washed beginning at tip of penis. Used circular motion, cleaned around head of penis.   _____ _____ _____

    c.   Washed down shaft toward scrotum. Did not repeat washing area without changing to clean area on washcloth.   _____ _____ _____

    d.   After washing penis, replaced foreskin if necessary.   _____ _____ _____

    e.   Washed around scrotum and inner thighs. Turned client to side and washed anal area and buttocks.   _____ _____ _____

4.   Made client comfortable.   _____ _____ _____

    a.   Removed equipment and gloves, and performed hand hygiene.   _____ _____ _____

    b.   Covered client and positioned for comfort.   _____ _____ _____

•   Performed completion actions.   _____ _____ _____

Additional Comments:

Name _____   Specific Skill Performed _____

Date _____   Attempt Number _____

Instructor _____   PASS _____   FAIL _____

Performance Checklist 31-3: Helping the Client With a Tub Bath or Shower

	S	U	Comments
1. Performed preliminary actions.			
2. Assessed client's capacity for self-care. Assessed tolerance for activity, cognitive state, and musculoskeletal function.			
3. Made sure that bathroom was prepared and that tub or shower was clean. Placed disposable mat or towel on floor by tub or shower. Adjusted room temperature so client was not chilled during bath.			
4. Put on clean gloves.			
5. Assessed client's ability to access bathroom. Transported or accompanied client to bathroom.			
6. Kept client covered with bath blanket while preparing water and transporting.			
7. Provided privacy for client by placing "occupied" sign on door.			
8. Tested water temperature before client got into tub or shower. If used bathtub, filled it no more than half full of warm water (40.5° C or 105° F).			
9. Provided assistance for client while client entered tub or shower.			
10. Assessed whether client could safely bathe without assistance. If client could remain unattended, showed client how to use call signal and safety bars. Explained which faucet controlled hot water, and placed all bath supplies within easy reach.			
11. If client was left unattended, checked every 5 to 10 minutes to determine if help was needed.			
12. If client was unable to bathe independently, remained with client at all times. Assisted as needed with bathing; encouraged client to do as much of bath as possible.			
13. Washed any areas that client was unable to reach. Assisted female client to shave legs and/or axilla if desired.			
14. Watched closely for signs of dizziness or weakness while client was in tub or shower and immediately on exiting.			
15. Drained water from tub. Helped client out of tub or shower. Assisted with drying.			
16. Assisted with grooming and dressing in clean pajamas or gown. Removed gloves, and performed hand hygiene.			
17. Helped client return to room.			
18. Assessed client's tolerance for procedure.			
19. Left bathroom clean. Discarded soiled linen. Cleaned tub or shower according to agency policy.			

20. Documented client's response to activity.   _____ _____ _____

•   Performed completion actions.   _____ _____ _____

Additional Comments:

Name _____ Specific Skill Performed _____

Date _____ Attempt Number _____

Instructor _____ PASS _____ FAIL _____

Performance Checklist 31-4: Making an Occupied Bed

	S	U	Comments
1. Performed preliminary actions.			
2. Organized environment, and positioned client to expose half of bed.			
a. Performed hand hygiene.			
b. Closed door or curtain for privacy.			
c. Made sure rail on opposite side was up and locked.			
d. Positioned bed at comfortable working height.			
e. Lowered head and knee position to flat if tolerated.			
f. Lowered rail on nearest side of bed.			
g. Loosened top linen.			
h. Placed open bath blanket on top of spread. Removed spread, top sheet, and blanket in one movement, at same time pulling bath blanket over client. If top linens are to be reused, folded and placed in a chair.			
i. Placed any linen that was not to be reused in laundry hamper or linen bag. Avoided contact with uniform. Held at arm's length while removing from bed to linen hamper.			
j. Loosened bottom sheet on near side of bed. Had client roll to opposite side of bed. Adjusted pillow under head.			
3. Made half bed from top to bottom.			
a. Fan-folded dirty bottom sheet and draw sheet, and tucked under client's back and buttocks as tightly as possible.			
b. Placed clean bottom sheet on bed. Started with bottom edge even with foot end of bed, with center fold in middle of bed. Unfolded to top and allowed extra length to hang over top. Tucked end of sheet under mattress and mitered corner. If contour sheets were used, fitted elastic edges under top and bottom corners of mattress.			
c. Fan-folded clean sheet to middle of bed. Made roll of linens as flat as possible.			
4. Placed draw sheet on top of bottom sheet. Placed folded edge at top of client's shoulders.			
a. Placed center fold along center of bed.			
b. Fan-folded top layer toward client.			
c. Tucked excess under mattress along with bottom sheet.			

    d.   Smoothed out wrinkles. _____ _____ _____

    e.   If incontinence pad was used, fan-folded it and placed
        on top of linens near client's back. _____ _____ _____

5. Made second half of bed. _____ _____ _____

    a.   Raised side rail, and moved to opposite side of bed. Lowered
        side rail on that side. Helped client turn onto clean sheets. _____ _____ _____

    b.   Removed dirty linens. Folded toward center or one end of
        bed. Held linens away from body, and placed in dirty
        linen bag or hamper. _____ _____ _____

    c.   Pulled clean linens over exposed half of bed. _____ _____ _____

    d.   Tucked in bottom sheet. _____ _____ _____

    e.   Tucked draw sheet, moved from middle, to top, to bottom.
        Adjusted lift pad. _____ _____ _____

6. Put on top sheet and spread. _____ _____ _____

    a.   Helped client move back to center of bed. _____ _____ _____

    b.   Placed top sheet over client with seam side up, center
        crease at center of bed. Unfolded sheet from head to toe. _____ _____ _____

    c.   Had client grasp top sheet while pulling soiled sheet or
        bath blanket from under clean sheet. _____ _____ _____

    d.   Placed blanket, and spread evenly over top sheet. Made sure
        that they were even on both sides. _____ _____ _____

    e.   Made mitered corners at foot of bed with top sheet, blanket,
        and spread together. _____ _____ _____

    f.   Pulled top sheet, blanket, and spread into a pleat over
        client's toes. _____ _____ _____

    g.   Cuffed spread, blanket, and top sheet at head of bed;
        allowed adequate sheet to cover client's shoulders. _____ _____ _____

7. Changed pillowcase. _____ _____ _____

    a.   Grasped closed end of clean pillowcase at center point
        and inverted case over hand. _____ _____ _____

    b.   Grasped pillow and inverted case with same hand; used
        other hand to pull case over pillow. _____ _____ _____

8. Returned bed to its low position. Placed call light within
    client's reach. _____ _____ _____

9. Positioned client for comfort. _____ _____ _____

10. Performed hand hygiene, and documented care. _____ _____ _____

•   Performed completion actions. _____ _____ _____

Additional Comments:

Name _____ Specific Skill Performed _____

Date _____ Attempt Number _____

Instructor _____ PASS _____ FAIL _____

Performance Checklist 31-5: Making an Unoccupied and a Surgical Bed

	S	U	Comments
1. Performed preliminary actions.	___	___	_____

MAKING AN UNOCCUPIED BED

	S	U	Comments
2. Organized environment.	___	___	_____
a. Raised bed to a comfortable working height.	___	___	_____
b. Lowered side rails.	___	___	_____
3. Removed soiled linens. Folded soiled surfaces inward, and placed in hamper.	___	___	_____
a. Removed bedspread and blanket; folded and placed in chair if to be reused. If soiled, placed in hamper or linen bag. Removed pillow from pillowcase.	___	___	_____
b. When handling soiled linens, always held them away from body.	___	___	_____
4. Made one side of bed at a time. Then moved to other side.	___	___	_____
a. If bottom sheet was contour sheet, placed elastic bands under top and bottom corners of mattress and tucked along sides. If bottom sheet was not contour sheet, unfolded it lengthwise and placed vertical crease at center of bed; unfolded sheet, smoothed wrinkles, and made mitered corner at head of bed.	___	___	_____
b. Tucked side in along mattress.	___	___	_____
c. If client needed draw sheet, centered draw sheet on bed and unfolded toward opposite side; tucked under mattress. If needed, folded sheet into a pull sheet or placed absorbent pad in center of drawsheet.	___	___	_____
d. Moved to other side of bed. Removed linen with soiled side in. Held bundle of linen away from body, and placed in linen bag or hamper.	___	___	_____
e. Pulled linen to side. Tucked top of sheet, bottom end of sheet, and draw sheet.	___	___	_____
5. Placed top sheet, blanket, and spread over bed.	___	___	_____
a. Left a cuff at top of spread.	___	___	_____
b. Mitered corners all together at foot of bed.	___	___	_____
6. Prepared bed for client to return.	___	___	_____
a. Made toe pleat.	___	___	_____
b. Fan-folded linen to foot of bed to create an open bed.	___	___	_____

   c.   Changed pillowcase.   _____ _____ _____

   d.   Returned bed to its low position.   _____ _____ _____

   e.   Positioned call light.   _____ _____ _____

   f.   Disposed of soiled linen.   _____ _____ _____

7.   Performed hand hygiene, and documented care.   _____ _____ _____

MAKING A SURGICAL BED

1.   Made bed as an unoccupied bed.   _____ _____ _____

2.   Folded bottom and top edges on near side to opposite side, making a triangle.   _____ _____ _____

3.   Picked up center point of triangle, and fan-folded linen to side of bed.   _____ _____ _____

4.   Left bed in high position.   _____ _____ _____

5.   Changed pillowcase and left pillow at foot of bed or on chair.   _____ _____ _____

6.   Moved all objects away from bedside to leave room for stretcher.   _____ _____ _____

•   Performed completion actions.   _____ _____ _____

Additional Comments:

Name _____   Specific Skill Performed _____

Date _____   Attempt Number _____

Instructor _____   PASS _____   FAIL _____

Performance Checklist 31-6: Providing Oral Hygiene

	S	U	Comments
1. Performed preliminary actions.	___	___	___
2. Prepared for procedure.	___	___	___
a. Assessed client's ability to participate in procedure.	___	___	___
b. Donned clean gloves.	___	___	___
c. Positioned client in high or semi-Flower's position or in a lateral side-lying position.	___	___	___
3. Placed towel under client's chin and over upper chest.	___	___	___
4. Moistened toothbrush with small amount of water and applied toothpaste.	___	___	___
5. Either gave toothbrush to client for brushing or brushed client's teeth.	___	___	___
a. Asked client to open mouth wide, and held an emesis basin under client's chin.	___	___	___
b. Positioned the toothbrush at 45-degree angle to gum line.	___	___	___
c. Directed bristles of toothbrush toward gum line, and brushed from gum line to crown of each tooth, making sure to clean all surfaces.	___	___	___
d. Used back-and-forth strokes, cleaning biting surfaces of teeth.	___	___	___
e. Gently brushed client's tongue.	___	___	___
f. Had client rinse mouth with water and expectorate into emesis basin.	___	___	___
6. Had client rinse with mouthwash if desired.	___	___	___
7. Flossed client's teeth.			
a. Cut 10-inch piece of floss and wound ends around middle finger of each hand.	___	___	___
b. Held floss tightly and used "sawing" motion to get floss between bottom teeth.	___	___	___
c. Cut fresh floss and repeated process on upper teeth.			
d. Had client rinse mouth and expectorate into emesis basin.	___	___	___
e. Dried mouth and helped client to comfortable position.	___	___	___
8. Removed equipment, performed hand hygiene, and made client comfortable.	___	___	___
• Performed completion actions.	___	___	___

FOR AN UNCONSCIOUS CLIENT

1. Performed preliminary actions.   _____ _____ _____

    a. Donned clean gloves.   _____ _____ _____

    b. Placed client in a side-lying position.   _____ _____ _____

    c. Placed bulb syringe or suctioning equipment nearby in case
        client needs to be suctioned.   _____ _____ _____

    d. Placed towel or waterproof pad under client's chin.
        Placed an emesis basin under chin as well.   _____ _____ _____

3. Cleaned client's teeth and mouth.   _____ _____ _____

    a. Used padded tongue blade to open client's mouth.   _____ _____ _____

    b. Swabbed inside of mouth, tongue, and teeth with moist,
        padded tongue blade or swab.   _____ _____ _____

    c. Brushed client's teeth.   _____ _____ _____

    d. Rinsed client's mouth using a very small amount of water
        that could be readily suctioned from mouth.   _____ _____ _____

    e. Lubricated client's lips with petroleum jelly.   _____ _____ _____

4. Removed equipment and gloves, performed hand hygiene,
    and documented care.   _____ _____ _____

5. Left client dry and comfortable.   _____ _____ _____

    •   Performed completion actions.   _____ _____ _____

FOR DENTURES

1. Prepared for procedure as in step 1 for conscious client;
    donned clean gloves.   _____ _____ _____

    a. Asked client to remove dentures. If this was not possible,
        placed gauze square on front of upper denture. Grasped front
        teeth between thumb and forefinger, pulled down gently
        until suction that held upper dentures in place was loosened.
        Loosened lower dentures by lifting up and out.   _____ _____ _____

2. Cleaned dentures according to client's usual routine or
    instructions on cleaning product.   _____ _____ _____

    a. Soaked in denture cleanser. If unavailable, used warm water
        and gauze square or toothbrush to clean.   _____ _____ _____

    b. Brushed denture with soft-bristle brush.   _____ _____ _____

    c. Rinsed under warm water.   _____ _____ _____

3. Brushed gums and tongue and rinsed mouth.   _____ _____ _____

4. Helped client replace denture.   _____ _____ _____

5. Used denture adhesive according to package directions if
    client desired.   _____ _____ _____

6. Cleaned work area, and made client comfortable. Documented care.   _____ _____ _____

•   Performed completion actions.   _____ _____ _____

Additional Comments:

Name _____ Specific Skill Performed _____

Date _____ Attempt Number _____

Instructor _____ PASS _____ FAIL _____

Performance Checklist 31-7: Shampooing the Client in Bed

	S	U	Comments
1. Performed preliminary actions.			
2. Prepared for procedure.			
a. Placed waterproof pads under client's head and shoulders.			
b. Removed pins, clips, or barrettes from client's hair. Undid braids and brushed hair thoroughly.			
c. Placed bed in its flat position.			
d. Placed a shampoo board or inflated basin under the client's head.			
e. Draped a towel over client's shoulders and padded shampoo board with folded washcloth if using.			
f. Uncovered client's upper body by folding linens down to waist level. Placed bath blanket over client's chest.			
g. Placed washcloth over client's eyes.			
h. Placed receptacle in position to catch water.			
3. Shampooed client's hair.			
a. Donned gloves if appropriate.			
b. Used water pitcher and poured water over hair until it was thoroughly wet. Ensured that water was comfortably warm.			
c. Applied small amount of shampoo. Using fingertips, gently worked it into lather over entire scalp. Worked from hairline to neckline.			
4. Rinsed hair with warm water, and reapplied shampoo if needed. Repeated until hair was "squeaky clean" when hair shafts were rubbed.			
5. Applied small amount of conditioner if desired. Rinsed according to conditioner instructions.			
6. Made turban by wrapping towel around client's head. Patted or towel-dried until hair was free of excess moisture.			
7. Changed client's gown and linens if they were wet.			
8. Combed, dried, and styled client's hair.			
9. Helped client to assume comfortable position.			
10. Removed all equipment, and left environment clean.			
• Performed completion actions.			

Additional Comments:

Name _____   Specific Skill Performed _____

Date _____   Attempt Number _____

Instructor _____   PASS _____   FAIL _____

Performance Checklist 31-8: Shaving the Client

	S	U	Comments
1. Performed preliminary actions.	_____	_____	_____
2. Prepared for procedure.	_____	_____	_____
a. Placed client in sitting position, either in a bed or chair.	_____	_____	_____
b. If using safety razor, applied warm, wet towel to client's face before beginning to shave.	_____	_____	_____
c. Applied thick layer of soap or shaving cream to client's face.	_____	_____	_____
3. Shaved with even strokes in direction of hair growth while holding skin taut and motionless.	_____	_____	_____
4. Used damp washcloth to remove excess shaving cream. Inspected for areas that may have been missed. Applied after-shave lotion if desired.	_____	_____	_____
5. Cleaned area, made client comfortable, performed hand hygiene, and documented care.	_____	_____	_____
• Performed completion actions.	_____	_____	_____

Additional Comments:

Name _____   Specific Skill Performed _____

Date _____   Attempt Number _____

Instructor _____   PASS _____   FAIL _____

Performance Checklist 31-9: Performing Foot and Nail Care

	S	U	Comments
1. Performed preliminary actions.			
2. Prepared for procedure.			
a. Donned gloves if necessary.			
b. Helped client to sit in chair if possible. If client could not sit in chair, elevated head of bed.			
c. Filled basin half full of warm water (100° to 104° F).			
d. Tested temperature with bath thermometer or asked client to test water.			
e. Placed waterproof pad under basin.			
3. Placed client's foot or hand in basin. Washed with soap and allowed to soak for about 10 minutes.			
4. Rinsed foot or hand thoroughly with washcloth. Removed foot or hand from basin, and placed it on towel.			
5. Dried foot or hand thoroughly but gently, being especially careful to dry between digits.			
6. Emptied basin, refilled with warm water, and repeated with other foot or hand.			
7. While second foot or hand was soaking, provided nail care for first hand or foot.			
a. Carefully cleaned under nails with cotton-tipped applicator. Used orange stick to remove debris. Pushed cuticle back with orange stick. Was careful to avoid injury to skin under nail rim.			
b. Began with large toe or thumb, clipped nails straight across. Clipped small sections at a time, starting with one edge and working across. Filed and shaped each nail with emery board or nail file.			
c. After completing manicure or pedicure, applied lotion to client's feet or hands.			
8. Helped client to comfortable position, removed all equipment, performed hand hygiene, and documented care.			
• Performed completion actions.			

Additional Comments:

Name _____ Specific Skill Performed _____

Date _____ Attempt Number _____

Instructor _____ PASS _____ FAIL _____

Performance Checklist 31-10: Assisting an Adult Client With Eating

	S	U	Comments
1. Performed preliminary actions.	___	___	_____
2. Prepared client and environment.	___	___	_____
a. Explained procedure.	___	___	_____
b. Assisted client with urinary or bowel elimination before feeding.	___	___	_____
c. Assisted client to perform hand hygiene and possibly complete oral hygiene.	___	___	_____
d. Placed meal tray on overbed table so client could view it.	___	___	_____
e. Checked tray for client's name, diet, and completeness of dietary items. Checked tray against diet order and client's identification bracelet.	___	___	_____
3. Positioned client appropriately.	___	___	_____
a. Assisted client to supported upright position or to chair.	___	___	_____
b. Placed client in lateral position if unable to sit.	___	___	_____
c. Sat next to client to assist with feeding.	___	___	_____
4. Assisted client to degree necessary.	___	___	_____
a. Encouraged client to eat as independently as possible.	___	___	_____
b. Described location of foods on plate for visually impaired client using a clock face analogy.	___	___	_____
c. Prepared food items by removing food covers, applying condiments, cutting foods, and pouring liquids as needed.	___	___	_____
d. Asked client about preferences for order of eating foods.	___	___	_____
e. Monitored temperature of beverages to ensure not too hot or too cold.	___	___	_____
f. When assistance was necessary, fed small amounts at a time, allowing ample time for chewing and swallowing.	___	___	_____
g. Provided liquids at client request, or after three to four mouthfuls of one food.	___	___	_____
h. Did not hurry, and created a pleasant environment.	___	___	_____
5. At completion of meal, made client comfortable.	___	___	_____
a. Assisted client to clean mouth and hands.	___	___	_____
b. Positioned client for comfort and semi-upright to prevent regurgitation if needed.	___	___	_____
c. Removed meal tray from bedside area.	___	___	_____

6. Documented food and fluid intake as well as adverse symptoms
   (e.g., nausea, fatigue). Reported insufficient dietary intake to nurse. _____ _____ _____

- Performed completion actions. _____ _____ _____

Additional Comments:

Name _____   Specific Skill Performed _____

Date _____   Attempt Number _____

Instructor _____   PASS _____   FAIL _____

Performance Checklist 32-1: Performing Range-of-Motion Exercises

	S	U	Comments
1. Performed preliminary actions.	_____	_____	_____
2. Explained procedure to client, and assessed client's ability to assist with exercises.	_____	_____	_____
3. Used head-to-toe approach if moving joints of the entire body through range of motion.	_____	_____	_____
4. Supported client's body part by cradling or cupping above and below joint being moved.	_____	_____	_____
5. Put joint through its complete ROM, but did not force it beyond where it would comfortably move.	_____	_____	_____
6. Observed client for tolerance, including pulse rate and discomfort, if any. Did not exercise to the point of causing pain.	_____	_____	_____
• Performed completion actions.	_____	_____	_____

Additional Comments:

Name _____   Specific Skill Performed _____

Date _____   Attempt Number _____

Instructor _____   PASS _____ FAIL _____

Performance Checklist 32-2: Helping a Client Get Out of Bed

	S	U	Comments

WITHOUT A TRANSFER BELT

1. Performed preliminary actions.

2. Placed bed in lowest position, and raised head of bed.

3. Placed chair or wheelchair at 45-degree angle to bed on client's strongest side.

4. Used good body mechanics to help client to full sitting position while swinging client's leg over edge of bed in single, smooth motion. Supported client's upper body as client came to sitting position.

5. Supported client in sitting position on side of bed with feet dangling.

6. If client was able, had client place hands on nurse's shoulders or on mattress on either side of body.

7. Placed hands under client's arms. Placed knees in front of client's knees, and helped client to rise to a standing position.

8. Pivoted with client toward chair, being careful not to dislodge equipment or lines.

9. Used good body mechanics to lower client into chair or wheelchair slowly. Repositioned client in proper body alignment. Made client as comfortable as possible.

WITH A TRANSFER BELT

1. Placed transfer/gait belt around client's waist (after completing steps 1 to 5 above).

2. Stood in front of client, and grasped transfer belt on both sides of client toward the back. Assessed whether or not client had strength to stand. When client was ready, helped to standing position by rolling client's body and arms upward, pulling client with transfer belt.

3. Pivoted client toward chair, and lowered client slowly into it.

4. Had client reach for arm rests, if available, while lowering into chair.

• Performed completion actions.

Additional Comments:

Name _____   Specific Skill Performed _____

Date _____   Attempt Number _____

Instructor _____   PASS _____ FAIL _____

Performance Checklist 32-3: Using a Mechanical Lift

	S	U	Comments
1. Performed preliminary actions.	_____	_____	_____
2. Obtained functioning lift, and moved it into client's room. Locked wheels on both bed and chair.	_____	_____	_____
3. Placed one- or two-piece sling under client by turning client onto side, placing sling along back, and assisting client to roll onto sling. Ensured that sling supported client's shoulders and buttocks.	_____	_____	_____
4. Placed bed in low position. Securely attached sling to lift. Had client cross arms across own chest.	_____	_____	_____
5. Raised lift to elevate client enough to clear bed.	_____	_____	_____
6. Moved lift until client was aligned with chair. Locked wheels, released pressure valve, and lowered client slowly into chair.	_____	_____	_____
7. Kept sling under client, and positioned client into comfortable and functional body alignment.	_____	_____	_____
• Performed completion actions.	_____	_____	_____

Additional Comments:

Name _____   Specific Skill Performed _____

Date _____   Attempt Number _____

Instructor _____   PASS _____   FAIL _____

Performance Checklist 32-4: Supporting the Ambulating Client

	S	U	Comments
1. Performed preliminary actions.	_____	_____	_____
2. Applied gait belt around client's waist, and helped client to standing position as outlined in Performance Checklist 32-2.	_____	_____	_____
3. Stood beside and slightly behind client, and walked with client while holding onto back of belt.	_____	_____	_____
4. If client had intravenous pole, assisted client to push pole while walking.	_____	_____	_____
5. If client was weaker on one side than the other, walked on client's weak side while grasping belt and guiding posture.	_____	_____	_____
6. If client was especially weak (or this was the first time ambulating), asked another person to help to support the client. Had another assistant follow with a wheelchair in case the client became too weak to stand.	_____	_____	_____
7. If client started to fall, did not try to prevent fall by supporting client's weight with own body. Rather, helped client to fall safely, without injury to client or to self.	_____	_____	_____
8. As client started to fall, moved feet so nurse's stronger leg was somewhat behind other leg.	_____	_____	_____
9. At same time, used transfer belt to pull client toward the nurse, allowing client to slide against caregiver, supported, as client was eased onto the floor.	_____	_____	_____
10. Stayed with client until help arrived. Assessed client for injury before trying to move client.	_____	_____	_____
11. Documented events leading up to fall, client's assessment, notification of physician, and any action taken.	_____	_____	_____
• Performed completion actions.	_____	_____	_____

Additional Comments:

Name _____   Specific Skill Performed _____

Date _____   Attempt Number _____

Instructor _____   PASS _____   FAIL _____

Performance Checklist 32-5: Walking With Crutches

	S	U	Comments
1. Performed preliminary actions.	_____	_____	_____
2. Inspected prescribed crutch or crutches to make sure that rubber tips were in place.	_____	_____	_____
3. Reinforced importance of arm exercises, such as flexing and extending arms, body lifts, and squeezing a rubber ball.	_____	_____	_____
4. Checked that crutches were correct length.	_____	_____	_____
a. Had client stand.	_____	_____	_____
b. With crutch tip and client in basic crutch stance (tripod position), checked that distance between axilla and top of crutch was at least "3 fingers" or 1 or 2 inches (2.5 to 5 cm) wide.	_____	_____	_____
5. Taught client how to balance using tripod (triangle) position by placing crutches 6 inches (15 cm) in front of feet and out laterally about same distance.	_____	_____	_____
6. Checked with physician or physical therapist to determine which gait client needed (four-point, three-point, or two-point).	_____	_____	_____
a. For a four-point gait, had client follow this series of steps:	_____	_____	_____
(1) Moved right crutch forward about 6 inches (15 cm).	_____	_____	_____
(2) Moved left foot forward.	_____	_____	_____
(3) Moved left crutch forward.	_____	_____	_____
(4) Moved right foot forward.	_____	_____	_____
b. For a three-point gait, had client follow this series of steps:	_____	_____	_____
(1) Moved both crutches and weaker leg forward.	_____	_____	_____
(2) Moved stronger leg forward.	_____	_____	_____
c. For a two-point gait, had client follow this series of steps:	_____	_____	_____
(1) Moved left crutch and right foot forward at same time.	_____	_____	_____
(2) Moved right crutch and left foot forward at same time.	_____	_____	_____
7. Taught client how to ascend stairs.	_____	_____	_____
a. Instructed client to step up with stronger leg first.	_____	_____	_____
b. Instructed client to shift weight to the strong leg and move crutches and weaker leg onto same step.	_____	_____	_____
c. Instructed client to repeat steps a and b until stairs were negotiated, with crutches always supporting the weaker or affected leg.	_____	_____	_____

8. Taught client how to descend stairs. _____ _____ _____

    a. Instructed client to shift weight to stronger leg and move crutches and weaker leg onto lower step. _____ _____ _____

    b. Instructed client to shift weight to crutches and move stronger leg onto that step. _____ _____ _____

    c. Instructed client to repeat steps a and b until stairs were negotiated, with crutches always supporting the weaker or affected leg. _____ _____ _____

9. Taught client how to get in and out of chair. _____ _____ _____

    a. Instructed client to stand in front of chair making sure back of stronger leg was against chair. _____ _____ _____

    b. Instructed client to transfer crutches to weaker side and hold them by the handbar. _____ _____ _____

    c. Instructed client to grasp arm of chair with the hand on the stronger side, lean forward, flex knees and hips, and lower body into chair. _____ _____ _____

    d. To get out of chair, instructed client to move to edge of chair, and position stronger foot to support weight when arising. _____ _____ _____

    e. Instructed client to hold both crutches by the handbar using the hand on the weaker side and holding the arm of the chair on the stronger side. _____ _____ _____

    f. Instructed client to push down on crutches and armrest to push body out of chair. _____ _____ _____

• Performed completion actions. _____ _____ _____

Additional Comments:

Name _____   Specific Skill Performed _____

Date _____   Attempt Number _____

Instructor _____   PASS _____   FAIL _____

Performance Checklist 33-1: Turning and Moving a Client in Bed

	S	U	Comments
1. Performed preliminary actions.	___	___	___
2. Before turned or moved a client in bed or transferred to a stretcher, locked the bed's wheels and assessed client's condition.	___	___	___
a. Could client assist?	___	___	___
b. Where contractures present, did joints require special handling?	___	___	___
c. Could client tolerate having head of bed lowered?	___	___	___
d. Was the assistance of a colleague required.	___	___	___

TURNING A CLIENT ALONE

	S	U	Comments
1. Lowered head of bed and knee gatch until bed was flat; raised bed to comfortable working height.	___	___	___
2. Moved client to one side of bed.	___	___	___
a. Slid arms under client's shoulders and back, and moved client's upper body to one side of bed.	___	___	___
b. Slid arms under client's hips, and slid hips to the side.	___	___	___
c. Moved client's feet and legs to side of bed.	___	___	___
3. Crossed client's arms across chest, and crossed legs at the ankle. Positioned a pillow or wedge at head or foot of the bed to place behind client's back after turning.	___	___	___
4. Placed one hand on client's shoulder and other hand on client's hip. Rolled client toward self.	___	___	___
5. Turned client far enough forward to be able to release one hand, and positioned pillow or wedge behind client's back.	___	___	___
6. If necessary, went to opposite side of bed and pulled client's hips toward center of bed to make position more stable. Checked for proper positioning.	___	___	___

TURNING A CLIENT WITH ANOTHER NURSE

	S	U	Comments
1. Placed bed in flat position and at comfortable working height, and moved client to one side of bed.	___	___	___
a. If client was on turning sheet, nurses stood on opposite sides of bed and grasped top and bottom of sheet.	___	___	___
b. If client was not on turning sheet, both nurses stood on same side of bed.	___	___	___

- One nurse slid own arms under client's shoulders, while the other slid arms under client's hips.   _____ _____ _____

- On the count of three, both nurses slid client to one side of bed.   _____ _____ _____

2. Bent client's knee on the side opposite to which client is turning.   _____ _____ _____

- Folded client's arms over chest.   _____ _____ _____

- Positioned self on one side of bed with another nurse positioned on other side of bed.   _____ _____ _____

3. Turned client.   _____ _____ _____

   a. If client was not on turning sheet, nurse positioned on side of bed toward which client was turning placed one hand on client's shoulder and other hand on client's hip. Pulled client's shoulders and hip toward self.   _____ _____ _____

   b. If client was on turning sheet, used sheet to pull client's hips and shoulders in direction of turn.   _____ _____ _____

   c. At same time, nurse on opposite side of bed slid hands under client's bottom hip, pulled hip toward self, and placed a pillow at client's back.   _____ _____ _____

4. Placed pillow between client's legs.   _____ _____ _____

5. Ensured that client was properly positioned.   _____ _____ _____

6. If client's condition demanded that nurse maintain anatomic alignment of spine during procedure, used three nurses to keep spine straight.   _____ _____ _____

7. After turning client, documented that client was turned and position assumed.   _____ _____ _____

MOVING A CLIENT UP IN BED

1. Before moving client up in bed, determined whether nurse could do it alone or whether help was needed from another nurse. If planned to move client alone, determined whether to stand at side of bed or head of bed. Lowered head of bed as far as client could tolerate.   _____ _____ _____

   a. For one nurse to move client up in bed from side of bed: _____ _____ _____

   - Had client bend knees and place feet flat on bed.   _____ _____ _____

   - Placed one hand under client's back and one under thighs, close to hips.   _____ _____ _____

   - Told client to push with legs on the count of three, and slid client up toward head of bed.   _____ _____ _____

   b. For one nurse to move client from head of bed: _____ _____ _____

   - Started by removing headboard from bed.   _____ _____ _____

   - Placed bed in a slight Trendelenburg position.   _____ _____ _____

   - Used a turning sheet if possible; if not, slid hands under client's shoulders, and pulled client toward head of bed.   _____ _____ _____

2. If client had good upper-body strength, used trapeze to move client up in bed. _____ _____ _____

   a. Placed trapeze over bed. _____ _____ _____

   b. Had client bend knees and place feet flat on bed to push. _____ _____ _____

   c. Had client hold on to trapeze and pull with arms to lift hips slightly off bed. _____ _____ _____

   d. With hips lifted, had client push with legs. _____ _____ _____

   e. Assisted by placing hands under client's thighs, close to hips. _____ _____ _____

3. If client was too heavy, solicited help from a colleague. _____ _____ _____

   a. Stood on opposite sides of client's bed. _____ _____ _____

   b. Had client bend knees and place feet flat on bed. Both nurses grasped turning sheet with one hand at level of client's shoulders and other hand at level of client's hips. _____ _____ _____

   c. On count of three, had client push with legs as nurses slid torso up in bed. _____ _____ _____

4. After moving client up, raised head of bed and checked position. _____ _____ _____

5. Documented that client was repositioned and position assumed. _____ _____ _____

MOVING A CLIENT FROM A BED TO A STRETCHER

1. Determined that client was unable to move from bed to stretcher independently. _____ _____ _____

   a. Ensured that two caregivers were positioned on each side of stretcher. _____ _____ _____

   b. Designated one person to ensure that client's head was protected during move, while another ensured that feet were protected. _____ _____ _____

     • Locked wheels on both bed and stretcher. _____ _____ _____

     • Positioned bed and stretcher next to each other without any gaps between them. _____ _____ _____

2. Used a sheet to make transfer easier. _____ _____ _____

   a. Untucked sheet from client's bed. _____ _____ _____

   b. Grasped sheet under client's shoulders while another nurse on same side grasped it at client's hips and legs. Nurses on opposite side grasped sheet at shoulder and hip level. _____ _____ _____

   c. On a count of three, all nurses slid client onto stretcher. _____ _____ _____

3. As an alternative, used transfer board. _____ _____ _____

   a. Two nurses standing on same side of bed turned client away from stretcher. _____ _____ _____

   b. Placed transfer board where client was lying, and turned client back onto board. _____ _____ _____

    c.   Pulled board onto stretcher with client on it. _____ _____ _____

    d.   Turned client again to remove board. _____ _____ _____

4.   Raised side rails on outside of stretcher. Moved between bed and stretcher, and raised remaining side rails. _____ _____ _____

5.   If stretcher could not be positioned adjacent to bed, but was positioned at a right angle to the bed, used three-person lift to transfer client. _____ _____ _____

    a.   Positioned three nurses on same side of bed. _____ _____ _____

    b.   Slid hands and arms under client's head and shoulders. Another nurse slid hands under client's back and buttocks, and a third nurse slid hands under legs and thighs. _____ _____ _____

       •   On a count of three, nurses simultaneously lifted client. _____ _____ _____

    c.   Walked as a unit to rotate and transfer client to stretcher. _____ _____ _____

6.   Covered client with sheet. _____ _____ _____

   •   Supplied client with pillow, and raised head of stretcher if needed. _____ _____ _____

   •   Fastened safety strap over client. _____ _____ _____

   •   Put side rails up. _____ _____ _____

•   Performed completion actions. _____ _____ _____

Additional Comments:

Name _____   Specific Skill Performed _____

Date _____   Attempt Number _____

Instructor _____   PASS _____ FAIL _____

Performance Checklist 33-2: Applying Antiembolism Stockings

	S	U	Comments
1. Performed preliminary actions.	___	___	___
2. Checked physician's order.	___	___	___
3. Placed client supine in bed with legs horizontal for 15 minutes before first application.	___	___	___
4. Measured client's legs to determine correct stocking size.	___	___	___
a. For calf-length stockings, measured calf circumference and distance from foot to knee.	___	___	___
b. For thigh-length stockings, measured calf and thigh circumference and distance from foot to thigh.	___	___	___
5. Placed stocking on client's foot.	___	___	___
a. Inserted one hand into top of stocking and slid it down as far as heel pocket.	___	___	___
b. Grasped center of heel pocket, and turned stocking inside out down to heel area.	___	___	___
c. Carefully slid stocking onto foot and ankle, ensuring that client's heel was centered in heel pocket.	___	___	___
6. Pulled body of stocking firmly up client's ankle and calf, ensuring that no wrinkles formed.	___	___	___
7. Checked client's toes for pressure.	___	___	___
8. Repeated procedure with other leg.	___	___	___
9. Assessed client to ensure that stockings were functioning properly without wrinkles and not rolling down.	___	___	___
a. Made sure stockings had no wrinkles.	___	___	___
b. Prevented stockings from rolling down.	___	___	___
c. Removed stockings at bath times and before bed to provide skin care and perform skin and neurovascular assessment.	___	___	___
10. Documented size and length of stockings, time applied, condition of client's skin, any client complaints, and times stockings were removed and reapplied.	___	___	___
• Performed completion actions.	___	___	___

Additional Comments:

Name _____   Specific Skill Performed _____

Date _____   Attempt Number _____

Instructor _____   PASS _____   FAIL _____

Performance Checklist 33-3: Using a Sequential Compression Device

	S	U	Comments
1. Performed preliminary actions.	____	____	_____
2. Checked physician's order.			
3. Placed client in a supine position with legs horizontal.	____	____	_____
4. Applied antiembolism stockings.	____	____	_____
5. Measured circumference of client's upper thigh.	____	____	_____
6. Opened inflatable sleeve on the flat bed, cotton side up, and placed client's leg on sleeve.	____	____	_____
7. Wrapped sleeve snugly around client's leg, beginning with side that did not contain tubes. Fastened sleeve with Velcro fasteners.	____	____	_____
8. Connected tubing on sleeve to the compression controller.	____	____	_____
9. Followed physician's orders in setting controller to correct amount and time of compression. After turning it on, observed to make sure unit was working properly.	____	____	_____
10. Removed client's antiembolism stockings three times daily, and perform skin care and skin and neurovascular assessment.	____	____	_____
11. Documented date and time sleeves were applied and assessment findings.	____	____	_____
• Performed completion actions.	____	____	_____

Additional Comments:

Name _____ Specific Skill Performed _____

Date _____ Attempt Number _____

Instructor _____ PASS _____ FAIL _____

Performance Checklist 34-1: Endotracheal Suctioning

	S	U	Comments
1. Performed preliminary actions.	____	____	_____
2. Identified need for suctioning.	____	____	_____
a. Wet gurgling respirations with nonproductive cough.	____	____	_____
b. Bubbling rhonchi.	____	____	_____
c. Nasotracheal or tracheostomy tube.	____	____	_____
3. Gathered equipment.	____	____	_____
4. Determined whether or not to use sterile or clean technique (sterile in acute care; clean in home setting).	____	____	_____
5. Explained procedure to client to get cooperation.	____	____	_____
6. Set up equipment.	____	____	_____
a. Turned on suction (80 to 120 mm Hg for adult, 80 to 115 mm Hg for child, 60 to 100 mm Hg for infant).	____	____	_____
b. Opened sterile saline, and placed cap inverted on clean surface.	____	____	_____
c. Opened suction kit.	____	____	_____
d. Carefully picked up plastic or cardboard container to hold saline, squeezed to open, and set aside.	____	____	_____
• Poured solution into container.	____	____	_____
e. Put on sterile gloves.	____	____	_____
f. Picked up sterile catheter with dominant hand, and picked up nonsterile suction tubing with nondominant hand.	____	____	_____
g. Connected catheter to tubing, keeping dominant hand and suction catheter sterile.	____	____	_____
h. Tested suction with sterile saline.	____	____	_____
7. Instructed partner to hyperventilate lungs with 100% oxygen.	____	____	_____
a. If client did not have an artificial airway, instructed client to take several deep breaths.	____	____	_____
b. If client had an endotracheal tube or tracheostomy, used an Ambu bag to give 2 to 3 deep breaths.	____	____	_____
8. Inserted suction catheter via nasopharynx, endotracheal tube, or tracheostomy tube.	____	____	_____
• Refrained from applying suction during catheter insertion.	____	____	_____
• Applied intermittent suction on removing catheter; limited suction time to 10 seconds.	____	____	_____

9. Hyperventilated lungs to reoxygenate client. _____ _____ _____

   a. If client was able or not intubated, had client take several slow, deep breaths or _____ _____ _____

   b. Used Ambu bag attached to ET tube or tracheostomy tube or used face mask if client not intubated. _____ _____ _____

10. Assessed results, repeated if needed. Did not withdraw catheter from nose until finished suctioning trachea. Cleared catheter by suctioning saline or water before repeating procedure. Assessed amount and character of sputum and decreased ronchi. _____ _____ _____

• Performed completion actions. _____ _____ _____

Additional Comments:

Name _____   Specific Skill Performed _____

Date _____   Attempt Number _____

Instructor _____   PASS _____   FAIL _____

Performance Checklist 34-2: Administering Oxygen

	S	U	Comments
1. Performed preliminary actions.	_____	_____	_____
2. Assembled equipment. Checked physician's order for delivery device and liter flow.	_____	_____	_____
a. No smoking sign and removed all smoking materials from room.	_____	_____	_____
b. Humidification device.	_____	_____	_____
c. Nasal cannula.	_____	_____	_____
d. Simple face mask.	_____	_____	_____
e. Face mask with nonrebreathing oxygen reservoir bag.	_____	_____	_____
f. Venturi mask.	_____	_____	_____
g. Face tent.	_____	_____	_____
3. Set up system.	_____	_____	_____
• Inserted flowmeter into oxygen source.	_____	_____	_____
• Attached connecting tube and oxygen delivery device; added extra tubing if needed.	_____	_____	_____
• Checked function of system after establishing oxygen flow.	_____	_____	_____
• Observed for bubbling in water used for humidification.	_____	_____	_____
4. Placed oxygen delivery device on client, and made client comfortable. Relieved client concurs about oxygen.	_____	_____	_____
• Adjusted strap comfortably around client's head.	_____	_____	_____
• Prevented pressure behind ears.	_____	_____	_____
• Used a water-soluble lubricant if needed to relieve irritation to external nares.	_____	_____	_____
5. Reassessed client and system (signs and symptoms of oxygen deficit, liter flow, humidity, position of device).	_____	_____	_____
• Performed completion actions.	_____	_____	_____

Additional Comments:

Name _____   Specific Skill Performed _____

Date _____   Attempt Number _____

Instructor _____   PASS _____ FAIL _____

Performance Checklist 34-3: Cleaning a Tracheostomy

	S	U	Comments
1. Performed preliminary actions.	_____	_____	_____
2. Determined if procedure should be clean or sterile.	_____	_____	_____
3. Gathered equipment.	_____	_____	_____
4. Prepared client. Suctioned tracheostomy or had client cough. Removed soiled dressing using standard precautions.	_____	_____	_____
5. Set up sterile field. Using outer wrapper of kit, donned sterile gloves.	_____	_____	_____
• Poured hydrogen peroxide into one basin and normal saline into another.	_____	_____	_____
6. Unlocked and removed inner cannula following curve of tube; without moving outer tube, placed inner cannula in hydrogen peroxide.	_____	_____	_____
7. Cleaned inner cannula with brush or pipecleaner; rinsed in normal saline. Replaced inner cannula, and locked it into position.	_____	_____	_____
8. Cleaned tracheostomy site.	_____	_____	_____
• Used saline to clean skin.	_____	_____	_____
• Used hydrogen peroxide to clean external tube.	_____	_____	_____
• Used gauze or cotton-tipped applicator, according to amount of secretions, using gentle pats or strokes.	_____	_____	_____
9. Changed tracheostomy ties and applied dressing.	_____	_____	_____
• Protected tracheostomy from accidental removal by having second person hold tracheostomy during change of ties.	_____	_____	_____
• Ensured that ties were tight enough so that one finger can be slipped under tie.	_____	_____	_____
10. Evaluated results of procedure, condition of skin, cleanliness of tube, and client comfort.	_____	_____	_____
• Performed completion actions.	_____	_____	_____

Additional Comments:

Name _____   Specific Skill Performed _____

Date _____   Attempt Number _____

Instructor _____   PASS _____ FAIL _____

Performance Checklist 35-1: Administering Blood

	S	U	Comments
1. Performed preliminary actions.	____	____	_____
2. Verified that blood was ready in blood bank.	____	____	_____
3. Assessed client for allergies or previous reactions to blood.	____	____	_____
4. Followed institution's procedure for consent forms.	____	____	_____
5. Measured vital signs.	____	____	_____
6. Prepared equipment.	____	____	_____
7. Obtained blood from blood bank.	____	____	_____
8. Verified with another registered nurse that the following information was correct:	____	____	_____
• Client's name and identification number on blood bank slip matched client's identification bracelet.	____	____	_____
• Blood bank slip and unit of blood contained the same blood type, donor number, and expiration date.	____	____	_____
9. Donned gloves.	____	____	_____
10. Primed tubing.	____	____	_____
a. Closed all clamps on Y-tubing.	____	____	_____
b. Inserted spike on tubing into normal saline.	____	____	_____
c. Opened clamp and primed arm of tubing, drip chamber tubing below chamber.	____	____	_____
d. Clamped tubing.	____	____	_____
e. Gently rotated unit of blood.	____	____	_____
f. Inserted second spike into port on unit of blood.	____	____	_____
g. Opened clamp and primed arm of tubing to the drip chamber.	____	____	_____
h. Closed clamp.	____	____	_____
11. If client did not have an IV, performed venipuncture with 18- or 19-gauge catheter.	____	____	_____
12. Opened clamp on normal saline and infused 50 mL slowly; closed normal saline clamp.	____	____	_____
13. Opened clamp on blood, and regulated at keep-open rate. Maintained rate for 15 minutes while staying with client.	____	____	_____
14. Monitored vital signs, and observed for signs of transfusion reaction per institution protocol.	____	____	_____

15. Reset drip rate to rate prescribed, if client had stable vital signs and no signs of transfusion reaction. Continued to monitor vital signs and response to transfusion.   _____ _____ _____

16. Completed transfusion by flushing line with normal saline, clamping tubing, and disconnecting.   _____ _____ _____

17. Completed transfusion record, and returned designated portion of form and empty bag to blood bank.   _____ _____ _____

18. Placed designated portion of form in client record.   _____ _____ _____

19. Completed documentation date, type, and identification number of product; time started and ended, and client response.   _____ _____ _____

• Performed completion actions.   _____ _____ _____

Additional Comments:

Name _____   Specific Skill Performed _____

Date _____   Attempt Number _____

Instructor _____   PASS _____   FAIL _____

Performance Checklist 35-2: Adult Cardiopulmonary Resuscitation

	S	U	Comments
1. Assessed client for responsiveness.	_____	_____	_____
2. Called for help or activated emergency response system if client unresponsive.	_____	_____	_____
3. Ensured that client had an open airway.	_____	_____	_____
a. Positioned client on back on hard flat surface with arms at sides if possible.	_____	_____	_____
b. Opened airway using head tilt–chin lift method or jaw-thrust maneuver.	_____	_____	_____
c. Removed visible food or vomitus from mouth if present.	_____	_____	_____
4. Determined whether or not client was breathing.	_____	_____	_____
a. Looked to observe if chest rose and fell.	_____	_____	_____
b. Positioned ear over client's mouth and nose. Listened for exhaled air, and felt for air movement from breathing on own cheek.	_____	_____	_____
5. Administered 2 breaths if client not breathing within 10 seconds.	_____	_____	_____
a. Used thumb and index finger of hand resting on client's forehead to pinch nose closed for mouth-to-mouth.	_____	_____	_____
b. Used hand resting below client's chin to hold mouth closed for mouth-to-nose.	_____	_____	_____
c. Took a normal breath, and closed lips around client's mouth or nose.	_____	_____	_____
d. Gave two effective breaths, inhaling between breaths if not using a bag-valve mask.	_____	_____	_____
e. After delivering each breath, turned head and positioned ear over client's mouth and nose to listen for exhaled air.	_____	_____	_____
6. Checked for a pulse for 5 to 10 seconds at the client's carotid artery.	_____	_____	_____
a. Located carotid pulse using 2 to 3 fingers in groove between trachea and neck muscles.	_____	_____	_____
b. If pulse felt, continued rescue breathing at 10 to 12 breaths per minute (1 breath every 5 to 6 seconds).	_____	_____	_____
c. Began compressions if no pulse felt and client not breathing.	_____	_____	_____
7. Placed hands in correct position for chest compressions.	_____	_____	_____
a. Placed heel of one hand on lower half of sternum, just above xiphoid process.	_____	_____	_____

b. Placed heel of second hand over first so that hands were parallel, and raised or intertwined fingers leaving only heels of hands resting on chest.

c. Locked elbows and kept arms straight. Positioned shoulders directly over client's sternum.

8. Administered chest compressions.

a. Used enough force to depress chest 1½ to 2 inches on an adult. Released pressure fully on sternum between compressions to allow chest to return to normal position.

b. Delivered compressions at a rate of 100 per minute.

c. For 1 or 2 person rescue, gave 2 breaths followed by 30 compressions.

d. Opened airway and delivered 2 effective rescue breaths (1 second each).

e. Found proper hand position and began 30 more compressions at rate of 100/min.

f. Performed 5 cycles of 30 compressions and 2 breaths.

g. Reassessed client after 45 cycles of 30 compressions and 2 breaths.

- Checked for return of carotid pulse for 3 to 5 seconds.

- If absent, resumed CPR with chest compressions.

- If present, checked breathing.

- If breathing absent, performed rescue breathing at 10 to 12 breaths/min and monitored pulse.

- Coordinated efforts with a second rescuer who arrived on the scene.

h. Opened airway after 30 compressions and began rescue breathing, giving two rescue breaths. Instructed second rescuer to take over chest compressions.

- Allowed second rescuer to deliver 30 compressions before giving 2 more breaths.

i. Stated to interrupt CPR when emergency team arrived only for intubation and connection to 100% oxygen by bag-valve mask.

Additional Comments:

Name _____ Specific Skill Performed _____

Date _____ Attempt Number _____

Instructor _____ PASS _____ FAIL _____

Performance Checklist 36-1: Back Massage

	S	U	Comments
1. Performed preliminary actions.	_____	_____	_____
2. Determined if client needed or could tolerate a back massage.	_____	_____	_____
3. Prepared client for procedure.	_____	_____	_____
a. Raised bed to a comfortable working height.	_____	_____	_____
b. Lowered side rail, and helped client into prone or semiprone position.	_____	_____	_____
c. Exposed client's back, shoulders, upper arms, and sacral area. Covered rest of body with blanket.	_____	_____	_____
4. Applied a generous amount of prewarmed lotion to area or provider's hands.	_____	_____	_____
5. Administered back massage.	_____	_____	_____
a. Started with firm, circular strokes at the small of the back. Using both hands, stroked firmly to the shoulders. Repeated 8 to 10 times.	_____	_____	_____
b. Massaged over neck and shoulders using friction strokes at the base of the skull and kneading the shoulder muscles. Repeated 8 to 10 times.	_____	_____	_____
c. Moved down both sides of vertebral column using circular strokes, Repeated 3 to 5 circles in each area, ending with the lumbar region.	_____	_____	_____
d. Focused on small of back; used effleurage from center of spine, out in all directions.	_____	_____	_____
e. Repeated steps a to d with tapotement.	_____	_____	_____
f. Used effleurage from side to side; started at top and moved down back; repeated one to three times.	_____	_____	_____
g. Finished effleurage as in step a.	_____	_____	_____
h. Gradually slowed stroke and decreased pressure until hands were no longer touching client.	_____	_____	_____
6. Wiped off excess lotion and assisted with putting on gown or pajamas if needed.	_____	_____	_____
• Performed completion actions.	_____	_____	_____

Additional Comments:

Name _____   Specific Skill Performed _____

Date _____   Attempt Number _____

Instructor _____   PASS _____ FAIL _____

Performance Checklist 38-1: Inserting a Hearing Aid

	S	U	Comments
1. Performed preliminary actions.	___	___	___
2. Checked that battery was operating.	___	___	___
3. Inspected hearing aid.	___	___	___
4. Turned down volume, inserted ear mold into ear canal, and secured the rest of the aid in place according to the design.	___	___	___
5. For a behind-the-ear hearing aid, secured battery device behind client's ear. Avoided kinking connecting tube.	___	___	___
6. Slowly turned up volume while speaking to client in a normal tone of voice. Asked client when volume was comfortable.	___	___	___
7. If feedback occurred, checked for a problem.	___	___	___
• Performed completion actions.	___	___	___

Additional Comments:

Name _____   Specific Skill Performed _____

Date _____   Attempt Number _____

Instructor _____   PASS _____   FAIL _____

Performance Checklist 38-2: Ear Lavage/Irrigation

	S	U	Comments
1. Performed preliminary actions.	_____	_____	_____
2. Examined ear canal with an otoscope to assess for intact tympanic membrane and otitis media.	_____	_____	_____
3. Explained the procedure, and instructed client to avoid any sudden movements.	_____	_____	_____
4. Checked temperature of irrigant.	_____	_____	_____
5. Selected irrigating device.	_____	_____	_____
6. Covered client's shoulder. Tipped client's head to the side to be irrigated and asked client to hold emesis basin.	_____	_____	_____
7. Placed tip of irrigation device just inside external meatus with tip still visible. Straightened auditory meatus.	_____	_____	_____
8. Directed fluid toward posterior wall of ear canal.	_____	_____	_____
9. Performed steady irrigation. Did not use more than 70 mL of solution at one time.	_____	_____	_____
10. Periodically examined ear canal with otoscope to determine patency and cerumen removal.	_____	_____	_____
11. Tilted head to drain excess fluid from ear. Dried ear canal gently with cotton-tipped applicator.	_____	_____	_____
• Performed completion actions.	_____	_____	_____

Additional Comments: